FUNDAMENTALS OF ORTHOGNATHIC SURGERY

Second Edition

FUNDAMENTALS OF ORTHOGNATHIC SURGERY

Second Edition

editors

Malcolm Harris

Warwick University Medical School, UK

Nigel Hunt

University College London, UK

Imperial College Press

ICP

Published by

Imperial College Press
57 Shelton Street
Covent Garden
London WC2H 9HE

QM LIBRARY (WHITECHAPEL)

Distributed by

World Scientific Publishing Co. Pte. Ltd.

5 Toh Tuck Link, Singapore 596224

USA office: 27 Warren Street, Suite 401-402, Hackensack, NJ 07601

UK office: 57 Shelton Street, Covent Garden, London WC2H 9HE

British Library Cataloguing-in-Publication Data
A catalogue record for this book is available from the British Library.

FUNDAMENTALS OF ORTHOGNATHIC SURGERY (2nd Edition)

ISBN-13 978-1-86094-993-7
ISBN-10 1-86094-993-2
ISBN-13 978-1-86094-994-4 (pbk)
ISBN-10 1-86094-994-0 (pbk)

Typeset by Stallion Press
Email: enquiries@stallionpress.com

Printed in Singapore by B & JO Enterprise

Contributors

Peter Ayliffe
FDSRCS, FRCS (OMFS)
Consultant Oral and Maxillofacial Surgeon
Great Ormond Street Hospital for Children
and University College London Hospital NHS Trust
Honorary Senior Lecturer
Institute of Child Health, University College London, London

Mohammad Anwar Bamber
PhD, BA, MSSCh, FIMPT, MBRCP, LFHom, ILTM
Senior Maxillofacial Instructor
Department of Oral and Maxillofacial Surgery
University College London Eastman Dental Institute, London

Kieran M. Coglan
MB FRCS (Ed.), FFDRCSI
Consultant Oral and Maxillofacial Surgeon
Barts and the London NHS Trust/
Princess Alexandra Hospitals NHS Trust
NHS Trust, London

Susan Cunningham
PhD, MSc, BChD, FDS RCS (Eng), MOrth RCS, FDS (Orth) RCS
Senior Lecturer and Honorary Consultant
Unit of Orthodontics
University College London Eastman Dental Institute, London

Oonagh Griffin
BSc (Hons) SRD
Senior Specialist Dietician
Barts and the London NHS Trust

Dan Harris
MBBS, BSc, MRCS, FCEM
Consultant Accident and Emergency Physician
Kingston Hospital, Kingston upon Thames

Malcolm Harris
DSc, MD, FRCS (Edin), FDSRCS
Emeritus Professor
University College London
Postgraduate Dental Education Unit
Warwick University Medical School, Coventry

Nigel Hunt
PhD, MSc, BDS, FDS RCS (Eng), FDS RCS (Ed), FDS RCPS,
DOrth, MOrth RCS
Chairman of Division of Craniofacial and Developmental Sciences
Head of Unit of Orthodontics
University College London Eastman Dental Institute, London

Santdeep H. Paun
FRCS (ORL-HNS)
Consultant Rhinologist and Facial Plastic Surgeon
Barts and the London Hospital Trust, London

Edwin Payne
Chief Technical Instructor
Division of Craniofacial Developmental Sciences
University College London Eastman Dental Institute, London

Paul Thomas
DMD, MS
Senior Research Fellow
Units of Orthodontics and Maxillofacial Surgery
University College London Eastman Dental Institute, London

Preface and Acknowledgements

This is the second edition of this broad-based craft book which was originally published in 1991 by Malcolm Harris and Ian Reynolds shortly after Ian's untimely death. It is intended to be a basic manual for undergraduate and postgraduate students as well as trainees in surgery and orthodontics. It is also hoped to be of value to the professions complimentary to medicine and dentistry and especially technical and nursing staff.

The last 15 years have seen numerous advances in diagnostic technology and computer planning software as well as technical developments in both orthodontics and maxillofacial surgery. As a consequence, there are new sections dealing with computerised cephalometrics and digital image morphing software written by Paul Thomas, the psychological aspects of facial deformity and orthognathic surgery by Susan Cunningham, distraction osteogenesis by Kieran Coghlan, rhinoplasty by Santdeep Paun, and ankylosis of the temporomandibular joint. Many sections of the book have been completely rewritten or revised, including the chapter on orthodontic mechanics. Peter Ayliffe has revised the section on cleft lip and palate management. Anwar Bamber has updated his chapters on laboratory technical aspects with a contribution by Edwin Payne. Oonagh Griffin has rewritten the nutrition chapter and Dan Harris has modernised the complications section.

Many of the drawings from the original text have been retained and were by Mohamed Nour Awang and David Banks. Helen McParland has provided new illustrations for the rhinoplasty chapter and Daljit S. Gill and Cristina Nacher for Chapter 7. The authors also wish to acknowledge the clinical contributions, illustrated cases and useful comments by Nayeem Ali, Daljit Gill, Stephen Jones, Samantha Hodges, Tim Lloyd, Mike Mars, and Allan Thom. Finally, we wish to thank Karen Burke for her secretarial assistance and Gemma Harris for her invaluable editing. The illustration for the cover was provided by Alfred Tsang and Jason Cheng and created by Dr. Kai-Hung Fung.

We both must express our gratitude for the patience and support of our wives Naomi and Susan.

Contents

1

General Assessment

Introduction

The overall management of a patient with facial deformity requiring orthognathic surgery is both an art and a science. The management must be based on a team approach. Whilst the team may vary according to local circumstances, the optimum would consist of an orthodontist, an oral and maxillofacial surgeon, a liaison psychiatrist or clinical psychologist, a specialist in restorative dentistry, supported by a maxillofacial technician. A speech therapist is essential for cleft cases and plastic surgery expertise should also be available on an individual patient basis. Whilst a patient may be referred to any of the above specialists, it is important that all patients follow an agreed care pathway to ensure patient satisfaction with the outcome. Unfortunately the patient's personal concerns may be overlooked and it is imperative that as part of the initial consultation, patients are encouraged to state precisely what specific aspects of their facial features and or dentition they would like corrected, for what reason and the length of time that they have sought treatment. Research has shown that clinicians and the general public differ in their perception of an ideal face. Whilst the patient can be guided to what constitutes an ideal facial appearance, it is vital that the clinician does not lose sight of the patient's underlying concerns. The motivation behind the request for treatment is also very important and special consideration is required when marked psychological factors appear to influence both the diagnosis and the treatment.

Combined orthodontic/surgical treatment goals are:

- Improve facial aesthetics
- Improve dental aesthetics
- A functional, balanced and stable occlusion
- A satisfied patient.

The management protocol for facial deformity should comprise the:

- History
- Clinical examination
- Investigations
- Initial diagnosis
- Treatment plan
- Presurgical orthodontics
- Final treatment plan
- Surgery
- Postsurgical orthodontics
- When appropriate, restorative dentistry, psychological intervention or support and speech therapy will be required.

History

The purpose of the history is to identify the patient's orofacial problems and their cause. This may be a family trait, congenital deformity, or trauma in infancy or adolescence. It is useful to ask the patient to draw up a problem list in order of priority of the specific features they wish to have corrected and for the clinician to note where the drive for treatment has arisen. For example, a patient may complain of having a prominent chin, which they have noticed ever since adolescence and for which they have frequently requested treatment through the general dental practitioner. This differs from the sudden desire to change minimal deformity as a response to a personal crisis. The long term success in terms of patient satisfaction is far better when driven by the patient than that of a patient seeking surgery driven by a parent, partner or close relative. The overall treatment goals must be to improve facial and dental aesthetics, and to provide a functional, balanced and stable occlusion but with the underlying premise that these satisfy the patient's reasonable wishes.

The Medical History

Most orthognathic patients are young and fit to undergo a general anaesthetic and prolonged surgery. Occasional disorders, which require specific attention include:

  i) haemophilia or similar clotting disorders which require pre- and intraoperative correction
 ii) acromegaly patients may be a cardiomyopathy risk
iii) antibiotic or analgesic idiosyncrasy or allergy
 iv) rheumatic or congenital heart valve lesions
  v) obstructive sleep apnoea should warrant a sleep study and specific assessment.

Body Dysmorphic Disorder (Formerly Dysmorphophobia)

A small but significant proportion of patients may present with varying degrees of concern about one or more aspects of their facial appearance without appropriate clinical signs. This may be a manifestation of a psychiatric disturbance now called Body Dysmorphic Disorder (formerly dysmorphophobia). This condition will create problems in surgical management as the patient is often dissatisfied with the final result. The condition raises the conflict as to whether one does,

i)   what the patient wants
ii) what the patient needs
iii) or nothing.

It is therefore worth considering in some detail. See Chapter 6.

Evaluation of the Patient

Patient Evaluation

* Clinical examination
* Radiographic examination
* Analysis of study models
* Psychological examination where appropriate.

Introduction

The full examination must include the simultaneous scrutiny of the patient, radiographs, cephalometry and study casts. The evaluation of the orthognathic patient should begin with a systematic examination of the patient's facial features from both the frontal perspective (vertical proportions) and the lateral profile (horizontal relations). It is important to consider the vertical facial proportions and their balance in relation to the patient's general build, and personality. Examples of patients who may not need surgery are: (i) a young female patient who possesses a vivacious and extrovert personality suited to a mild Class II malocclusion accompanied by a broad smile and marked incisor exposure and (ii) similarly, a well-built male may be suited to a mild Class III malocclusion with a minor degree of mandibular prognathism. It is also important to take into consideration the overall facial shape, as clearly there is extreme variation from a square shaped facial appearance to one of a long ovoid appearance. In the former case this may fit in well with a shorter stature whereas a longer face may be more suited to a tall individual. At the moment these decisions are based on experience and intuition.

Clinical Examination

The clinical examination should be undertaken with the patient comfortably seated with the Frankfort plane horizontal. Not only is it easy to visualise a line running from the inferior orbital margin to the upper end of the tragal cartilage, but this can be readily compared with the same horizontal plane on the lateral skull radiograph (cephalogram) and photographs.

Frontal Assessment

There are several important facial features to note. These include:

a) *The facial proportions*

The useful classic guide is to consider the face as having three equal vertical components (Figure 1.1): The distance from the hairline to the soft tissue bridge of the nose; from the soft tissue bridge of the nose to the alar base and from the alar base to the chin. It is also important to determine whether or not there is a relative excess or deficiency in the vertical height of either the maxillary or mandibular thirds.

b) *The alar base width*

Traditionally in a westernised population it is accepted that the alar base width, as measured from the lateral aspects of the alar cartilages of the nose, should be approximately equal to the intercanthal distance as measured between the inner canthi of the eyes (Figure 1.2). This measurement has importance when planning a maxillary impaction.

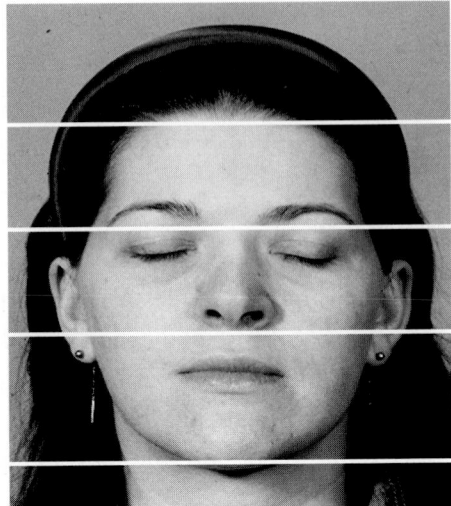

Figure 1.1   The superficial aesthetic proportions of the face can be divided into equal thirds. However the underlying cephalometric proportions of the upper to the lower facial height are 45:55 (see Figure 2.3).

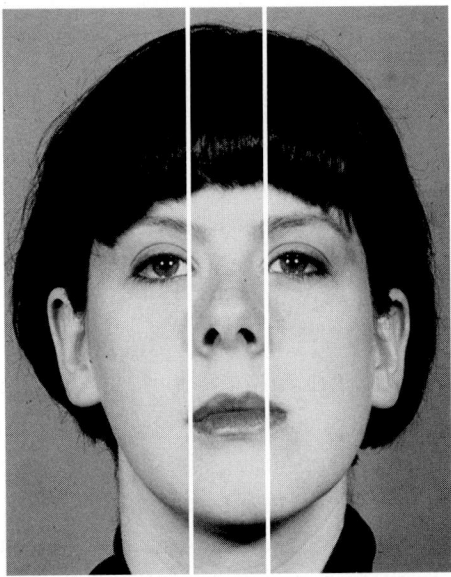

Figure 1.2   The alar base width should approximate the inner intercanthal distance.

c) *Incisor exposure (the lip — incisor relationship)*

For a patient with an average upper lip length of 20–25 mm, the standard exposure for orthognathic planning of the upper labial segment with the lips parted at rest should be 2–4 mm of the incisor crown. On smiling, the exposure should increase to the level of the gingival margin of the upper labial segment. This assessment is crucial when planning the ultimate vertical height of the mid face. Quite clearly the amount of incisor exposure should be inversely proportional to the length of the upper lip. (Figure 1.3). Where the upper lip length is very short then the patient would expect to show more of the upper incisors. Any attempt to reduce the incisor exposure in relation to a short upper lip will lead to an unaesthetic reduced middle face height. Similarly, with a long upper lip, the patient would be expected to show less or no upper incisor, both at rest and during facial animation. The lip incisor measurement should be done with the face at rest. Animation especially smiling will enhance the face and make planning difficult.

The harmony between the components of the lower third of the face is also important, in that the subnasale to the upper lip vermillion border should be a third of the total (i.e. half of the lower lip vermillion border to the soft tissue menton). In those cases where the lower third of the face appears overclosed, it is wise to re-evaluate both the upper lip length and the incisor exposure with the mouth open so that the lips are taken just out of contact.

d) *Facial asymmetry and centre line relationships*

It is important to note any asymmetry of the middle or lower third of the face, including the position and levels of the eyes. This may be facilitated by marking the midlines on the patient's face and also by analysing a clinical photograph or surface laser scan.

The patient's maxillary and mandibular dental midlines may not be coincident nor match their skeletal midlines (Figure 1.4).

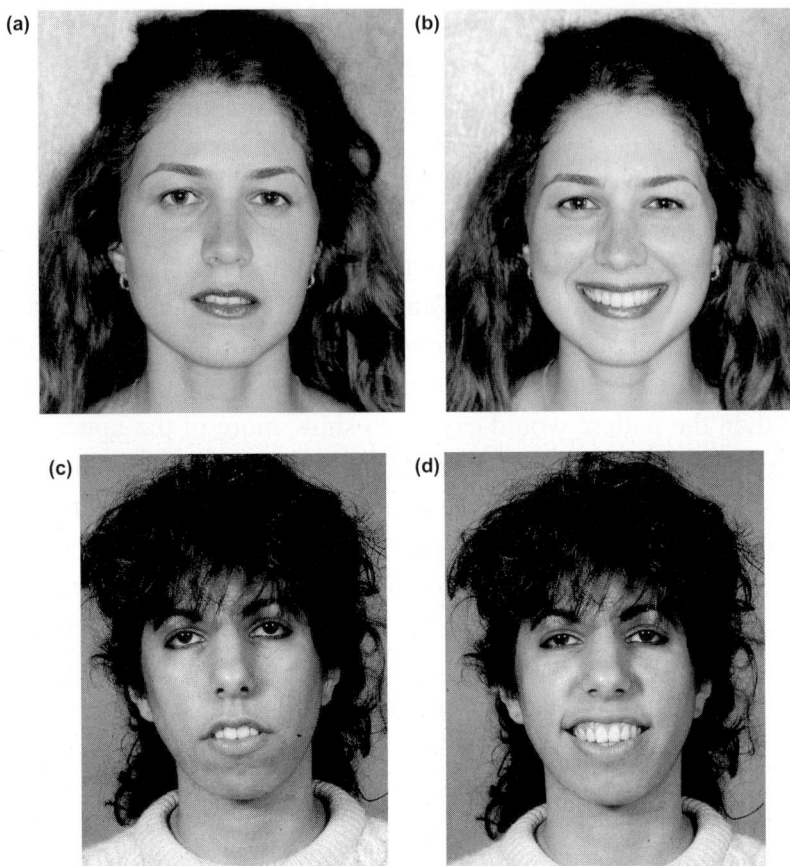

Figure 1.3   With an average upper lip length, a useful aesthetic proportion is (**a**) 2–4 mms of maxillary incisor crown visible with the lips apart at rest. (**b**) Increasing to the level of the gingival margin on smiling. (**c**) The excess incisor exposure of vertical maxillary excess at rest is important for the estimation of the required vertical impaction. (**d**) The aesthetic animated face makes this estimation difficult.

Generally where the maxillary dental midline is displaced to one side of the skeletal midline, there is an indication for orthodontic correction rather than attempting to rotate the maxilla in order to produce a dental midline coincident with the midface. Where a mandibular dental midline discrepancy is noted in relation to the

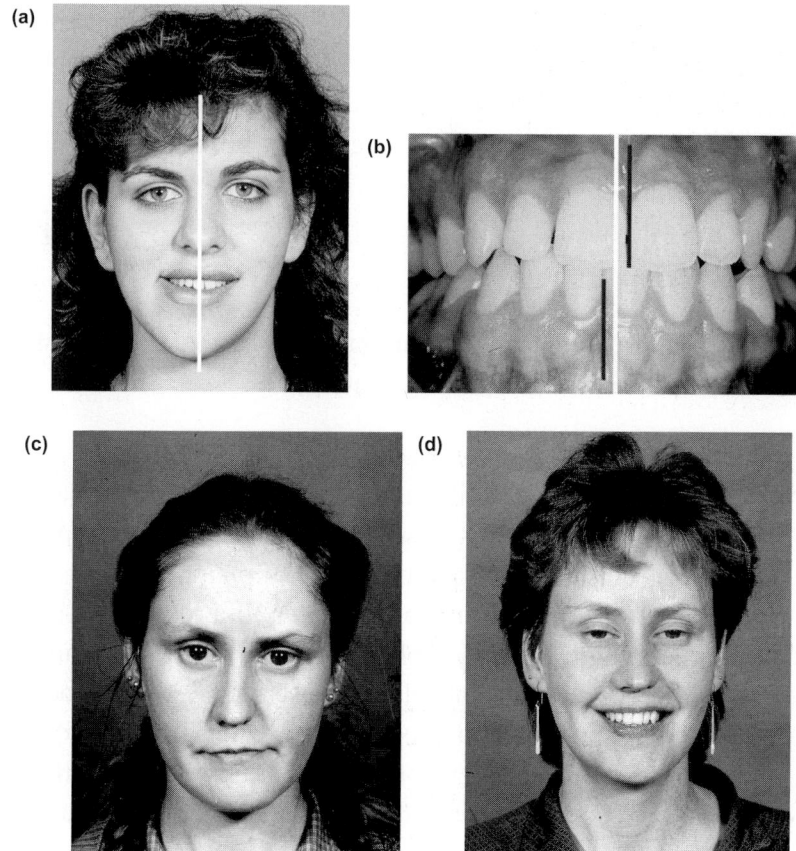

Figure 1.4 (a) The facial asymmetry of a left-sided hemimandibular elongation with the chin point displaced to the right. The lower dental midline mirrors the mandibular skeletal asymmetry and will be corrected as part of the surgery. (b) The maxillary dental midline is displaced to the left of a symmetrical maxilla and therefore should be corrected as part of the orthodontic preparation of the case. (c) Postural camouflage showing tilting of the head to level the lip line, in an asymmetrical face can give a false impression of orbital dystopia. (d) Levelling the occlusal plane with bimaxillary osteotomies also "levels" the eyes!

upper midline, it is important to determine whether it is coincident with a mandibular skeletal asymmetry or of purely dental origin. Where the skeletal asymmetry and dental midlines coincide the centre lines will be corrected as part of the surgical procedure.

Postural camouflage can be a problem with the asymmetrical face (Figures 1.4c and 1.4d). The patient with a marked occlusal cant habitually tilted the head to level the lip line giving the impression of orbital dystopia. This was corrected by bimaxillary levelling of the occlusal plane.

Profile Assessment

As with frontal evaluation it is important to work down the face from above to observe several key features.

a) *Relative protrusion of the maxilla and mandible*
    The relations of the maxilla and mandible to each other and to the skull base will be discussed in greater detail in Chapter 2. It is very common for patients to complain of a big chin, whereas it is the relationship of the maxilla to the skull base which is at fault, i.e. a hypoplastic maxilla related to a normal mandible. This can be clinically demonstrated by simply padding out the upper lip with soft wax or cotton wool (Figure 1.5) until the lip relationship and facial profile appear normal. Similarly, the surgical correction of a retrognathic mandible may be visualised

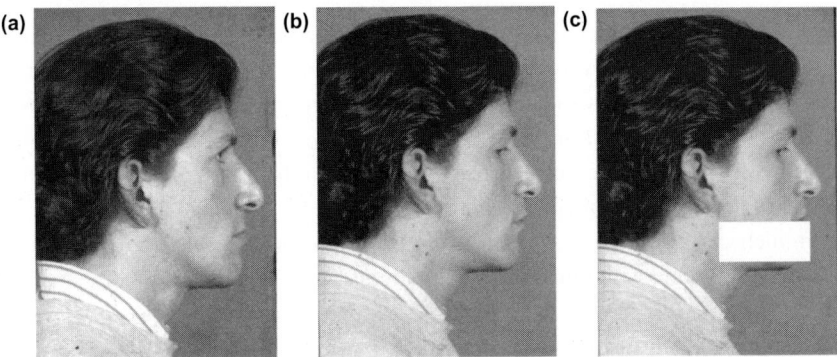

Figure 1.5 **(a)** Apparent mandibular prognathism. **(b)** Padding the upper lip suggests a maxillary advancement will harmonise the profile and maintain a "strong chin". **(c)** Masking the mandible facilitates judging the mid face.

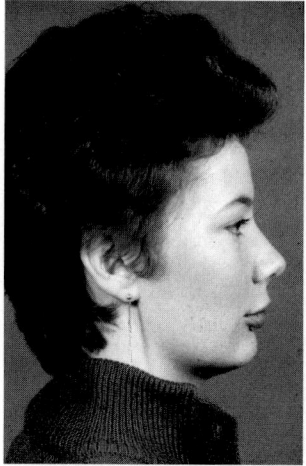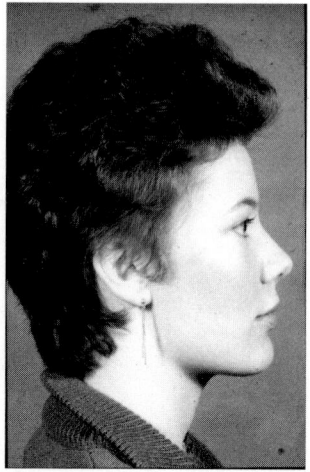

Figure 1.6 Forward posturing of the mandible will help to visualize the horizontal and vertical effects of a mandibular advancement to correct a marked Class II deformity.

by asking the patient to slide the mandible forwards (Figure 1.6). Most orthognathic cases require a combination of both maxillary and mandibular surgery and an easy assessment of the relative protrusion of the mid third and mandible can be made by assessing their position relative to the perpendicular to the Frankfort plane passing downwards through the soft tissue nasion. With normal facial proportions the soft tissue profile of the maxilla should be approximately 2–3 mm in front, and the soft tissue pogonion should lie 2 mm behind this facial plane (Figure 1.7). However the face can vary with ethnic norms, giving anterognathic, mesognathic or posterognathic profiles.

b) *Position of the infra-orbital margin*

A good indicator of middle third hypoplasia arises from the relative protrusion of the maximum convexity of the globe of the eye in relation to the infra-orbital margin. Ideally the globe should be just 2–3 mm in advance of the infra-orbital margin (Figure 1.8).

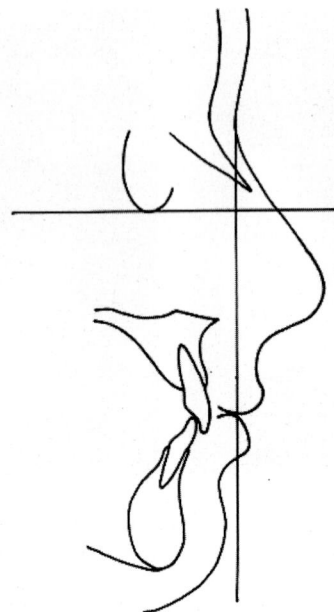

Figure 1.7 (a)   The relative protrusion of the mid third and mandible can be assessed by a perpendicular to the Frankfort plane passing downwards through the soft tissue nasion. With "normal facial proportions" the soft tissue profile of the maxilla should be 2–3 mm in front of the line and that of the mandible 2–3 mm behind.

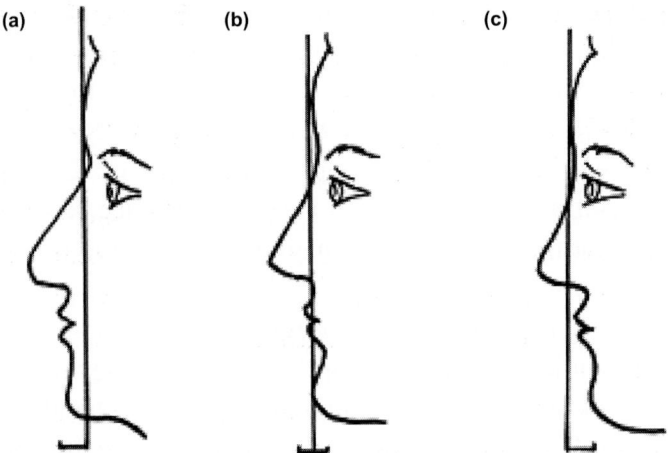

Figure 1.7 (b)   The "normal profile" can vary with concepts of beauty and ethnic variation as is seen above showing: **(a)** the anterognathic, **(b)** mesognathic, and **(c)** posterognathic norms.

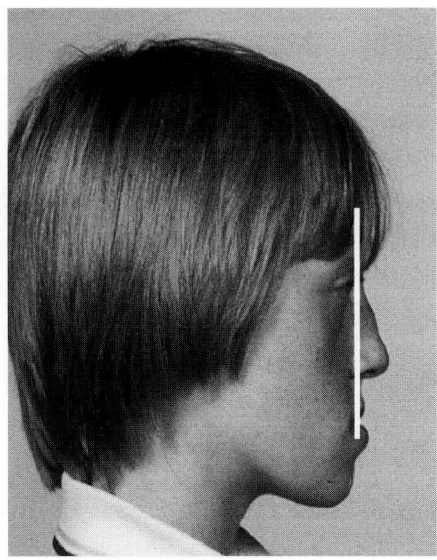

Figure 1.8   A patient with midface hypoplasia. Note the retruded infra-orbital margin relative to the globe of the eye, which should only be 2–3 mm in front of the orbital margin.

c)   *Nasal morphology*

The appearance of the nose will often change both relatively and anatomically with many osteotomies. For instance, an apparent large nose may appear more acceptable following a bimaxillary correction (Figure 1.9) due to the change in the adjacent soft tissue drape. Alternatively, a Le Fort I maxillary advancement and/or impaction will tend to raise the nasal tip and straighten a nasal hump unless modifications to the surgical procedure are included (Figure 1.10). Where a formal rhinoplasty is considered essential, it should always be undertaken as a separate surgical procedure once the changes produced by the jaw surgery have stabilised. See Chapter 12.

The importance of the nasolabial angle in the surgical planning process will be discussed in greater detail in Chapter 5. However it is important to record the nasolabial angle, which is the angle formed by the intersection of tangents to the lower border of the nose and upper lip. Ideally, in Caucasians this angle

(a) (b)

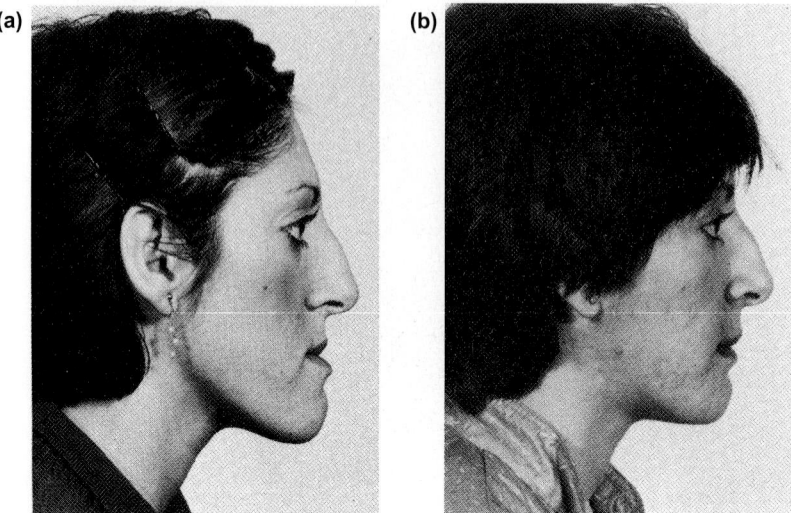

Figure 1.9   **(a)** The relative prominence of the nose seen preoperatively is diminished with a bimaxillary correction, **(b)** which has radically changed the adjacent soft tissue drape.

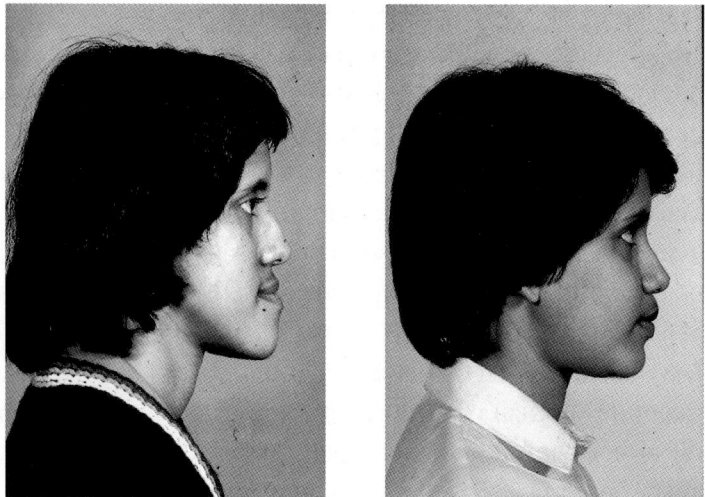

Figure 1.10   Maxillary impaction and advancement can raise the nasal tip.

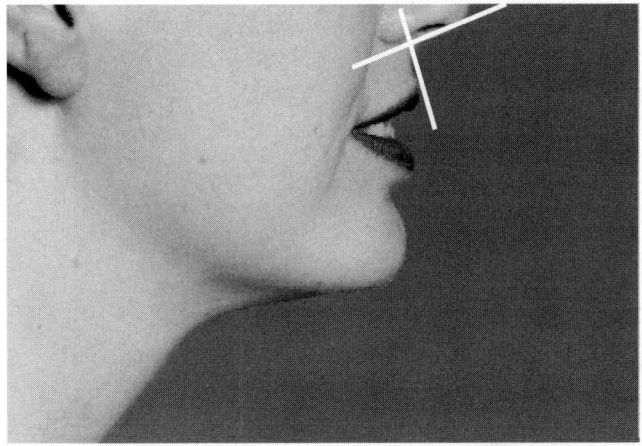

Figure 1.11 The nasolabial angle is assessed at the intersection of tangents to the columella (lower border) of the nose and the upper lip.

should be slightly greater than 90 degrees indicating optimum lip support (Figure 1.11).

d) *Morphology of the ears*

The ears, being first arch derivatives, may concurrently suffer with a gross facial deformity. The ear deformity associated with hemifacial hypoplasia (microsomia) will require reconstruction at a later stage (Figure 1.12). It is not uncommon for the external auditory meati to lie at unequal levels. This creates an asymmetrical facial artefact and difficulties when taking a facebow recording for transfer to the articulator. See Chapter 7. Bat ears appear to be an independent abnormality and do not seem to concern most adults.

e) *Chin depth*

When assessing the facial height in the frontal and sagittal plane, the lower facial third can be further subdivided into the upper lip which forms one-third, whilst the distance from the lower lip margin (stomion) to the chin margin (soft tissue menton) should comprise two-thirds of the lower facial height.

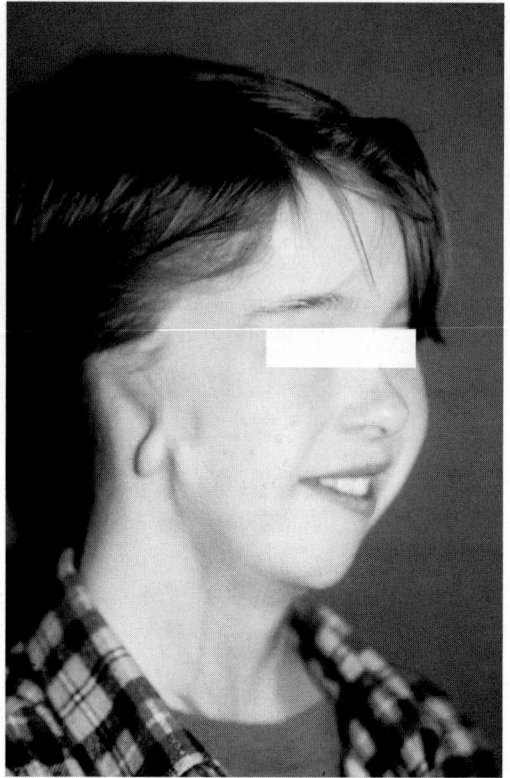

Figure 1.12   Severe ear deformity in a patient with hemifacial microsomia.

Taken together with the chin profile this is an important component for correcting jaw disproportion (Figure 1.13).

f)   *Chin-Throat angle*

Some patients request cosmetic surgery for an excess fat deposit in the throat region. This should be distinguished from a dewlap which is a fold of loose skin. As a consequence the fat gives a bulky contour below the chin. Surgery to setback the mandible may occasionally accentuate this build up of submental soft tissue, in which case liposuction or plastic surgery procedures may need to be incorporated into the postoperative surgical plan. However in the young patient the submental neck area usually remodels spontaneously after a setback.

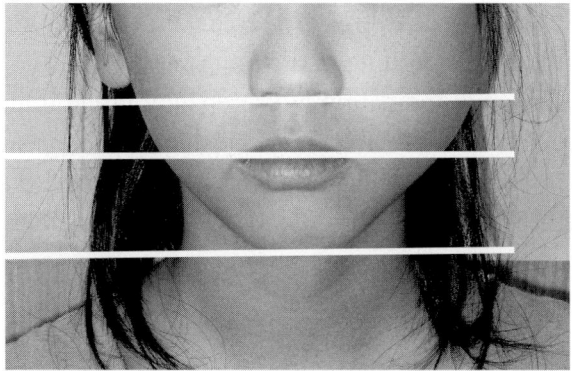

Figure 1.13   The upper lip length should be a third of the lower facial height.

Temporomandibular Joint Examination

Although there is no evidence of malocclusion or jaw deformity causing temporomandibular joint symptoms, it is important to record any abnormalities present in patients considering surgery. The examination of the joint should include observation of the path of opening and closure of the mandible, noting any clicking sounds whilst palpating the joints. If a click is present, it should be noted how this relates to the opening or closing cycle. Also, the extent of maximum opening should be recorded.

Intraoral Examination

A full intraoral dental examination must be carried out with the study models and radiographs.

1. Record the teeth that are present or unerupted and any that are impacted, carious, overerupted or periodontally involved. This is often overlooked.
2. The following orthodontic base line notes should include:
   a) A definition of the dental occlusion and dental base relationships.

b) Any dental centre line discrepancies relative to each other and the facial midline and chin point.

c) Any crossbite indicating a discrepancy in the transverse relations. This includes both anteroposterior and buccal crossbites. It is important to check and record whether there is any associated displacement or deviation of the mandible on closing. In the buccal segments, it is also important to note whether the segments have attempted to compensate for the discrepancy by tipping of the dentition.

d) The upper and lower incisor inclinations and in particular, compensatory changes due to the jaw disproportion, e.g. retroclined lower incisors and proclined upper incisors in a prognathous mandible.

e) The presence of crowding or spacing together with any tooth size discrepancies. Note also any tilting and rotation of teeth.

f) The levels and shape of the occlusal planes, both the anteroposterior curves of Spee, and the transverse occlusal plane. A wooden spatula placed across the transverse occlusal plane can help identify any cant in relation to extraoral structures, for example, the interpupillary line.

g) The depth of the overbite and whether it is complete or incomplete. The size of the overjet from the most prominent incisor should also be recorded.

h) Whether the maxillary intercanine width can accommodate the lower arch.

i) The arch form and the coordination of upper and lower arches.

3. Examine and record the tongue size and mobility, and the speech pattern.

4. Enlarged tonsils may jeopardise the patency of the airway. Adenoids are rarely a problem as they have usually regressed in size during early adolescence. However, remember that the micrognathic mandible will create an intubation problem for the anaesthetist.

5. Cleft cases require careful analysis of the cleft site and bony defects that will require grafting. Velopharyngeal competence should be examined by endoscopy and speech recorded by a speech therapist.

Investigations

Radiographs

1. A panoramic film, e.g. orthopantomograph shows at a glance:
    a) Any unerupted and impacted teeth.
    b) The shape and relative size of each half of the mandible, including the condyles, in two dimensions.
    c) The presence of any pathological condition such as impacted unerupted teeth, caries, periodontal disease, apical granulomas or cysts.
    d) The trabeculation pattern of the bone, especially at the lingula, which when visible is an indication of adequate thickness of the ascending ramus and ease with which the ramus can be split.
2. The true lateral skull radiograph is taken with the head in a reproducible position with the aid of a craniostat. The tube is set 1.5 m from the film so that the central parallel rays are used, producing a life-sized image with minimal distortion. Ideally the teeth should be in centric relation (retruded contact position), i.e. the mandible should be gently closed to the natural retruded cuspal contact position to approximate to the supine anaesthetised centric relation during surgery. However, the influence of centric occlusion and centric relation on planning will be discussed in Chapter 7.
3. A craniostat posteroanterior view of the skull helps to reveal facial bone asymmetry. However, remember that the head may be tilted in the craniostat if the external auditory meati are asymmetrically placed, giving a misleading image.

4. Long cone periapical films are essential for assessing the space between teeth when segmental surgery is required.
5. A maxillary occlusal radiograph defines the bone defect in cleft cases.
6. Major deformity is best visualised with a 3-dimensional CT scan.

If the patient elects to have surgery, a preoperative chest radiograph is required by some surgeons but is only justified where a costo-chondral graft is to be harvested.

Study Models (Casts)

Impressions are taken for study models, together with a careful inte-rocclusal record ("squash bite") so that the models can be trimmed in centric relation. This is done with the patient in a relaxed supine position. The models must show all the teeth present as well as the sulci. The patient's name, hospital number and the date of taking the impressions must be marked on them after trimming in a standard-ised manner (e.g. Angle or Tweed).

Initially two replicas are made of the originals and one set is mounted on an anatomical articulator using a facebow recording, although a simple plasterless articulator is suitable for those cases involving mandibular surgery alone. Model surgery is discussed in detail in Chapter 7.

In cases of posterior open bite, a plaster backing block may be required, although the majority of the planning will be undertaken on an articulator.

Photographs

The basic orthognathic series of colour images consists of (Figure 1.14):

i) Full face at rest and smiling.
ii) Right profile but both profiles with any asymmetry.
iii) Anterior teeth and right and left buccal segments in occlusion.

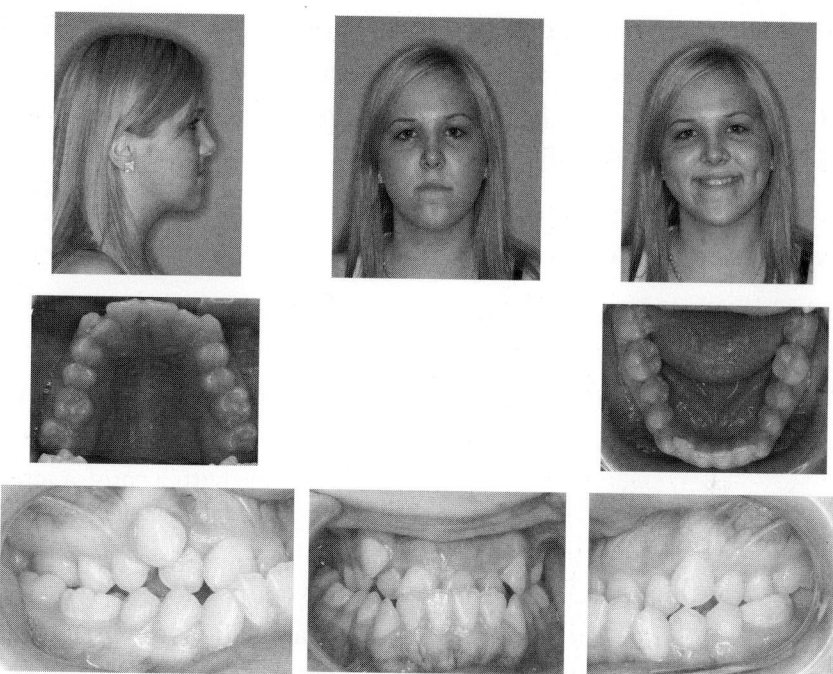

Figure 1.14   A basic orthognathic series of photographic records.

iv) Some also include occlusal views of the upper and lower dentition.

v) Cleft cases require a palatal view.

vi) Cleft and rhinoplasty patients also need an inferior view of the alar margins to capture problems of asymmetry.

In addition, some surgeons use black and white prints of the patient's profile for treatment planning but as the 1:1 object-image profile photograph is not exactly comparable to the lateral skull tracing, there is little value in superimposing them for planning purposes. These techniques have been largely superseded by the advent of digital imaging and the development of computer imaging and morphing software programmes which are used to simulate surgical changes (Chapter 3).

Photographs should be taken pre- and postoperatively as a surgical audit, for teaching and rarely for medico-legal reasons. If photographs are to be of value, hair must be retracted from the face and ideally moustaches and beards removed.

Lateral Skull Tracing

The "true lateral skull" radiograph is traced manually or digitised by computer for cephalometric analysis.

These will be discussed in detail in Chapter 3 and in the sections on deformities.

The Diagnosis

With many patients this can be readily stated, together with its surgical solution, at the first clinical examination; for example, "mandibular prognathism requiring a sagittal split osteotomy push-back". However, without more formal scrutiny, bimaxillary, orthodontic, restorative and periodontal problems will be overlooked.

Complex deformities require a detailed appraisal by the surgeon and orthodontist jointly, and even then a surgical solution may not suggest itself immediately. Hence it is useful to describe the case under the following headings, in the form of a "problem list".

1. The jaw relationship and facial proportions, including the nose and ears
2. Orthodontic diagnosis
3. Restorative, including periodontal problems
4. Speech
5. Psychological assessment.

2

Radiographic Analysis and Imaging

The standard radiographic views which are fundamental to orthognathic surgery planning consist of a panoramic screening radiograph, for example, an orthopantomogram, and a lateral skull radiograph taken in a cephalostat. In addition the posteroanterior skull radiograph may be used in cases where there is clinical evidence of asymmetry. More detailed radiographs, for example, long cone periapical views or an upper standard occlusal radiograph may be taken for clarification of specific areas of pathology. It is not uncommon for surgical patients to have previously undergone some form of orthodontic treatment and therefore it is important to ensure that the roots of the teeth are perfectly sound.

The Need

Cephalometric analysis is helpful in establishing the relations of:

1. The maxilla and the mandible to the base of the skull.
2. The maxilla to the mandible.
3. The maxillary teeth to the maxilla.
4. The mandibular teeth to the mandible.
5. The upper incisors to the lower incisors.

In order for these measurements and relationships to be meaningful it is important that the radiograph is taken in a standardised centric relation position (retruded contact position) with the patient's Frankfort Plane (the line from the lower border of the orbital rim to the upper border of the cephalostat ear post) horizontal. It is also important to ensure that the soft tissues are at rest when the radiograph is recorded.

Modern radiological guidelines require that intensifying screens should be used and that the radiographic beam has undergone appropriate collimation so as to avoid excessive exposure of structures considered unnecessary in the planning process.

Ethical approval is also required for repeated radiographs used for research purposes.

The Tracing

A sheet of clear, matt acetate paper is fixed securely with adhesive tape to the lateral skull radiograph placed on a horizontal viewing box. The radiographic image is enhanced by tracing in a darkened room with any peripheral light from the viewing box masked off. Many operators will have their preferred landmarks and analyses but the following outlines and points are commonly registered (Figure 2.1).

Outlines:

1. The soft tissue profile including glabella, nasion, nasal tip, upper lip, lower lip and the soft tissue chin.
2. The inner outline of the sella turcica, the anterior aspect of the nasal bones together with the frontonasal suture and the outline of the lower bony margin of the orbit.
3. The maxillary outline, upper incisors and upper first molar.
4. The mandibular outline with the mandibular incisors and first molar and articulare. As a result of superimposition it is often difficult to identify the head of the condyle but it is easy to register the articulare where the posterior margin of the ramus crosses the cranial base. In general, where bilateral landmarks

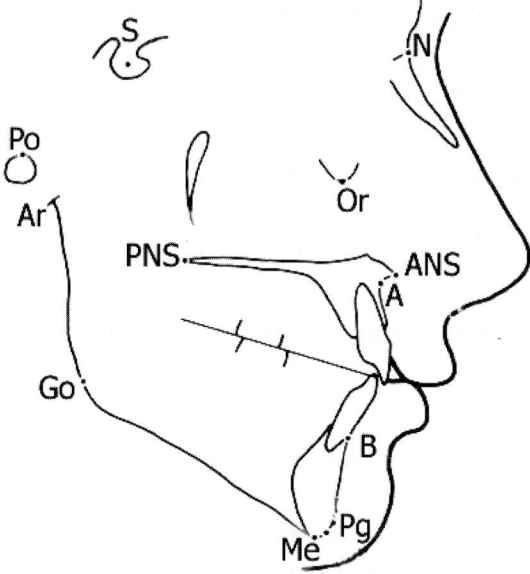

Figure 2.1   Cephalometric outlines and landmarks: A, point A; ANS, anterior nasal spine; Ar, articulare; B, point B; Go, gonion; Me, menton; N, nasion; Or, orbitale; PNS, posterior nasal spine; Pg, pogonion; Po, porion; S, sella.

present two images, the average of the two should be drawn. The exceptions to this are those cases where there is an obvious asymmetry of the mandible, which has resulted in two distinct lower borders to the mandible. From the point of view of measurement, it is normal practice to take the lower border which conforms to the normal side of the face, as assessed clinically.

Points:

- S Sella: The centre of the sella turcica determined by visual inspection.
- N Nasion: The anterior point of the frontonasal suture.
- ANS. Anterior nasal spine: Where the tip of the anterior nasal spine deviates markedly upwards or downwards, it is taken as

the mid-point of the upper and lower spine outlines where it is 2 mm wide.

- PNS. Posterior nasal spine.
- Point A. The deepest midline point on the maxillary alveolus outlined between the anterior nasal spine and the maxillary alveolar crest.
- Point B. The deepest midline point between the mandibular alveolar crest and pogonion.
- Me Menton: The most inferior point on the lower border of the bony symphysis.
- Pg Pogonion: The most anterior point on the bony symphysis.
- Go Gonion: Is determined by bisecting the angle formed by tangents to the lower and posterior borders of the mandible. It is the point where the bisector cuts the angle of the mandible.
- Ar Articulare: The intersection of the posterior border of the ramus and the temporal bone.
- Co Condylion: The superior point on the condylar head.
- Or Orbitale: The most inferior point on the orbital margin.
- Po Porion: The upper margin of the bony external auditory meatus. The upper margin of the condylar head (Co) may also be used as it is often more easily determined.
- UMC. The tip of the mesio-buccal cusp of the upper first permanent molar.
- LMC. The tip of the mesio-buccal cusp of the lower first permanent molar.
- UIA. The tip of the post prominent maxillary incisor root apex.
- UIE. The most prominent maxillary incisor crown edge.
- LIE. The most prominent mandibular incisor crown edge.
- LIA. The tip of the most prominent mandibular incisor root apex.

The following lines are then drawn (Figure 2.2):

- S-N (the anterior cranial base).
- S-Ar.

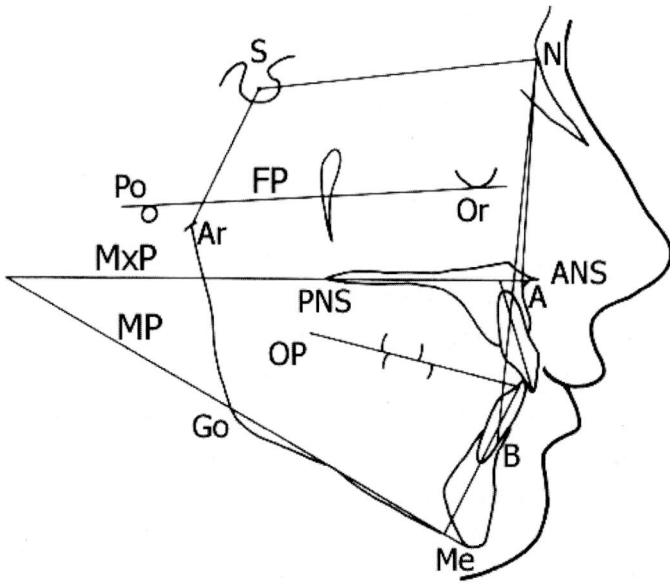

Figure 2.2 The planes and angles. Using the cephalometric points the following planes are constructed; SN plane (SN), mandibular plane (MP), maxillary plane (MxP) and Frankfort plane (FP). The long axes of the maxillary and mandibular incisors are considered relative to the maxillary and mandibular planes respectively. The important cephalometric angles can be readily derived from these points and planes. For key, see Table 2.1.

- N-A.
- N-B.
- Or-Po (the Frankfort plane-FP).
- ANS-PNS (the maxillary plane-MxP).
- Me-Go (mandibular plane-MP).
- Long axes of the upper (UI) and lower (LI) incisors.
- The occlusal plane (OP) is drawn through the outline of the buccal segment teeth, including the premolars. However, it may be difficult to determine the outline of the molars due to super-imposition. Therefore for simplicity, the tips of the upper and lower mesial cusps (UMC and LMC) and the upper and lower distal cusps only are drawn.

The Analysis

The accuracy when undertaking a cephalometric tracing of a radiograph by hand and its analysis only permits linear and angular measurements to be expressed to the nearest whole millimetre or degree. The values obtained can then be compared with the population normal values to determine the patient's problems (Tables 2.1–2.3). It is important to appreciate that they will vary with age, sex and ethnic origin. Table 2.1 presents the mean angular cephalometric values based on a Caucasian population. As can be seen from these tables, there is considerable variation for all values.

Although cephalometric analysis is helpful in providing information for diagnosis and treatment planning, it has to be borne in mind that the ultimate goal is not necessarily to achieve ideal values near to the mean but to produce a proportional and harmonious facial structure. To that end, where there are

Table 2.1   Mean angular cephalometric values (Caucasians)

Measurement	Mean $^0 \pm$ SD
SNA	81 ± 3
SNB	78 ± 3
ANB	3 ± 2
SN/MxP	8 ± 3
SN/MP	35 ± 4
FP/OP	8 ± 4
NSAr (saddle angle)	125 ± 5
SArGo (articular angle)	140 ± 6
ArGoMe (gonial angle)	128 ± 7
MxP/MP	27 ± 4
UI/MxP	109 ± 6
UI/LI	130 ± 6
LI/MP	93 ± 6

For explanations of abbreviations, see text.

Table 2.2   Mean linear cephalometric values (Caucasians)

Measurement		Mean mm ± SD
Facial Heights		
Total anterior	TAFH (N-Me)	124 ± 8
Lower anterior	LAFH	68 ± 8
Total posterior	TPFH (S-Go)	79 ± 6
Lower posterior	LPFH	34 ± 5
	Ar – Go	54 ± 4
Lower anterior face height ratio	LAFH/TAFH%	55 ± 2
Lower posterior face height ratio	LPFH/TPFH%	44 ± 1
Dentoalveolar Heights		
Lower posterior	LPDH (LMC-MP)	38 ± 3
Lower anterior	LADH (LIE-MP)	40 ± 2 (females)
		44 ± 2 (males)
Upper anterior	UADH (UIE- MxP)	33 ± 3
Upper posterior	UPDH (UMC-MxP)	28 ± 3

For explanations of abbreviations, see text.

Table 2.3   Angular cephalometric values (Negroes and Chinese)

Measurement	Value ^{0}	
	Negroes	Chinese
SNA	85	83
SNB	80	80
ANB	5	3
MxP/MP	28	28
UI/MxP	118	113
LI/MP	98	96

For explanation of abbreviations, see text.

These figures may be used for Negro and Oriental patients instead of those in Table 2.1 but should be regarded as a broad guide, rather than an exact ideal, bearing in mind that numbers in some surveys are small and may be the average of a wide range. Because of natural incisor proclination, the aesthetic nasolabial angles are invariably acute, i.e. significantly less than the Caucasian range.

discrepancies between clinical observation and cephalometric values, the analysis of the clinical presentation is always more important.

Vertical Values

Vertical cephalometric analysis is of great value in orthognathic planning.

Linear

The total anterior face height (TAFH) is the sum of the upper anterior face height (UAFH), measured from nasion to the maxillary plane, and the lower anterior face height (LAFH), maxillary plane to menton. The lower anterior face height is usually $55 \pm 2\%$ of the total anterior face height.

Posterior face height is similarly measured from sella to gonion using the maxillary plane to divide the upper posterior face height (UPFH) from the lower posterior face height (LPFH). The lower posterior face height being approximately $43 \pm 1\%$ of the total posterior face height (Figure 2.3).

The anterior dentoalveolar heights are measured from the incisal edges of the upper and lower incisors (UIE and LIE) to the maxillary plane and mandibular plane respectively. It should be noted that these measurements reflect the components of the lower face height. In other words, if the lower anterior face height value is high, then the upper and lower anterior dentoalveolar heights (UADH and LADH) will also be increased, except in some cases of anterior open bite.

The upper and lower posterior dentoalveolar heights (UPDH and LPDH) can be recorded from the tips of the mesial cusps of the upper and lower molars (UMC and LMC) to the maxillary and mandibular planes respectively.

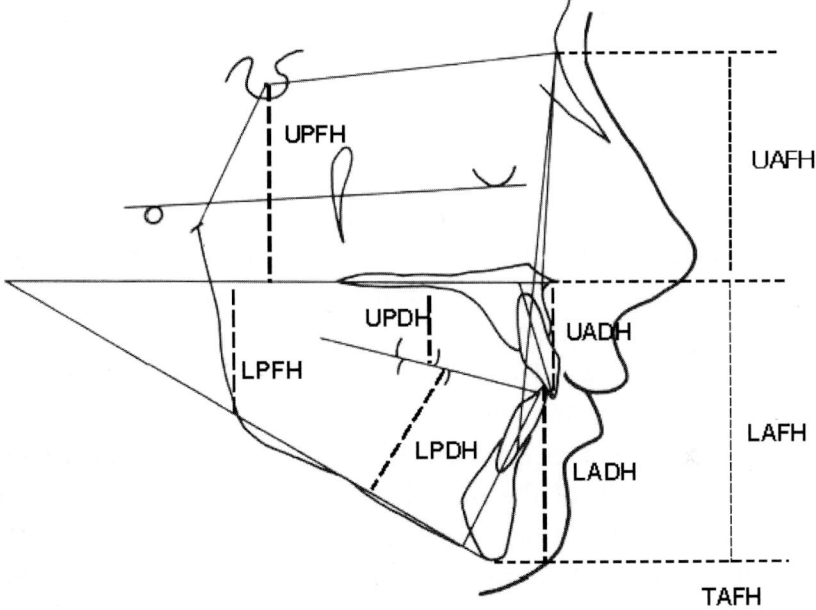

Figure 2.3   Linear measurements for the vertical dimensions. See Table 2.2 for details.

Angular

The relationship of the anterior and posterior face heights is reflected by the angles between the skull base and the maxillary and mandibular planes.

The angle of the maxillary to the mandibular plane (MxP/MP) is normally 27 ± 4°. This angle is important because as with the posterior face height measurement, it reflects the surgically important pterygomasseteric sling length (muscle, fascia and ligaments). For instance, a patient with a high angle, i.e. greater than 35°, tends to have a relatively short posterior face height and therefore posterior musculo-ligamentous height. Any attempt to stretch this posterior connective tissue by rotating the anterior body of the mandible upwards, in an anticlockwise direction, around a fulcrum produced by the posterior molar occlusion, is doomed to failure and will lead to early surgical relapse.

Anteroposterior Relationships

In clinical practice anteroposterior lengths are rarely measured or used to relate the jaws to each other. It has become conventional to study the angular relationship of the jaws to the cranial base (SN). Orientation to the Frankfort plane is also used to compare these structures. However, in extremes of skeletal variation some angular measurements may be misleading. A typical example is the problem of SNA and SNB to analyse the anteroposterior relationship of the maxilla to the mandible (Figure 2.4). In the normal Class I patient, SNA is 81° with a standard deviation of 3°, and the normal maxillary-mandibular relationship (ANB) is 3°. An increased ANB angle suggests a Class II relationship, whereas a negative ANB angle suggests a Class III case. However, variations in the positions of N will influence both the SNA and SNB. For example, with a shorter anterior cranial base length (SN) increasing SNA by 10° alters the ANB angle to 7° giving the impression of a skeletal Class II jaw relationship (Figure 2.4). These variations, due to an "abnormal" SNA, may be corrected by subtracting 0.5° from the ANB angle for every degree by which SNA exceeds the normal value of 81°. In the above example, applying the conversion would reduce the apparent ANB angle from 7° to 2°. Conversely, where the SNA is below the normal value of 81°, 0.5° should be added to the ANB angle for every degree that SNA is below the normal figure. This conversion is only possible providing the SN/MxP values are within the normal range of $8^0 \pm 3^0$. If the SN/MxP value is outside this range then alternate analyses of the anteroposterior skeletal pattern should be employed as detailed in cephalometric specific texts.

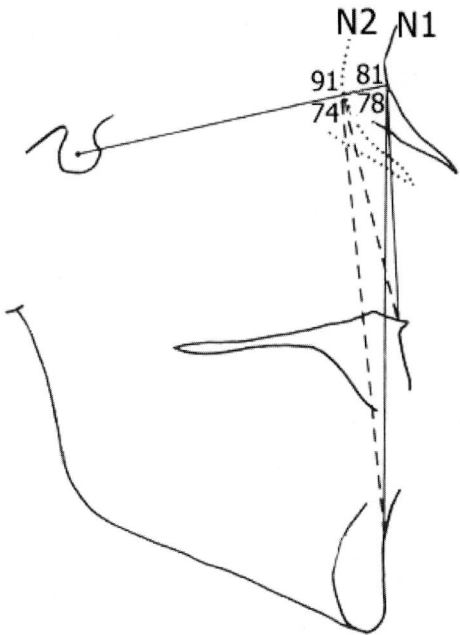

Figure 2.4   Cephalometric idiosyncrasies. The tracing shows how variations in skull base length (SN) can influence the angular values relating to A point and B point. With SNA 81° and SNB 78°, ANB is 3° indicating a Class I skeletal pattern (continuous line). With an unchanged jaw relationship, a shorter skull base SN (from N1 to N2) changes the SNA and SNB angles, i.e. SNA 91°, SNB 74° and ANB becomes 7°, suggesting a Class II skeletal pattern (broken line).

*Analysis of the Incisor Angulations to the Maxillary
and Mandibular Bases*

Skeletal deformity with its disturbed muscular skeletal pattern will lead to changes in the angles of the upper incisor to the maxillary plane (UI/MxP) and the lower incisor to the mandibular plane (LI/MP) adding a degree of secondary deformity (dental compensation) to any underlying skeletal discrepancy (Figure 2.5). Thus with a mandibular prognathism the lower incisors tend to be retroclined

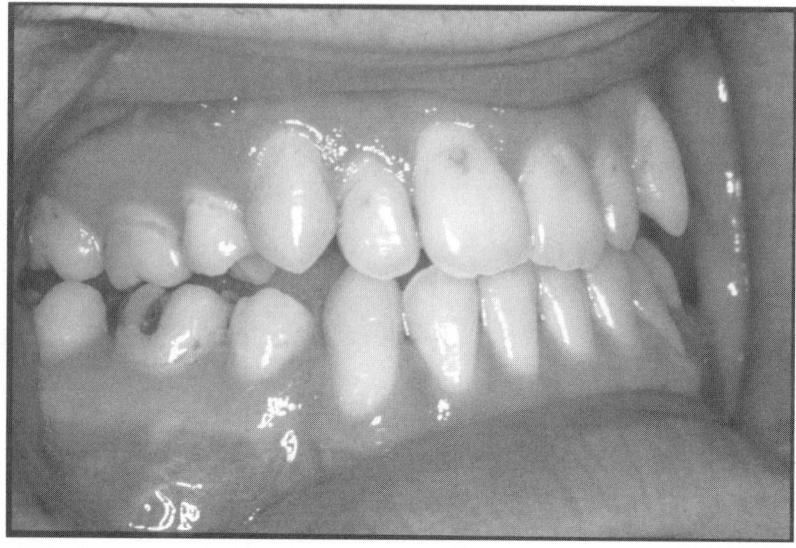

Figure 2.5   Dental compensation in a Class III case with proclination of the maxillary incisors and retroclination of the mandibular incisor teeth. See also Figures 4.8 and 4.9.

and the maxillary incisors proclined. In some severe Class II deformities the lower lip may become trapped behind the maxillary incisors with the effect that the upper incisors may actually procline, whilst the lower incisors may be retroclined. This "compensation" requires correction, i.e decompensation, as part of the overall treatment plan.

The Surgical Application of Cephalometry

Caution must be used in the interpretation of precise linear measurements such as the anterior face height. Measurements from different samples can vary by as much as 10 mm. This problem is diminished when the components are expressed as a percentage. In addition, too many measurements may cause confusion, defeating the purpose of the analysis. However, the exercise is an important means of studying the clinical problem. The geometry can also be checked by the use of diagnostic templates.

Various templates to be matched to the patient for age and sex have been developed from population studies. The Bolton ("unisex") template, provides a simple means of diagnosis when superimposed over the cranial base and calvarium of the patient's lateral skull radiograph or tracing (Figure 2.6a). The Jacobson templates are alternatives, which provide racial separation (Figure 2.6b). This direct method of diagnosis may be particularly attractive to those who find cephalometrics confusing. However, a template should not be considered in any way a treatment goal but rather an aid in establishing the exact areas of discrepancy.

Computerised Cephalometrics

Many computer software packages are now available which with direct digitisation of radiographs, store the data as co-ordinates. Computerised cephalometrics have the advantage that any number of identical copies of the computerised tracing can be produced, and superimpositions can be achieved readily by incorporating normal template tracings into the data bank. But they also have the disadvantage of removing the "personal touch". Many operators still prefer undertaking a hand tracing as it gives a greater appreciation of any difficulties of a particular case, identified during the planning process. Computerised cephalometrics are discussed in detail in Chapter 3.

Posteroanterior Radiograph Tracings

The major use of posteroanterior skull radiograph tracings is for the identification of facial asymmetries. By constructing a series of horizontal and vertical reference planes the exact extent of the asymmetry can be readily demonstrated (Figure 2.7).

(a)

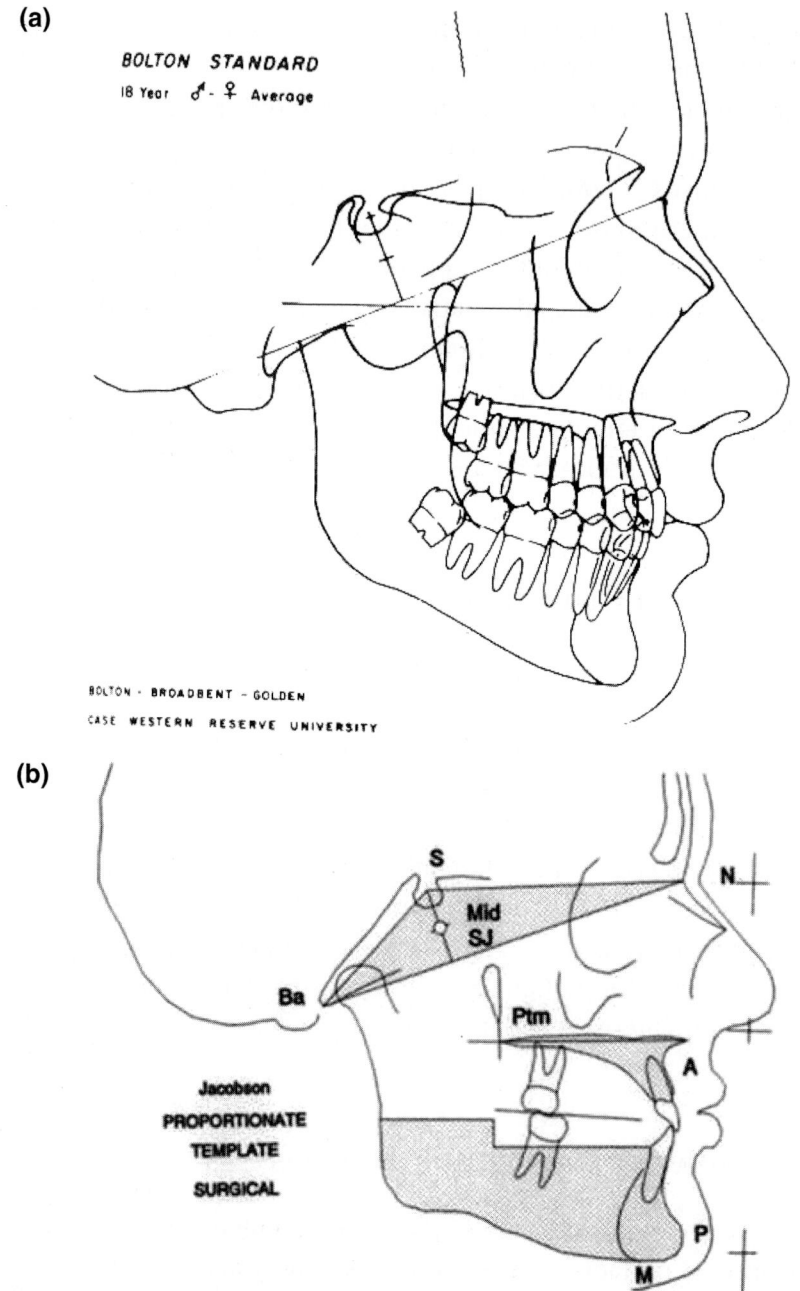

Figure 2.6   **(a)** Bolton standard template. **(b)** Jacobson proportional template.

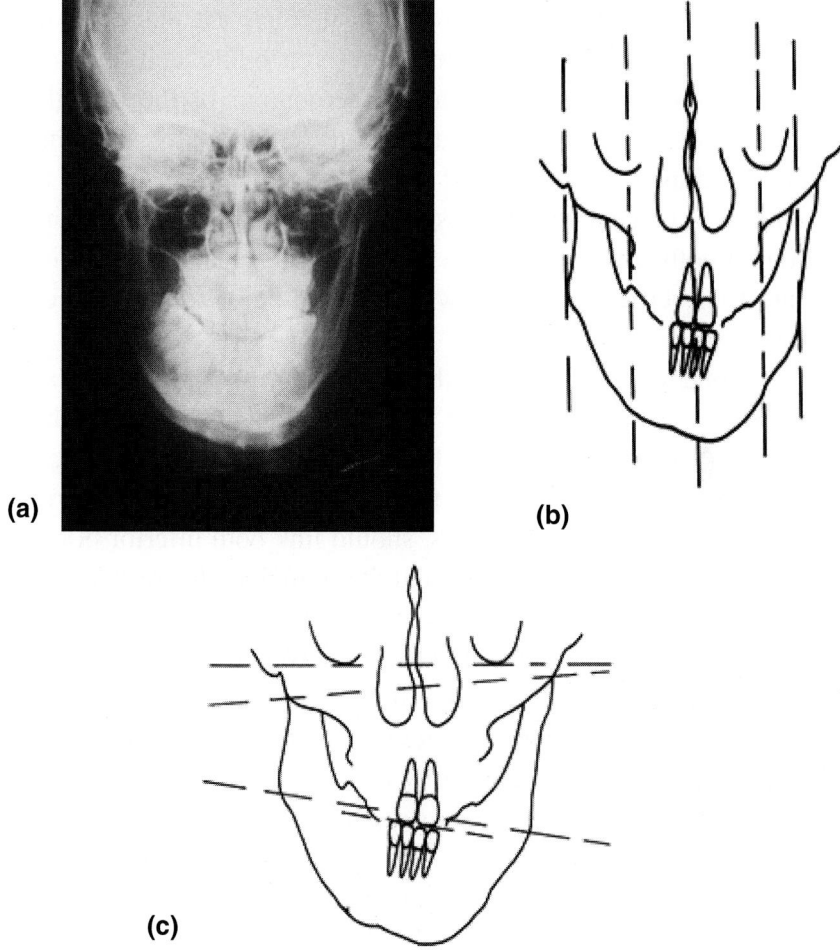

(a)

(b)

(c)

Figure 2.7 (a) Posteroanterior cephalogram used in the assessment of facial asymmetry. Vertical (b) and horizontal (c) reference lines give an indication of the site of the asymmetry. See text for details.

In the vertical plane it is normal to draw a median reference line passing through the centre of the nasal bones, through the majority of the nasal septum (unless there is gross deviation) and this line when extended inferiorly should coincide with the midline of the upper central incisors, midline of the lower central incisors and the midpoint of the chin. Two more vertical reference planes should then be drawn, parallel to the median reference line, and forming a tangent to the most lateral point of the contour of the maxillary tuberosity region. Moving further laterally, additional vertical lines should be drawn, again parallel to the median reference line, and passing as a tangent to the most lateral point of the gonial angle region on both sides of the face. As such the face has been divided up into four vertical segments which should be of equal transverse width.

A second series of lines is then drawn in the horizontal plane. The horizontal reference plane should be taken as a line which passes as a tangent to the lower border of the infra-orbital margins, and ideally this should intersect the median vertical plane at a right angle. The second and third lines, should link both inferior borders of the right and left tuberosities and the gonial angles respectively, revealing any horizontal discrepancies. Finally, lines drawn across the incisal edges of the upper and lower incisors represent the upper and lower occlusal planes as seen in the PA view.

Through a combination of these vertical and horizontal reference lines the exact source of bony and dental asymmetries can be identified. This form of analysis is particularly useful in identifying the presence and extent of any cants to the occlusal plane but is dependent on an accurately positioned cephalogram.

Orthopantomogram Tracing

Tracing of the orthopantomogram is not undertaken as part of routine assessment. However, when considering asymmetries in the lower border of the mandible a full tracing of the radiograph may prove useful. An example of a tracing is seen in Figure 2.8 where a tracing of the normal side of the radiograph has been superimposed on the abnormal side using the occlusal plane as a guide. The discrepancy of the mandibular borders can be seen readily (Figure 2.8b). In marked cases of mandibular asymmetry, a procedure

(a)

(b)

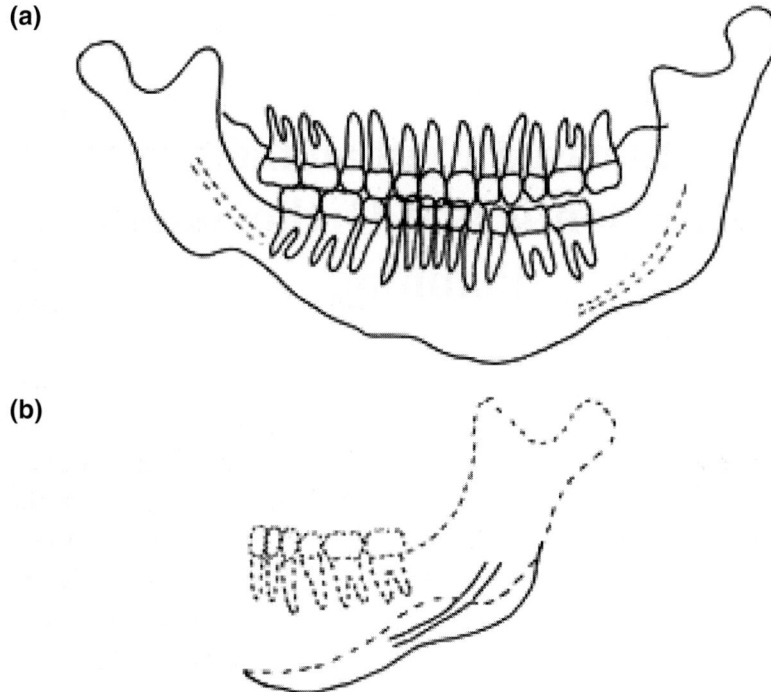

Figure 2.8 **(a)** Orthopantomogram tracing of a patient with hemimandibular hyperplasia. **(b)** The "normal" side tracing has been superimposed over the "abnormal" side, using the occlusal plane as a reference, indicating the extent of bone removal necessary to achieve a symmetrical lower border to the mandible and that repositioning of the dentoalveolar nerve would be required.

to reduce the lower border of the mandible may be considered. This tracing can give information as to the extent of the bone to be removed and whether or not the inferior dental nerve is likely to need repositioning. The advent of CADCAM milling machines linked to three-dimensional CT scans have largely superseded this method of planning, however, tracing the orthopantomogram provides a simple approach when such techniques are unavailable.

3

Computerised Cephalometrics for Orthodontic and Orthognathic Planning

Although the basic cephalometric methodology has remained unchanged for many years the application of information technology, to store, display and manipulate cephalometric images has evolved so that;

i)   Analysis is significantly faster and more reliable when compared to manual measurement.
ii) Reformation of data enables the simulation of treatment alternatives.

These benefits are seen with direct digital imaging in which the X-ray beam is recorded by photoelectric sensors, such as charged coupled devices, or by a storage phosphor emulsion which is scanned and read by a laser diode (light source). These images require a reduced radiation exposure and can be read as a soft copy on a monitor or a hard copy printed out on transparency film or paper. Indirect digital imaging methods include copying the backlit radiograph film with a digital camera or by computer entry with a flatbed scanner. Both systems provide multiple advantages such as ease of storage, manipulation and enhancement, duplication and the possibility of automated landmark identification.

Regardless of the method used to produce the digital image, the data storage and display are very different from conventional film.

Images on a monitor display are composed of a matrix of discrete units called picture elements or pixels. The spatial resolution or clarity of the image is directly proportional to the number of pixels. More pixels mean a sharper image but it also requires the manipulation and storage of more information. The contrast of a digital radiograph is determined by the number of shades of grey which can be displayed. This is known as the bit depth which is determined by the means (algorithm) used to process the image. For example, in a 6-bit image each pixel will have 64 possible values, ranging from black (0) to white (63). An 8-bit image would be able to show 256 shades of grey and 12-bit images can show 1024 shades. Most dental radiology applications use 8-bit images but newer technologies are available that allow for 12- and 16-bit images.

A limiting factor when viewing digital images is the monitor itself. Typical monitors have 72–96 pixels per inch (ppi) display resolution and are capable of 625 digital (raster) lines. The full potential of any image with higher resolution can only be displayed with clarity after being printed as a hard copy. For digital images equal to film quality, a monitor capable of displaying 2048 raster lines would be needed. In addition to being expensive, it is difficult for computers to refresh (handle) this number of lines without creating a "flicker" in the image.

Digital images are further limited by the monitor's contrast capabilities. Analogue films have an almost infinite or continuous greyscale. As stated, most dental digital images are viewed with only 256 shades of grey. The problem is compounded by the fact that digital images are often displayed more brightly than with analogue film which tends to reduce the already inferior greyscale resolution. It is important to bear in mind that the number of shades of grey or bit depth needed is dependent on what is being diagnosed from the image.

Once the spatial resolution and contrast have been optimised, the capacity of the human eye becomes the limiting factor. The smallest detail the human eye can resolve is approximately 0.1 mm by 0.1 mm. Therefore, we are unable to appreciate more detail in

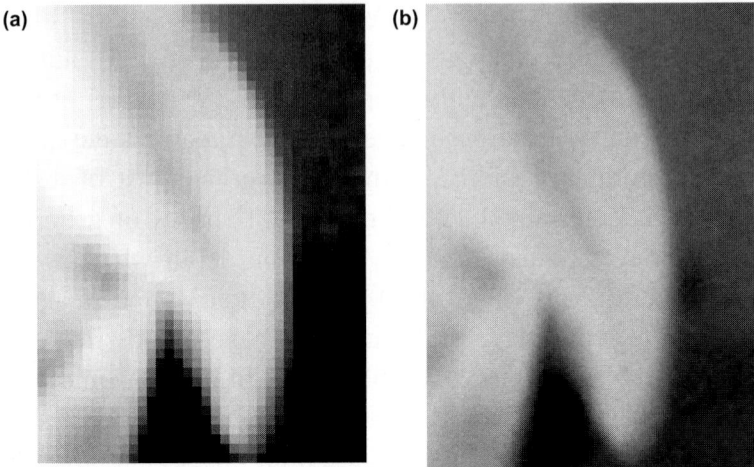

(a)   **(b)**

Figure 3.1 These digital images are identical except for spatial resolution. **(a)** The left image has a pixel dimension of 0.084 × 0.084 which is at the limit the human eye can resolve. **(b)** The pixel dimension of the image on the right is 0.35 × 0.35. Note the fuzzy appearance with loss of definition.

any image with a smaller pixel size. Conversely, images with pixels of a much larger size, for example 0.7 mm by 0.7 mm, may seem blurred (Figure 3.1). A pixel size of 0.1 mm should be equal to X-ray film when identifying landmarks on cephalometric radiographs.

Digital imaging technology is becoming the standard of care. The advantages of storage, portability, ease of duplication, manipulation and communication outweigh the disadvantages. However, with these advantages come responsibilities. The ease of data manipulation opens the opportunity for record tampering. The ease of duplication and portability create problems of confidentiality. The DICOM (digital imaging and communication in medicine) Standards have been developed to attain compatibility and to ensure workflow efficiency between imaging systems and other information systems. The standards also address security in record transmission and storage as well as record "locking" or digital signatures. The dedicated clinician must be vigilant of changes in hardware, software and responsibilities for their use.

Treatment Planning with Digital Images

Orthognathic treatment planning requires some method of predicting the anticipated outcome. In clinical practice this has been based on experience and intuition. Digital simulation is based on a tracing prepared from landmarks identified on a standardised lateral cephalometric radiograph. The dental and skeletal structures are moved to correct the malocclusion and the predicted soft tissue response is based on data collected from a retrospective analysis of previous treatment tempered with clinical experience. This process helps the clinician to anticipate and understand the dental and surgical movements needed (Figure 3.2). The simulation gives the patient and family a glimpse of the aesthetic change. Various terms have been given to this process including VTO (visualised treatment objective) and STO (surgical treatment objective). These simulations are almost always limited to a profile view due to the lack of data and the technical limitations associated with PA cephalometry. Surface laser scans and photogrammetry provide alternative techniques to overcome this limitation.

Although acetate tracings are adequate for most clinicians, patients may view them as arcane. To improve patient understanding efforts have been made to incorporate a photographic likeness into the process. Initially, this was limited to a photographic montage created by rearranging cut-outs of profile photographs. The computer has streamlined the process so that cephalometric data can be digitally entered, stored and recalled for analysis or manipulation. The graphic reproduction of tracings is done using a plotter which is basically a computer driven felt-tip marker. Early software programmes were limited to the analysis of cephalometric landmarks which had been entered or "digitised" into the computer memory. Software engineering has produced programmes which allow repositioning of anatomical structures and treatment simulations. Although technologically refined it is very important to remember that the result is no better than the data used to predict the soft tissue response.

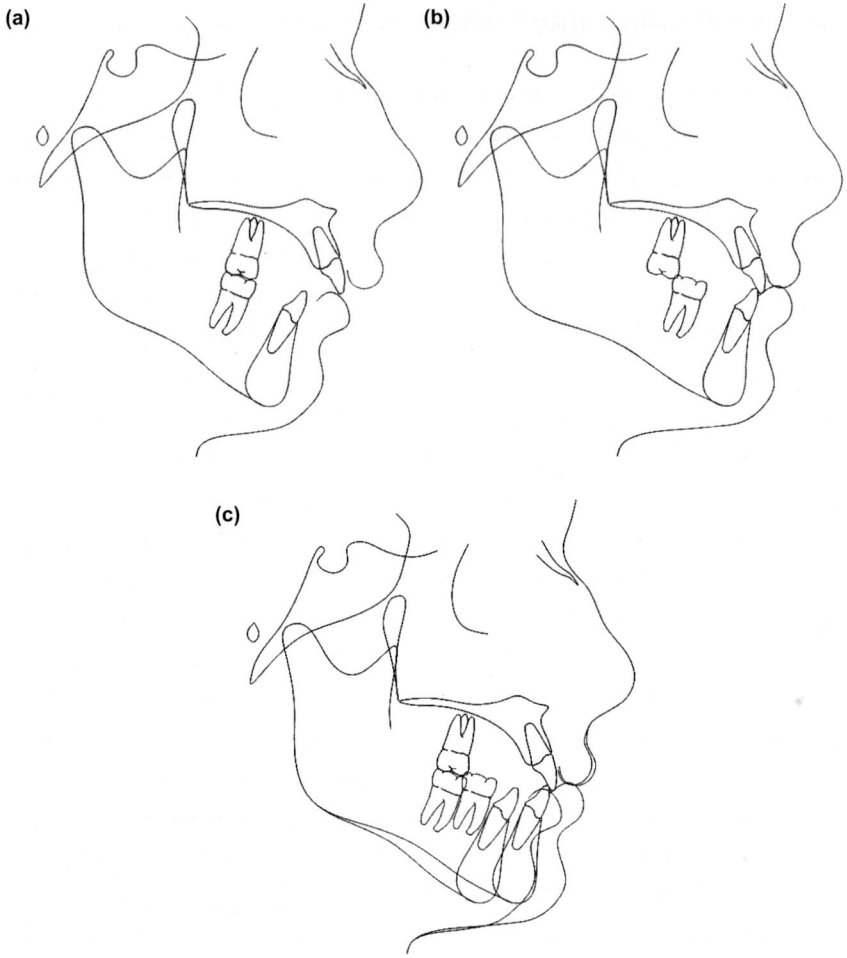

Figure 3.2   Simulation tracings can be done by hand on acetate or are computer generated. **(a)** The preoperative cephalometric tracing is altered to simulate the mandibular advancement **(b)**. **(c)** The superimposition graphically demonstrates the amount of movement needed for correction.

Patient Education

The breakthrough in treatment simulation for patient education came with the ability to manipulate patient's photographs, video images or slides which were "rasterised" (converted from analogue to digital form) prior to being linked to the cephalometric tracing. Although the result was still limited to a profile view, both patient and clinician had a representation which was much closer to a credible likeness.

Patients need to have the nature of their problem presented in a language they can understand. For both educational and a medico-legal reasons, those involved must understand the risk versus benefit of any treatment involving a change in appearance. Facial appearance is invariably the primary motivator for those seeking surgical correction but it may not necessarily be the principal underlying reason.

Some have voiced concerns regarding the use of digital imaging in patient communication suggesting the possibility of legal action if the treatment outcome does not approximate to the simulation. For this reason most vendors have a disclaimer on any printed copy of the image. Although there is no history of litigation related to disappointment over failure of the actual outcome to match treatment simulation, the need for good communication is paramount when patients have mild or moderate rather than severe aesthetic problems. These patients are in a borderline area where the alternatives could range from no treatment to surgical correction, with extractions and orthodontic compensation being a "compromise" option. It is generally easier for the patient and family to accept a surgical treatment plan when there is a severe dentofacial deformity. It is the middle-ground cases which require the greatest communication skills on the part of the orthodontist and surgeon to enable patients and or parents to select the management that best suits their needs.

The decision is crucial as the objectives for orthodontic compensation are the opposite to those for orthodontic preparation prior to orthognathic surgery. For example, the anterior teeth are compensated for the orthodontic solution but decompensated prior to surgery. Furthermore the extraction patterns differ between compensation and surgical preparation. The approach to levelling mechanics and space closure is also different with each option. Since it is difficult if not impossible to cope with a "change of heart" patient, all the information required to choose between the treatment options must be presented prior to the start of treatment. Digital treatment simulation is a valuable tool in making this decision. Treatment simulation may also be used immediately prior to surgery in the context of the final surgical planning.

Interactive Programmes

Digital imaging technology offers several options for planning and patient education. Interactive programmes are useful during the preliminary consultations. This type of software employs a mixture of still photographs, graphic art and multimedia which demonstrates specific problems and their potential solutions. The clinician can easily demonstrate the difference between orthodontic compensation and surgical correction using the illustrations from the programme (Figure 3.3). The artist's representations of treatment outcome can be stylised to demonstrate the trends in facial change seen with each option. If there is continued interest on the part of the patient and or family, full diagnostic records can be taken for analysis prior to developing an orthodontic/orthognathic problem list and the treatment simulation using the patient's data.

Simulation Programmes

Although the data entry approach varies among programmes, the following steps are common to each:

- The standard photographic series is directly entered with a digital camera or scanned into the computer from photographs or slides.
- The lateral cephalometric radiograph is imported into the programme via direct digital radiography or scanning with a transparency adapter.
- The conventional cephalometric analysis follows on-screen digitising the requisite landmarks for the protocol. Radiographs of marginal quality can be enhanced with a variety of graphic tools.

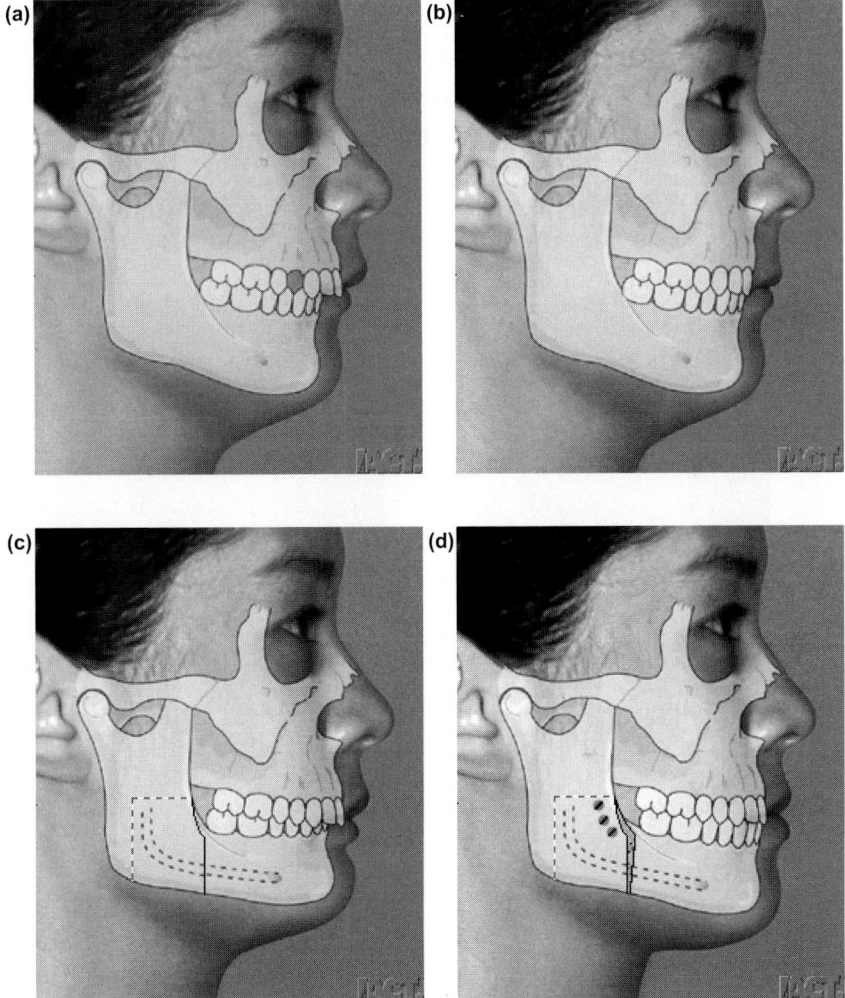

Figure 3.3 This multimedia programme demonstrates the contrast between correcting mandibular deficiency with orthodontic camouflage versus orthognathic surgery. Images (**a**) and (**b**) show extraction of the upper first premolars with subsequent retraction of the incisors and upper lip. Images (**c**) and (**d**) demonstrate the changes seen with surgical lengthening of the mandible. (courtesy of InterActive Communication & Training, 3300 Cahaba Road, Suite 101 Birmingham, AL 35253, USA).

- The resulting cephalometric tracing is manipulated to achieve "best fit" and superimposed on the profile photograph (Figure 3.4).
- Orthodontic and surgical movements can now be simulated using the linked image-tracing combination (Figures 3.4 and 3.5).

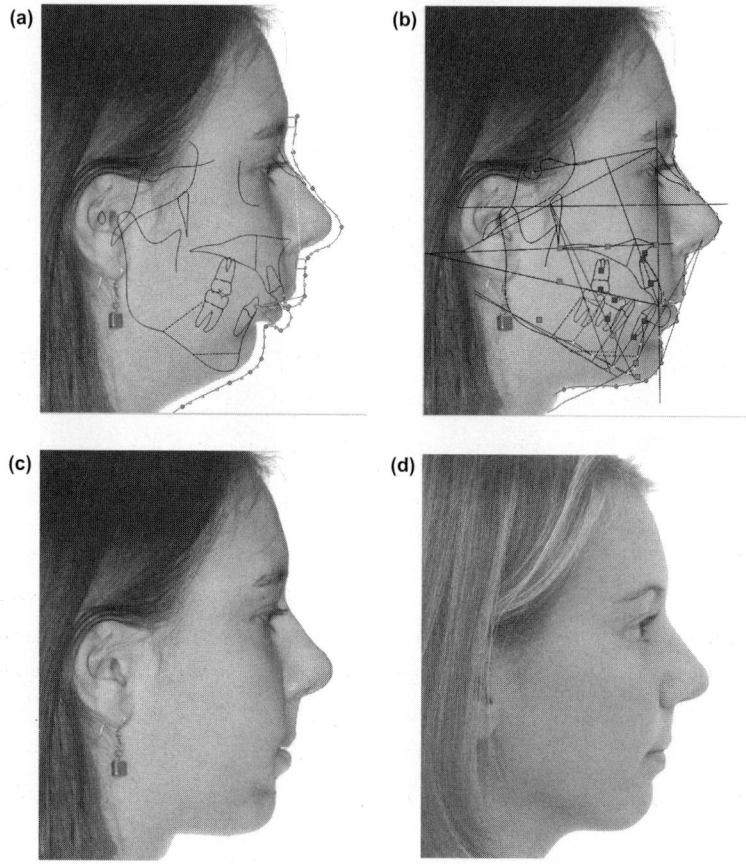

Figure 3.4   **(a)** Digital treatment simulation requires linking of the profile image with the tracing digitised from the lateral cephalometric film. The process is facilitated by having the head and soft tissue posture as identical as possible. The image-tracing pair **(b)** is manipulated with the software to simulate the surgical advancement of the mandible. The final simulation **(c)** is a close approximation of the actual outcome **(d)**. All software programmes have difficulty creating the natural contours of the lips and mentolabial fold.

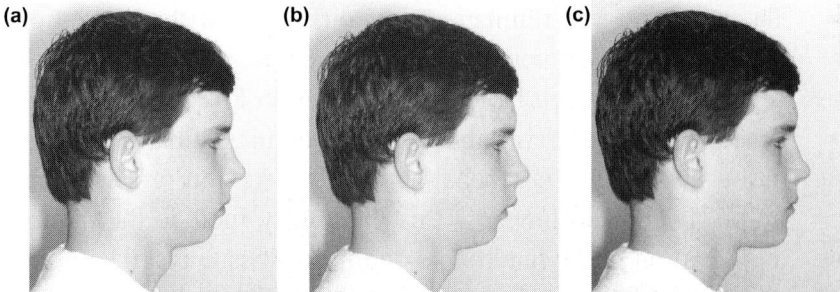

Figure 3.5   Treatment simulation software has been used to alter this patient's pre-treatment image **(a)** to portray the outcome of orthodontic camouflage **(b)** versus surgical mandibular advancement **(c)**. Compared to cephalometric tracings, these images are more easily understood by patients and their family.

- The soft tissue response from specific dental and skeletal movements is modelled by computer algorithms based on retrospective data from long-term studies of stability and treatment outcome.

Limitations

- Simulation is no better than the data on which it is based and which may be flawed by small sample size and heterogeneity, treatment instability, and errors in surgical management.
- Mean values are used to develop linear ratios which determine soft tissue movements relative to a skeletal landmark. The assumption is that the soft tissue response is a fixed percentage of skeletal movement, regardless of the extent of skeletal change. This approach fails to account for local variations due to muscle tone, soft tissue compression and tissue redundancy.
- Studies have shown that most programmes now produce reasonable simulations when the surgical movements are moderate, limited to the sagittal plane, and involve patients with competent lips and little eversion.

- These same programmes have difficulty with simulations involving vertical movements in patients with increased lip separation or a deep labiomental fold with lip redundancy.
- A second source of variability is the sophistication of the technique for linking the cephalometric tracing and profile photograph. Factors influencing this variability include the number and location of the landmarks on the soft tissue profile; and the ability to adjust for differences in the radiographic and photographic scales.
- The recognised differences in orientation between the radiograph and profile photograph invariably need some adjustment in linking.
- Finally, most programmes have image refinement tools which allow the clinician to adjust the simulation's soft tissue response according to personal experience with certain surgical movements. These adjustments introduce potential sources of inaccuracy but are often needed to correct the predicted lip posture.

4

Orthodontic Preparation

Timing and Duration

The objectives of presurgical orthodontic treatment are to enable maximal surgical correction of the deformity, to facilitate any segmental surgical procedures and to enable the production of an ideal stable occlusion. An essential feature of the treatment plan is to decompensate the dento-alveolar results of the jaw deformity and as such is very different from the "compensatory" approach of the pure orthodontic management of the case. Hence the need for careful consideration by the patient and clinicians as to the desired choice of treatment. The majority of orthodontic treatment is undertaken prior to surgery, although some prefer to undertake minimal orthodontic treatment prior to surgery leaving the major proportion to the postoperative phase. Both of these approaches have advantages and disadvantages. Extensive presurgical preparation is usually better accepted by the patient giving maximum compliance. However, the dental movements may be hindered by the underlying skeletal and soft tissue discrepancy. Conversely, although the orthodontic changes may be easier once a normal skeletal and soft tissue relationship has become established, prolonged postoperative orthodontics may not be tolerated by the patient and leads to poor patient satisfaction.

Presurgical Orthodontics

Presurgical preparation usually takes 18–24 months, whilst postsurgical refinement should be completed within 6 months of the operation.

The goals of presurgical orthodontics are to facilitate the surgery by:

- Alignment of the dentition.
- Levelling of the occlusal plane, either as a continuous arch or segmentally prior to surgical levelling.
- Incisor decompensation.
- Buccal segment decompensation.
- Coordination of the upper and lower arches.
- Providing a means of fixation.

Alignment of the Dentition — The Technology

Dental arch alignment requires 3-dimensional control of tooth position. Most use a pre-adjusted Edgewise appliance system with a slot dimension of .022" × .028" or variants upon this. The term pre-adjusted appliance refers to the bracket design such that adjustments are incorporated into the brackets to create a final position of the teeth with the correct mesiodistal angulation (tip), buccopalatal or buccolingual inclination (torque) and horizontal positions (in/out) relative to each other. Individual teeth within the dental arch therefore have specific adjustments built into their appropriate bracket (Figure 4.1). A variety of pre-adjusted systems are available each with minor variations in the tip and torque values. This is referred to as the bracket prescription. Segmental surgery requires the added facility of a double tube on the mandibular molars and/or a triple tube on the maxillary molars. The Tip-Edge™ appliance system is equally applicable to presurgical alignment although individual operators will have their preferred bracket prescription.

It is worthwhile considering the variations in bracket tip and torque required in specific cases. In an ideal occlusion, the crown of the lower incisor lies labial to the apex for ideal tooth inclination. In Class II cases where proclined lower incisor require decompensation, the use of MBT™ brackets with the 6^0 of additional lingual

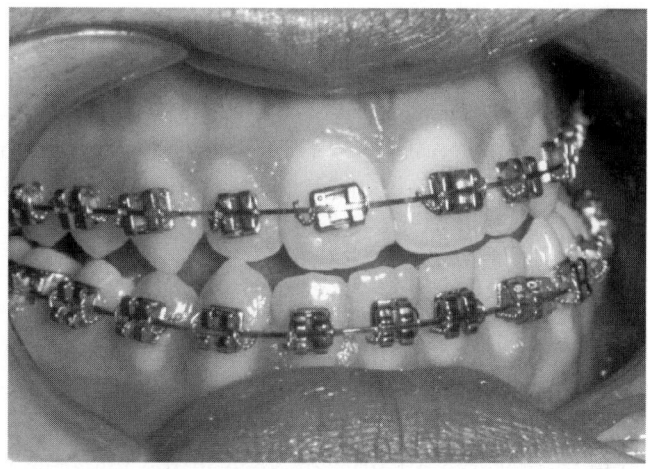

Figure 4.1   Pre-adjusted Edgewise appliances with individual brackets designed for specific teeth.

crown torque can aid the mechanics. Conversely, Super-torque™ brackets, with additional palatal root torque to the upper incisors, can be useful in correcting severely retroclined incisors in Class II division 2 cases. Mesiodistal tooth angulation (tip) becomes important when considering the preparation of a case for segmental surgery as it is important to facilitate the surgery (see below) by ensuring the roots adjacent to the osteotomy site are either parallel or slightly divergent. Again in an ideal functioning occlusion, the crown of the canine should lie mesial to the apex. Where the osteotomy cuts are to be made distal to the canines, the use of the canine bracket of the opposite side ensures that the tip incorporated into the bracket keeps the apices forward and out of the way of the surgical cuts.

The choice of archwire material and sequence is to a large extent, driven by operator preference. The use of modern "superelastic" nickel titanium wires is frequently beneficial for initial alignment. However, where the interbracket span is minimal, for example with mutually rotated lower incisors or premolars, the efficiency of these wires is reduced. In this situation, archwires with loops for flexibility may be preferable, for example .014" or .016" stainless steel or Titanium/Molybdenum (TMA) wires. Ultimately, heavy rectangular stainless steel archwires should be placed at the time of surgery (.019" × .028" or .022" × .028") for maximal tooth control and with the addition of hooks to facilitate fixation.

Arch Levelling

The decision as to whether to fully level the arches is very much dependent on the patient's facial height and the upper lip/incisor relationship. In Class II corrections, where the facial height is reduced, it is preferable to preserve a Curve of Spee in the lower arch so that when the mandible is advanced, the lower incisors slide down the cingulum plateau of the upper incisors thereby increasing the lower facial height (Figure 4.2). Although this may occur in some Class II division 1 cases, it is especially common in patients with Class II division 2 incisor relationships where the presurgical orthodontic preparation converts the incisors into a Class II division 1 pattern.

Following surgery this results in buccal segment lateral open bites with occlusal contact in only the incisor and terminal molar regions. This tripod of contacts is referred to as a "3-point landing". The lateral open bites (Figure 4.3) require closure as part of the postsurgical orthodontic phase of treatment (see Chapter 10).

In Class II cases where the intention is to avoid increasing the facial height, the lower arch should be levelled as part of the presurgical orthodontic preparation, or by segmental surgical procedures. With a shallow curve of Spee (approximately 2 mm), it may be possible to level the arches orthodontically through a combination of buccal segment extrusion, incisor intrusion and/or incisor proclination (Figure 4.4). Levelling the Curve of Spee without space will procline the lower incisors, and reduce the potential for mandibular advancement. If the intention is to maintain anteroposterior arch length, then premolar extractions will be required, especially if there is any crowding present (Figure 4.5).

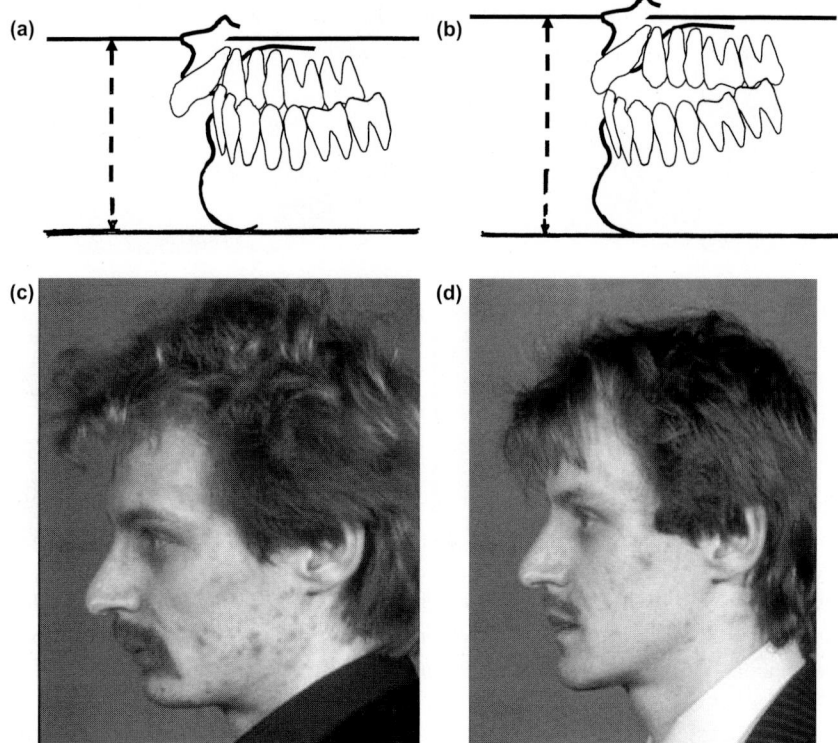

Figure 4.2 (a) and (c) Class II deep overbite cases, with an increased curve of Spee, facilitates an increase in anterior face height as the mandible is advanced (b) and (d). The resulting contact between the upper and lower incisors and the terminal molars of each side of the arch is referred to as a "3-point landing". Note the significant increase in lower facial height accompanying the advancement.

Segmental Levelling

a) *In cases of reduced vertical dimension*

In cases with a severe overbite the so-called "3-point landing" may produce lateral open bites which are too large to close by orthodontic extrusion of the premolars and canines. Many operators consider 2 mm of extrusion from each arch as the absolute maximum that can be achieved and remain stable without rebound. Beyond this, levelling

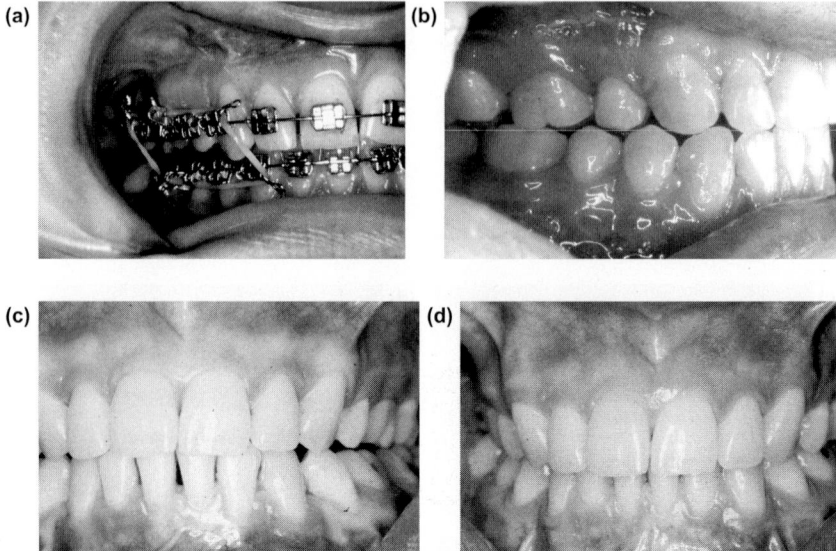

Figure 4.3   Following mandibular advancement the resulting lateral open bites can **(a)** be closed in the postoperative orthodontic phase **(b)** or may even close spontaneously **(c)** and **(d)**. See also Figure 4.16.

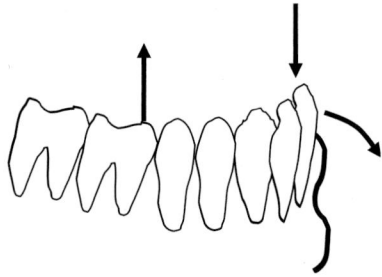

Figure 4.4   Orthodontic levelling of an increased curve of Spee can be achieved as a combination of premolar/molar extrusion, incisor intrusion or incisor proclination.

should be achieved through surgery, usually through a set-down of the lower labial segment with a mandibulotomy (see Chapter 9). Where there is a reverse Curve of Spee in the upper arch, as in some Class II division 2 cases, it may be necessary to undertake segmental surgery to both the upper and lower labial segments.

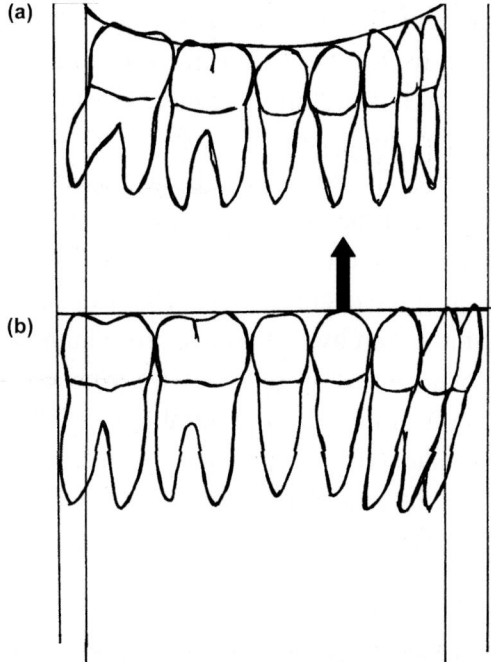

Figure 4.5   **(a)** Levelling the curve of Spee orthodontically will lead to **(b)** incisor proclination and an increase in arch length unless space is created through extractions.

With all segmental surgery cases, the presurgical orthodontics should facilitate the alveolar section by diverging the canine and premolar roots. The mesiodistal tip incorporated into the canine brackets is such that the root apex will align distal to the crown encroaching into the site of the surgical cuts. When planning cases for segmental surgery it may be desirable to use the right canine bracket on the left canine and *vice versa* in order to keep the roots away from the osteotomy site. The brackets can then be replaced with those of the correct side in the postsurgical period.

Segmental orthodontic levelling is designed to place the buccal segments at one level and the incisor segments at a different level. This can be achieved by three segmental archwires, two running in the buccal segments from premolar to molar on each side together with a third segment for the canine and incisors. This approach tends to produce a lack of control of the tooth positions and therefore a continuous arch is preferred, from molar to molar but with an anterior step for the canines and incisors.

In the latter case, the surgeon will cut the archwire across the osteotomy site at the time of surgery. Although the segments are immobilised using rigid internal fixation, it is essential to provide additional fixation at the occlusal level. This can be done with a prefabricated continuous archwire bent to the planned postoperative segments. However, insertion of this wire intraoperatively can be extremely time-consuming. It is preferable to use a rigid prefabricated horseshoe shaped 1.0 mm steel supplemental arch wire, engaged passively into double or triple tubes on the molars and secured by ligatures to the three archwire segments (Figure 4.6).

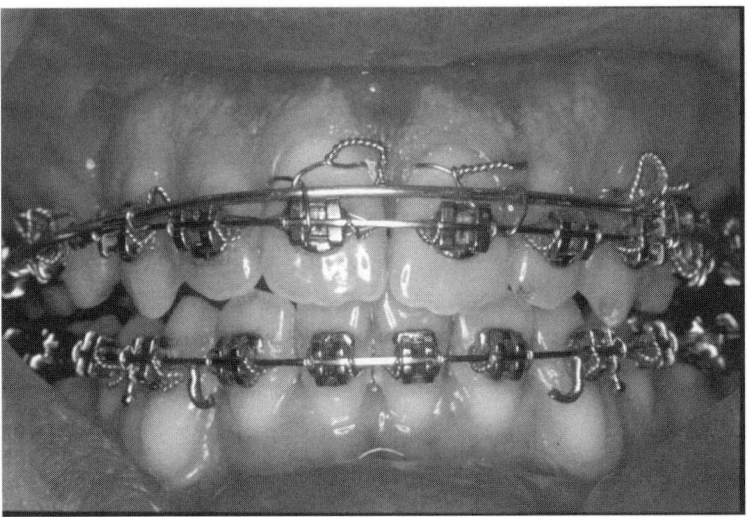

Figure 4.6   To control the occlusal relationship after segmental surgery the segmented arch (upper) is fixed at the occlusal level using a heavy 1mm stainless steel archwire. This is engaged passively into a headgear tube on the molar bands. Auxillary steel ligatures lash the segmented orthodontic archwire in the anterior and buccal segments to the heavy buccal arch.

Ultimately, the sectional arches can be replaced with a continuous archwire once the patient has recovered.

b) *In cases of increased vertical dimension*

In anterior open bite cases, the presurgical orthodontics must not be allowed to extrude the incisors as this is potentially unstable and will jeopardise the surgical correction. The presurgical orthodontics should accentuate the open bite through intrusion of the labial segments and extrusion of the buccal segments. In this way maximal surgical correction can be achieved and any post-surgical incisor change will ensure closure of the anterior open bite (Figures 4.7a and 4.7b).

Incisor Decompensation

In the majority of cases of severe antero-posterior disproportion, the soft tissues of the lips and tongue produce a secondary defor-mity of incisor inclination. In skeletal Class III cases, so-called

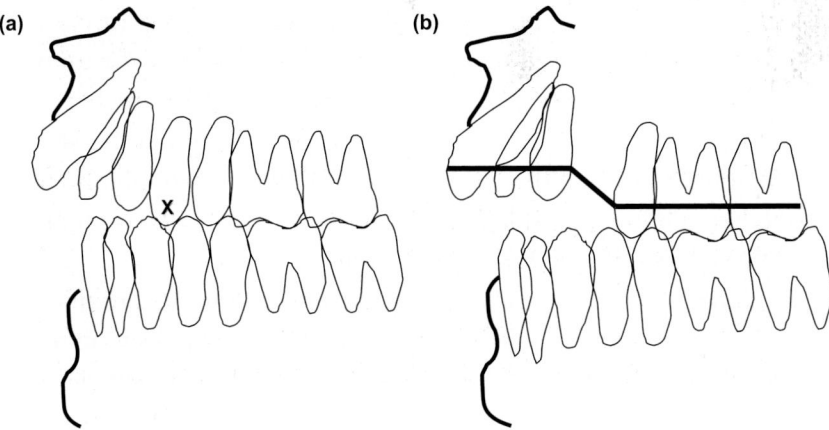

Figure 4.7   **(a)** and **(b)** Segmental orthodontic levelling of the Curve of Spee with a continuous archwire. The step in the archwire is designed to accentuate the anterior open bite by incisor intrusion and buccal segment extrusion. Any post-surgical rebound of the teeth will help maintain closure of the open bite.

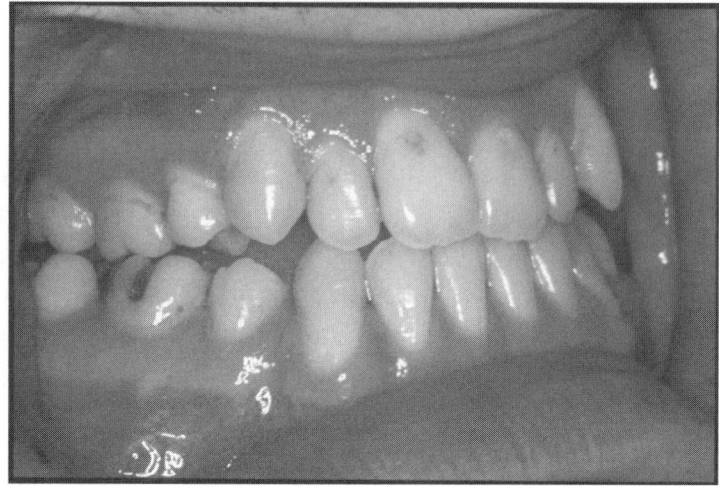

Figure 4.8   The secondary dental deformity of a prognathous mandible is the so called "compensation" with proclination of the maxillary incisors and retroclination of the mandibular incisor teeth.

compensation presents with proclined upper incisors and retroclined lower incisors (Figure 4.8). Presurgical preparation (decompensation) corrects the axial inclinations to maximise the mandibular setback (Figure 4.9). Although dictated by the amount of crowding, it is common for the lower arch to be treated non-extraction, aligning the labial segment by proclination. Care should be taken not to breach the labial alveolar plate, destroying the periodontal attachment, producing a dehiscence of the gingival margin. Periodontal grafting should be considered.

Severely crowded cases may need extractions to provide the space for arch alignment. With simultaneous decompensation of the lower incisors, the extractions of choice are the lower second premolars, assuming all teeth to be of good prognosis. This also adds to the anchorage balance in the lower arch through the incorporation of eight teeth in the anterior segment.

When using the pre-adjusted Edgewise brackets the orthodontist can take advantage of the mesiodistal tip incorporated into the

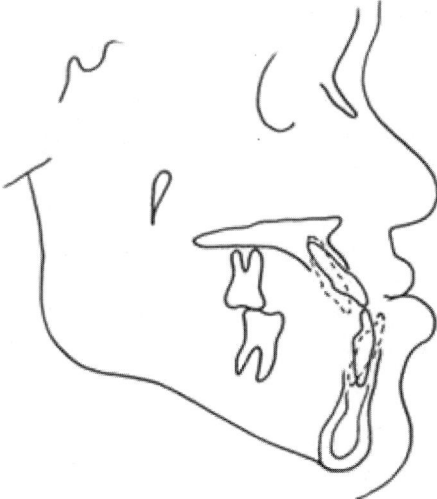

Figure 4.9 Dental "compensation" in a Class III case with proclination of the maxillary incisors and retroclination of the mandibular incisor teeth (continuous outline), compared with the ideal incisor inclination (broken outline) as seen on a lateral skull radiograph. The correction of the incisor angulation is termed decompensation.

canine bracket slot to aid lower incisor decompensation. During the alignment phase, the tip in the bracket would tend to throw the canine crown anteriorly, which in turn leads to proclination of the incisors (Figure 4.10a). Therefore the technique of "laceback" ligatures to the lower canine crown should be avoided (Figure 4.10b).

The upper incisors generally need to be retracted, a procedure, which may necessitate premolar extractions. In moderately crowded cases these will be the upper first premolars to aid the anchorage balance. In very mildly crowded cases, some would opt to move the upper arch distally using anchorage-reinforcing devices. In order to avoid the undesirable effects of the tip incorporated into the brackets, laceback ligatures should be employed during the aligning phase. The clinician may also use Class II directed interarch elastics to aid mutual decompensation of upper and lower arches.

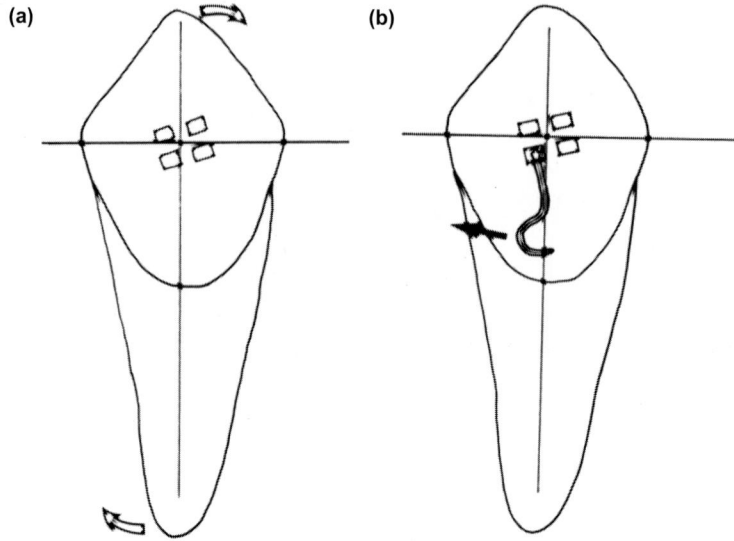

Figure 4.10   Once engaged with an initial aligning archwire, the mesiodistal tip incorporated into the mandibular canine bracket tends to throw the crown anteriorly **(a)** so aiding lower incisor decompensation in Class III cases. The technique of tying the crown back to the molar through the use of a "laceback" ligature **(b)** should be avoided in these cases.

Most cases with an anterior open bite, require a differential posterior impaction of the maxilla. The posterior maxilla is impacted by a greater amount than the anterior segment. The effect of this surgery is to retrocline the incisors (Figure 4.11). Hence when undertaking orthodontics in this situation, the presurgical preparation may intentionally leave the upper incisors slightly proclined.

Decompensation in Class II Cases

The soft tissue influence in Class II cases is variable nevertheless the goal is to place the incisor segments at the correct inclination to the dental bases. In the lower arch, the incisors may be proclined ("compensated"), in which case decompensation by retraction is

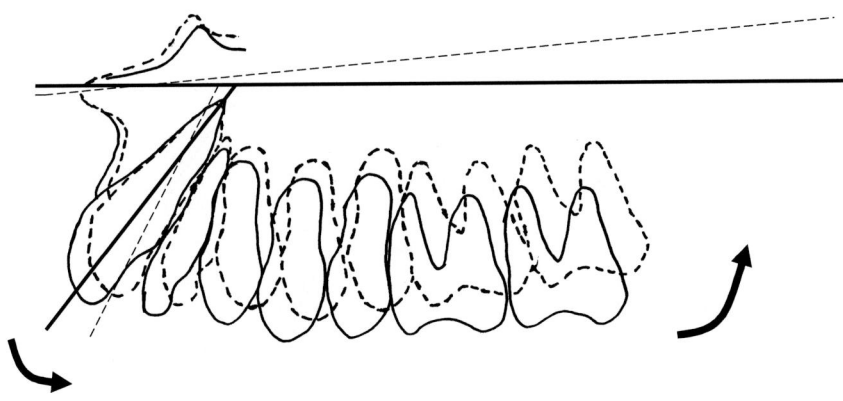

Figure 4.11   Impacting the maxilla posteriorly (dotted outline) has the effect of retroclining the maxillary incisors, and so presurgical orthodontics may intentionally leave the incisors proclined.

indicated and usually involves premolar extractions (Figure 4.12). As in the upper arch in Class III cases, laceback ligatures will aid decompensation.

In the maxillary arch, especially in patients with a low vertical dimension, the lower lip may become trapped palatal to the upper incisors which become proclined. Presurgical preparation will involve retraction of the upper incisors back to a normal inclination. If the proclined maxillary incisors are naturally spaced, retraction may be undertaken without the need to resort to extractions. However in many cases, especially where there is crowding, the loss of premolars is indicated.

Arch Coordination

Anteroposterior changes in skeletal relationships frequently require an alteration in the transverse widths of the arches for coordination,

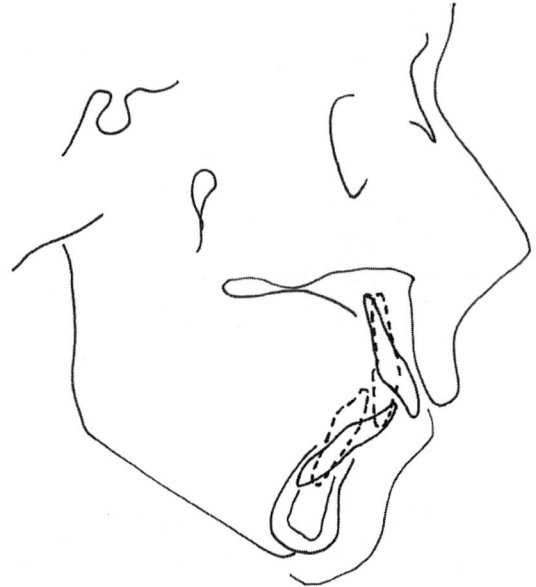

Figure 4.12   Decompensation in Class II cases will depend on the position of the incisors, which in most cases require retroclining in both upper and lower arches. Here shown as moving from the continuous to the broken outlines.

especially expansion of the upper arch. Whether this can be achieved by orthodontics alone, or through a combination of ortho-dontics and surgery depends upon:

- the amount of expansion required;
- the initial inclination of the buccal segment dentition;
- the relative degree of expansion required throughout the buccal segments.

Orthodontic expansion is achieved by tipping movement. Where the teeth are initially tipped palatally, uprighting will allow a good dental interdigitation, which is important for stability. Where the buccal teeth are either upright or even already flared buccally, further expansion will not produce a satisfactory stable occlusion. In such cases surgical expansion is required (see Chapter 9)

Methods of Orthodontic Arch Expansion

Quadhelix

The quadhelix appliance is the most frequently used appliance for expanding the maxillary dentition (Figure 4.13a). Although producing an overall tipping movement, it has the advantage of enabling differential expansion within the buccal segments.

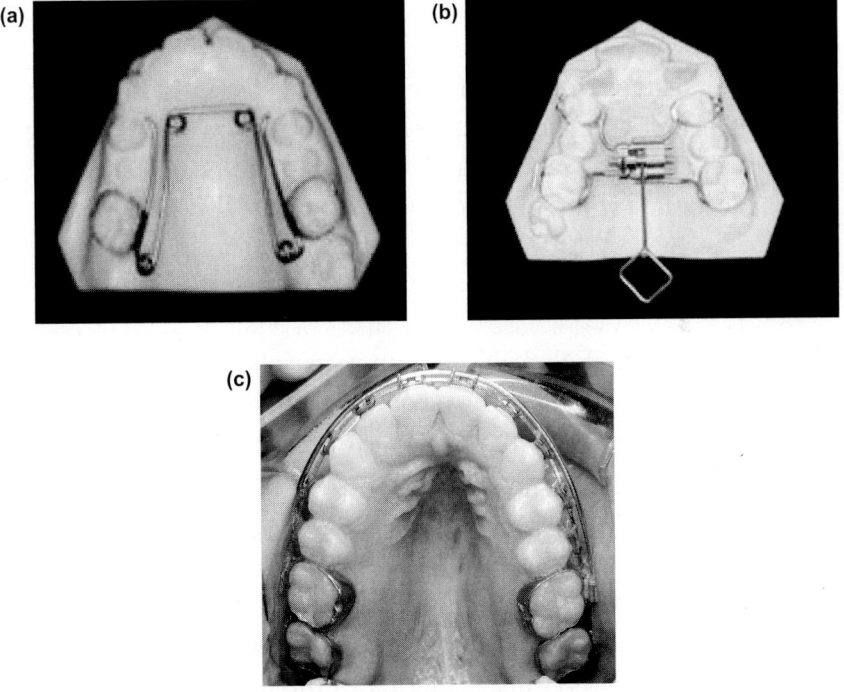

Figure 4.13 Examples of arch expansion methods: **(a)** quadhelix, **(b)** hyrax screw, and **(c)** auxillary expansion arch engaged in headgear tubes on molar bands.

Hyrax Screw

The hyrax screw (Figure 4.13b) is principally used for expansion prior to the fusion of the mid-palatal suture. The age at which this occurs may vary but it is usually complete by 21 years. Some suggest that the mechanism of expansion is more bodily movement rather than tipping in nature although this has been questioned.

Expansion Arch

Minor degrees of tooth movement can be achieved through expansion with a rectangular orthodontic archwire (usually of .018 × .025 minimum size). Use of a rectangular wire enables active buccal root torque to be placed in the buccal segments of the wire in order to achieve a positive overbite of the buccal cusps. Occasionally, the rectangular archwire can be used in conjunction with a 1mm rigid and expanded stainless steel arch fitted into the headgear tubes of the upper molars (Figure 4.13c).

Alternative Arch Expanders

The development of Nickel/Titanium materials has led to the marketing of an array of expansion devices which incorporate the shape/memory and superelasticity properties of these materials.

Monitoring Arch Coordination During Treatment

When preparing the arches for correction of Class II problems, testing of arch co-ordination in the transverse dimension can be achieved by simple forward posturing of the mandible. In Class III corrections the use of an acrylic template of the occlusal surfaces of the lower arch is invaluable. The template can be prepared by taking an alginate impression of the aligned lower arch and pouring cold cure acrylic resin into the occlusal portion of the impression.

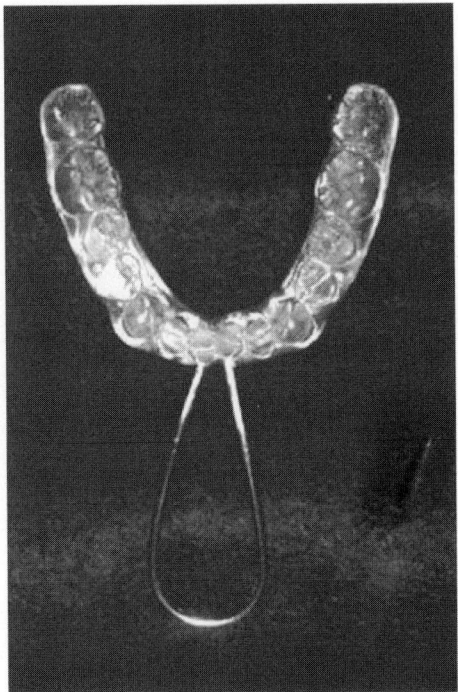

Figure 4.14.   An acrylic template of the aligned lower arch can be used to check coordination with the upper arch expansion at successive visits.

At successive visits, the template of the lower arch can then be occluded with the upper arch to check compatibility and avoid the need for repeated study models (Figure 4.14).

Facilitating Surgical Correction

Towards the end of the presurgical phase, upper and lower rectangular archwires should be in position and surgical hooks or soldered brass wires are added in the midline and throughout the buccal segments (Figure 4.15). These provide a means of attaching temporary intermaxillary fixation during surgery. They can also be used to attach seating elastics or intermaxillary elastics during the immediate postoperative period.

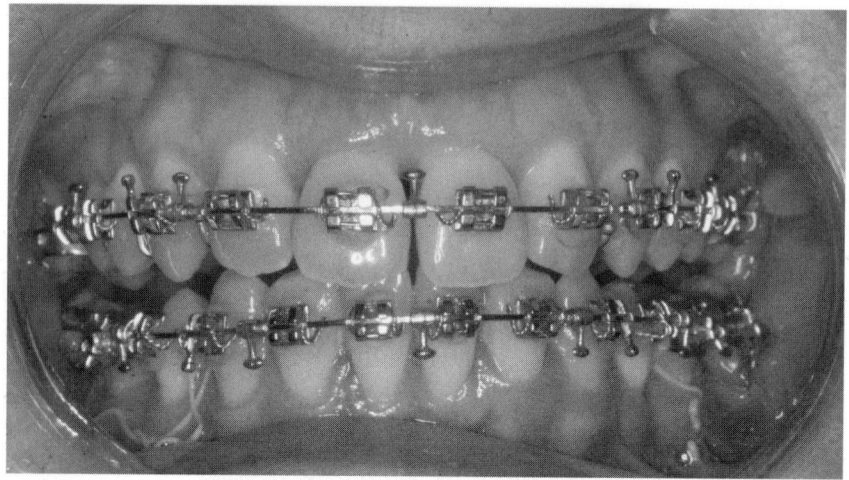

Figure 4.15   Rectangular archwires with surgical hooks. Note the archwires are engaged in the brackets using stainless steel ligatures.

Postsurgical Orthodontics

The goals of postsurgical orthodontics are to refine the occlusion, ensure a balanced occlusion and to plan the retention regime.

In cases of segmental surgery, where canine brackets have been reversed preoperatively, it is necessary to re-bond the canine brackets, placing brackets of the correct side in order to produce a normal canine angulation.

Postsurgical settling of a "3-point landing" usually involves a combination of flexible archwires together with vertical intra-oral seating elastics between the upper and lower arches (Figures 4.16a and 4.16b). Where the maxillary arch is level, a rigid upper rectangular archwire is maintained whereas a flexible wire, for example a braided steel wire, can be placed in the lower arch. When both arches need extrusion, the rectangular wires can be sectioned and seating elastics applied between the segments.

(a)

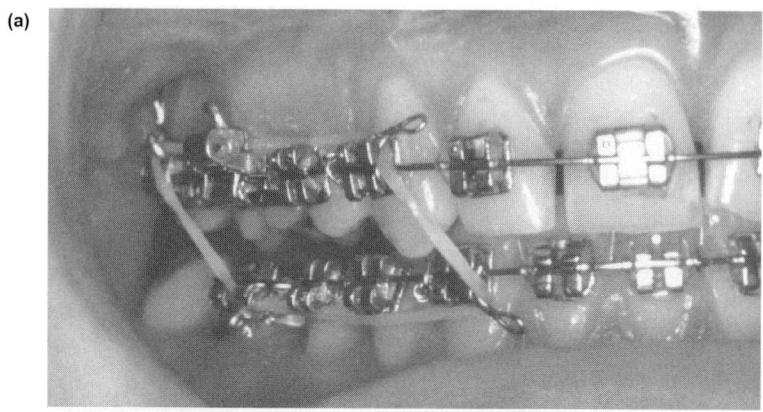

(b)

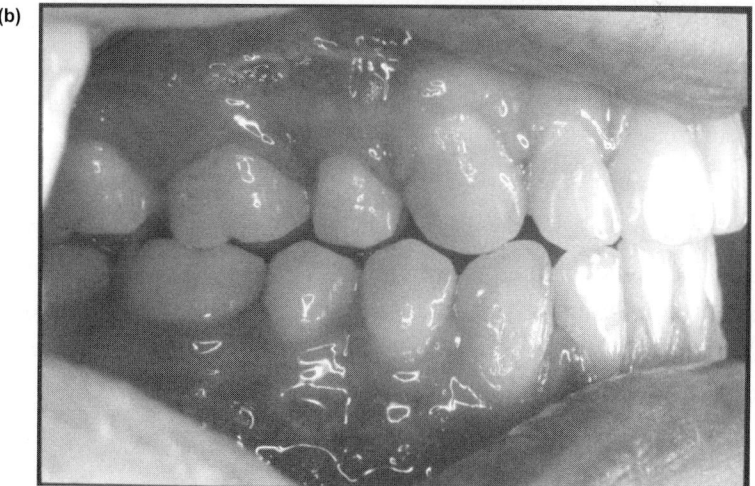

Figure 4.16 Closure of a lateral open-bite using postoperative intraoral elastics.

Retention

As in routine orthodontics, the tooth movements undertaken as part of orthognathic surgery require a period of retention following removal of the fixed appliances. This is to allow the alveolar bone and periodontal tissues to consolidate. Where there has been correction of

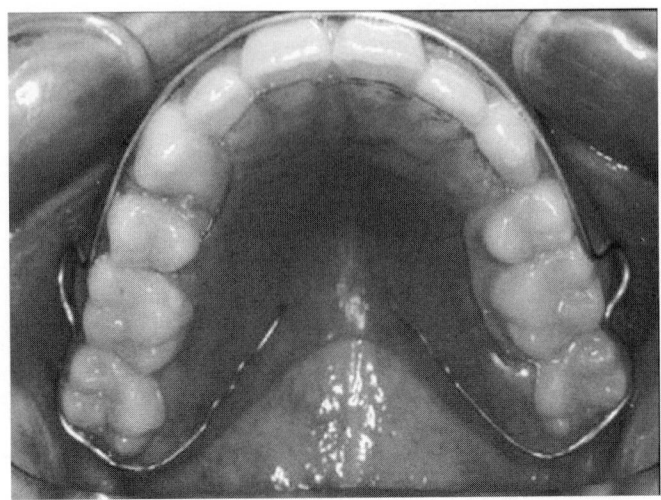

Figure 4.17   A removable retainer designed to avoid wirework passing through previously closed extraction sites.

incisor rotations or closure of large spaces, a permanent fixed bonded lingual or palatal retainer is employed. In other cases, a removable retainer of varying designs may be used. In general, it is good practice to avoid any retainer wirework passing through embrasures where extraction spaces have been closed (Figure 4.17).

5

The Definitive Treatment Plan

Treatment planning should only be undertaken after a thorough history and clinical examination of the patient, together with an analysis of the radiographs and study casts.

Planning the Maxillary Move

The key to successful surgery is to place the maxilla and the decompensated maxillary incisors in the optimum anteroposterior and vertical position in relation to the upper lip and face. The mandible is then placed in a Class I incisor relationship to the maxilla.

The profile of the seated patient is assessed with the Frankfort plane horizontal to decide the horizontal anteroposterior movement of the maxilla.

Changes of the naso-labial angle can be predicted with a moist cotton roll or soft pink wax. **The frontal view** is assessed by:

i) The ratio of the cephalometric upper to lower facial height — 45:55%.
ii) The incisor exposure with the lips parted at rest — will decide the vertical movement of the maxilla. Aesthetic exposure may vary from 1 to 4 mm. This is inversely proportional to the upper lip length which ranges from 18–24 mms.
iii) Excessive or unaesthetic incisor exposure is corrected with appropriate maxillary impaction.

iv) Where the upper lip is unduly short, the patient can show a greater amount of incisor. If not, the resulting midfacial appearance will be disproportionately small in the vertical dimension.

v) Rarely the patient has marked dento-alveolar hypoplasia and shows little or no incisor with a normal lip length. This is corrected with an inferior movement of the maxilla.

vi) Horizontal as well as vertical maxillary movements will affect the incisor exposure. Advancing the maxilla will lead to greater incisor exposure which will need to be adjusted for when considering the vertical move.

vii) Coronal occlusal cants and midline rotations must also be corrected.

viii) Moving the maxilla will also affect the nose. Vertical impaction widens the alar base and forward movements will elevate the nasal tip. Depending upon the initial appearance these changes may or not be desirable. If not, then a record should be made to provide a "cinch suture" across the lateral alar cartilages or to reduce the anterior nasal spine at the time of surgery.

ix) The inherent inaccuracy of the planning and surgical technique and the eye's inability to perceive small anatomical changes, determine that units of horizontal advancement should be no less than 3 mm. This also facilitates planning as a 3 mm minor advancement; a 6 mm intermediate; and a 9 mm major move. Cleft cases usually require 9 mm or more.

x) Similarly vertical moves of 2 mm for minor; 4 mm intermediate and 6 mm for major impactions are appropriate for all cases. These three categories also simplify the decision making process.

Planning the Mandibular Move

- Having planned where the maxilla is to be placed, the final step is to place the mandible in a Class I incisor relationship. This is built into the final wafer.

- If the definitive occlusion is not immediately possible because of the need for further orthodontics or restorative treatment, The wafer maintains the jaw relationship until orthodontics or restorative treatment can be commenced.
- The mandible will require autorotation, antero-posterior, vertical, rotational or rarely transverse movements.

Autorotation

Any changes in the vertical and horizontal position of the maxilla will necessitate a change in the vertical position of the mandible. This is mediated naturally through neuromuscular feedback mechanisms and the mandibular elevator muscles. Impacting the maxilla will lead to a shortening of the elevator muscles and will re-establish the freeway space. This closing autorotation of the mandible will also lead to a greater anterior prominence of the lower jaw.

Anterior Movements

Forward movement of the mandible to establish a Class I incisor relationship in Class II cases, will also increase lower face height. This is particularly the case with a deep overbite, when advancing the mandible without levelling the curve of Spee. The vertical facial height will increase and the everted lip will unroll and upright. If this change is desirable, the consequent lateral open bites need to be closed with postsurgical orthodontics to a stable position. If too severe for orthodontic closure, then surgery must incorporate a levelling of the occlusal plane with an anterior mandibulotomy procedure.

Posterior Movements

Mandibular setbacks will reduce the anterior facial height and evert the lip. Occasionally this may correct the occlusion but reduce the chin prominence which will require a paradoxical advancement.

Horizontal Rotation

These are required in asymmetry cases, for example hemimandibular elongation where the need is arch coordination especially with an adequate maxillary intercanine width.

Chin Position

Both anteroposterior and vertical movements of the mandible will affect the position of the chin. It is important that the chin be carefully assessed to avoid further surgery.

A common example is the need to correct a Class II division 1 malocclusion by a mandubular advancement which invariably leaves the patient with a deficient chin requiring a simultaneous advancement genioplasty.

With rare excess chin depth a combination of a vertical reduction and anterior sliding genioplasty helps provide a harmonious and balanced appearance.

Planning based on cephalometric assessment and the study model analysis.

Cephalometric Tracing Planning

The movements of the maxilla based on the clinical prediction of the incisor position, can then be repeated on a digital image or tracing of the patient's lateral cephalometric radiograph. Many still prefer to undertake this tracing procedure by hand although cephalometric software packages are available. When planning using hand tracing it is important to trace all the teeth in order to avoid missing potential premature contacts which may preclude the planned movements.

Having traced the revised maxillary position, the next step is to autorotate the mandibular tracing into the initial contact position. In reality, mandibular autorotation is not a simple hinge but a 3-dimensional movement with an envelope of adjustment within the temporomandibular joint. Despite this, it is useful to use as a 2-dimensional tracing despite its uncertainty as to the true centre of rotation. Some use the centre of the condyle, others use the point "condylion" whilst geometric constructions suggest that the point of rotation lies in the region of the mastoid air cells. Despite these differences the mandible in life appears to have an adequate envelope of condylar movement to adapt to crude planning geometry.

Assessment of the incisor position of the autorotated mandible is also important in determining if further adjustment of the maxillary position is required in order to establish a positive overbite.

1. With an anterior open bite autorotation leads to initial buccal segment contact. Closure of the residual anterior open bite by (anticlockwise) rotation of the mandible around this posterior pivot will lead to an elongation of the pterygo-masseteric sling and relapse. In such cases it is necessary to impact the posterior part of the maxilla differentially to that of the anterior maxilla. The extent of the differential impaction can be ascertained from the tracing.
2. With impactions for vertical maxillary excess, any minor incisor discrepancy on simple autorotation can be overcome by forward or backward adjusted movement of the maxilla. A significant discrepancy will require a bimaxillary procedure to ensure the incisor Class I relationship without compromising the upper lip incisor relationship.
3. Finally, the predicted profile can then be drawn on the composite planning tracing although this requires an estimate of the facial soft to hard tissue movements.

Imaging Simulations

The use of computerised software packages and the morphing of facial images as a means of planning the dental and surgical moves, together with the display of the predicted surgical outcome have been covered in Chapter 3.

6

The Psychopathology of Facial Deformity and Orthognathic Surgery

Introduction

The face has evolved as the most important of all human anatomical structures. It houses the principal receptors for sight, sound, taste and smell, has obvious and complex sexual significance, and the cerebro-neuromuscular means of expressing speech and emotion. Facial attractiveness is one of our most important social and psychological characteristics and the psychopathology of facial deformity is a complex spectrum extending from emotional problems in the normally integrated individual to manifestations of personality disorders, neurosis, depression and psychosis.

1. Social Aspects of Facial Deformity

Those who are blessed with an attractive face are frequently perceived as being more friendly, sensitive and successful than those who are unattractive. This unfair social advantage does not take into account overriding compensatory factors such as intellect, personality and motivation. Certain facial stereotypes are inappropriately portrayed as being associated with particular characteristics, for example a Class III malocclusion may be perceived as aggressive or a marked Class II as weak or stupid. Bat ears and large noses are similarly a source of teasing in childhood, thus creating a hypersensitive awareness, which may undermine self-esteem and self-confidence. There is also evidence that unattractive individuals are discriminated against in a wide range of situations from early life through to adulthood. Perceptions of facial attractiveness are said to vary from person to person and amongst different ethnic groups. Probably as a result of international media influence, this preference is changing in favour of the white western European stereotype of beauty.

We now appreciate that dentofacial deformity may be a severe handicap in many situations. This supports the view that the majority of patients requesting orthognathic treatment must suffer in some way the effects of discrimination or imagined discrimination in order to make them seek treatment which has inherent discomfort and risks. Therefore a psychological assessment of all orthognathic patients is a vital part of the planning procedure as it enables the identification of a wide range of psychological problems. It is vital to identify any of these problems before inappropriate planning decisions have been made. Ideally a liaison psychiatrist or clinical psychologist would undertake this role, however where constraints are placed on providing the optimum service, the orthodontist or orthognathic surgeon must be responsible for the initial screening and identify and refer those patients of particular concern.

2. The Psychological Assessment

The social and psychological acceptance of aesthetic orthognathic treatment has increased the demand for treatment. Despite this the treatment plan should be based not only on aesthetics and function, but also on the patient's perceptions of what they wish to obtain from treatment. Patients often perceive their facial appearance and in particular their profile, quite differently from clinicians. This emphasises the need for good communication from the outset when planning orthognathic procedures. The communication process is critical and will usually take several visits to accurately identify the patients' subjective problems and the changes they are seeking. The clinician must then decide whether these expectations can be met. Unfortunately, there is no validated proforma for quantifying inappropriate psychological characteristics. Despite this, the following standardised approach is essential to avoid overlooking problem areas and should be done on a one-to-one basis and not in a large multidisciplinary clinic, where patients may be reluctant to disclose personal details. A number of patients will require referral to a liaison psychiatrist or clinical psychologist for a more thorough assessment before proceeding further. This decision will be based on a multistage triage procedure.

A. In addition to patients in whom the clinician intuitively feels concerns, those to be considered for referral include patients with:

- A history of previous cosmetic surgery.
- Minimal facial deformity.
- Expectations that clearly exceed surgical feasibility.
- An obsessional concern with certain features.

B. There are a number of key interrelated questions which should be asked:

- *What is the main complaint?*
  This question establishes how the patient perceives their problem. The accuracy of the complaint is not important, for example the patient may feel they have a prognathic mandible when actually they have a retrognathic maxilla. However, they must be able to recognise the problem and be

relatively clear about it. Those who offer vague non-specific complaints such as "I just don't like my face" tend to make poor surgical patients compared with those who are clear about their complaint — "I think my chin sticks out and is not symmetrical".

- *What does the patient expect from treatment?*
  This is very important and the way this question is phrased can influence the response. It is helpful to ask "How do you think this treatment will affect your life?" Those patients who want to look better and feel more self-confident are classified as expecting primary gain from treatment and tend to be good surgical patients. Patients requiring psychological assessment prior to agreeing to treatment include those who: (i) are concerned with secondary gain such as promotion, a better job or new partner (ii) do not have any idea what they expect from treatment and (iii) are not able to verbalise their answers to these questions.

- *How long has he/she been concerned about their face? Why is he/she seeking treatment now?*
  Patients should always be asked how long they have had these concerns. Those who have become concerned only recently should again be assessed by a psychologist/psychiatrist as their worries may have been triggered by a recent life event such as redundancy, divorce, or bereavement. It is then appropriate to delay treatment until the patient has reached a more stable state before considering any intervention.

- *How does their dentofacial deformity interfere with their life?*
  A patient who can function in a normal way at work, socialise with friends and has developed a reasonable body image despite the facial deformity is likely to be satisfied following treatment. Those who have become reclusive as a result of their concerns must be investigated further, especially where

the extent of the deformity does not justify this abnormal behaviour pattern.

- *What is the main source of motivation?*

  The internally motivated patient usually has long standing inner feelings about their appearance, which impair their enjoyment of life, whereas the externally motivated patient is usually seeking treatment to please someone else (e.g. parent or partner). Externally motivated patients may require a change in their environment rather than orthognathic treatment. They require careful psychological assessment and counseling prior to consideration for treatment. Patients who are internally motivated usually make better candidates for orthognathic intervention.

- *Does the patient have family support?*

  This very important issue is frequently overlooked. Obviously patients should not be refused treatment if they have little family or social support. However, in this situation, the orthognathic team may need to offer more support than usual, particularly in the immediate pre- and postoperative periods when patients are at their most vulnerable. This is where a liaison nurse or social worker can play an extremely important role.

- *Has the patient previously sought treatment elsewhere?*

  Patients who embark upon numerous consultations (or "doctor shopping") often do so because they are dissatisfied with a previous rejection or a treatment plan which does not meet their unrealistic expectations. Other patients may already have undergone previous operations for dentofacial complaints. Such a history should be investigated fully, prior to agreeing to further intervention (see later section on BDD).

- *Has the patient received any medical treatment that may be of importance?*
  This is to determine whether the patient has undergone any previous psychiatric treatment. The diagnosis of psychiatric disorders is difficult for those with little or no psychiatric training but establishing the medication history can be an invaluable clue. Some clinicians find it useful to utilise screening questionnaires such as the Hospital Anxiety and Depression (HAD) scale or the Orthognathic Quality of Life Questionnaire (OQLQ), although such questionnaires are relatively limited in what they can tell you about the patient. The general medical history may also include conditions that make orthognathic treatment difficult or impossible, such as haemophilia, severe thallasaemia, acromegaly or osteoclast dysfunction bone dysplasias.

If any of these questions raise doubts the clinician should delay treatment for specialist assessment, to be followed by an interdisciplinary case conference. This delay will also help determine how keen the patient is to proceed with surgery.

3. Dissatisfaction with Treatment

The important measures of postoperative outcome and patient satisfaction are clinical audit to determine whether the treatment plan has been achieved. The majority of patients are satisfied with the outcome of orthognathic treatment even where there are minor discrepancies in the anatomical result. Careful management appears to be the key factor. Patients who experience less pain and numbness than expected, tend to be more satisfied and enjoy higher self-esteem than those who experience as much, or more pain and numbness than expected. This reinforces the need to inform patients of all possible problems they may encounter and give strong personal support if complications arise.

There are a number of other causes of postoperative dissatisfaction. The majority are due to an unfavourable interpersonal relationship with the clinician, rather than deficient technical skills or poor surgical outcome. Occasionally there is no obvious justification and the adverse reaction is the result of a psychological problem triggered by the surgery. Dissatisfaction may manifest itself in a number of ways including entering into litigation, obsessional behaviour, seeking additional surgical procedures, depression or even frank psychosis and physical aggression.

Most forms of post-surgical dissatisfaction can be avoided by careful patient assessment as described earlier, and realistic explanations of the procedure in terms of pain, swelling, speech, eating and time off work. It is now mandatory to include, in the process of informed consent, the possibility of the most common and important complications, which although self-evident are often overlooked. Not only should the information be given verbally but also reinforced with a detailed information leaflet. Most patients will remember only a small or selective part of what they are told in a clinic, especially when nervous. The principal clinic nurses should also be trained to inform and counsel all orthognathic patients pre- and postoperatively and where appropriate, advice should be provided for the immediate family, as this provides an additional person to remember the information being provided and ask questions.

It is important that the surgeon is vigilant in the postoperative phase and does not delegate aftercare to inexperienced junior staff. Many surgeons take for granted postoperative morbidity and are unaware of the psychological upheaval arising from the long anticipated change. Other patients may experience strong negative feelings when facing postoperative orthodontic treatment which should be kept to a minimum. Some patients experience debilitating postoperative clinical depression which once diagnosed must be immediately treated medically rather by ineffectual reassurance. A short course of anti-depressants will produce a marked improvement, but continued psychiatric care may be required. Frank psychosis is extremely rare because it may take the form of delusional states or violence, which need immediate attention with antipsychotic medication either through the hospital on-call psychiatrist or the patient's general medical practitioner.

Subjective Disorders of Appearance

Body Dysmorphic Disorder (BDD) Formerly Dysmorphophobia

Body dysmorphic disorder describes the patient with a persistent subjective feeling of ugliness or a physical defect which is minor and perhaps not even detectable by the clinician. This condition was formerly known as dysmorphophobia but is now termed BDD. In order to make this diagnosis, three criteria must be fulfilled:

- There is a preoccupation with a defect in the appearance. The defect is either imagined, or if a minor defect is present, the individual's concern is inappropriately excessive.
- This preoccupation causes significant distress to the patient and dominates all aspects of their life.
- The preoccupation is not accounted for by any other psychiatric disorder.

Presenting Features

The main feature of BDD is an obsession with an imagined or greatly exaggerated defect in the appearance. The area of concern may remain the same over a long period or change with time. It frequently affects the face, therefore orthodontists and maxillofacial surgeons should be fully aware of the presenting features.

BDD usually begins during adolescence with symptoms persisting over a number of years, but there is often a delay in seeking treatment. BDD patients have preoccupations which are distressing and time consuming. They may spend hours thinking about their "defect", studying it in the mirror or attempting to camouflage the area and may become housebound and even attempt suicide. A high proportion of patients avoid social relations and suffer impairment of their academic or work performance. Some experience suicidal ideation and exhibit aggressive behaviour.

BDD patients require early identification and careful assessment at their initial appointment. It is important not to risk making matters worse by drawing the patient's attention to other potential "defects". Referral letters are often misleading if the practitioner has uncritically accepted the patient's complaint. However, a history of innumerable referrals, with or without surgery, is a crucial marker of the condition. Some patients attempt to hide the problem unless specifically questioned and will avoid disclosing visits to other clinicians. In other cases they will demand constant reassurance about the supposed defect and often attend appointments with pictures, photographs or diagrams to show the problem or idealistic faces that they wish to emulate. BDD patients are frequently very well read and have researched the management of facial disfigurement on the internet, use medical terminology and "lead" the initial assessment so that the unwary clinician feels forced into undertaking treatment. It is vital that clinicians are aware of the inevitable poor outcome in carrying out unnecessary treatment for such persuasive patients.

The Body Dysmorphic Disorder Examination (BDDE) and the Body Dysmorphic Disorder Modification of the Yale-Brown Obsessive Compulsive Scale (BDD-YBOCS) may prove useful where a tentative diagnosis has been made. However the analysis and management from this point, requires a psychiatrist familiar with the condition.

Treatment Options

Surgery

BDD patients may constantly pursue surgical treatment for their "defect" and consult numerous surgeons in the hope of finding someone who is willing to operate on them. However, surgery rarely improves the situation and should only be considered when there is a detectable and remedial defect and the patient complies with psychiatric care. Unfortunately inappropriate surgery makes the condition worse with the patient frequently finding a new problem. The unsuspecting clinician may not only be faced with persistent dissatisfaction but also become the target of violence or litigation.

Pharmacological Treatment

Like all idiopathic conditions the medical management is empirical. The selective serotonin re-uptake inhibitors are currently the pre-ferred pharmacological treatment option for BDD patients. However, the lack of controlled clinical trials has made the assessment of pharmacological treatment in BDD uncertain. There is strong support for adjunctive cognitive behavioural psychotherapy.

Counselling and Psychological Therapy

A number of different psychological treatment options are available including cognitive behavioural therapy and systematic desensitisation. BDD symptoms seem to be significantly reduced in subjects who have undergone this form of therapy and studies have shown that the disorder appears to have been eliminated in 82% of cases immediately post-treatment and 77% at follow-up.

Ethnic Dysphoria

Dentofacial aesthetic norms vary between ethnic groups and when planning surgical changes special consideration should be given as to whether they are racially appropriate. Some ethnic patients, influenced by popular Caucasian features, may demand changes which are either unsuitable or unattainable. An example of this would be an African girl seeking a European profile (Figure 6.1). Her bimaxillary protrusion reproduces exactly the natural beauty of her tribal origin, seen in the classic sculpture of a Benin bronze. This could be altered with orthodontics or upper and lower segmental surgery but might not produce the aesthetic satisfaction the patient anticipated. The merits of change in such cases must be carefully discussed between patient, orthodontist, surgeon and psychologist. Where the dissatisfaction is marked the patient is best considered to be a case of BDD.

Gender Dysphoria

Gender dysphoria is an uncommon BDD variant in which the patient, usually a male, wishes to change gender. Where this is

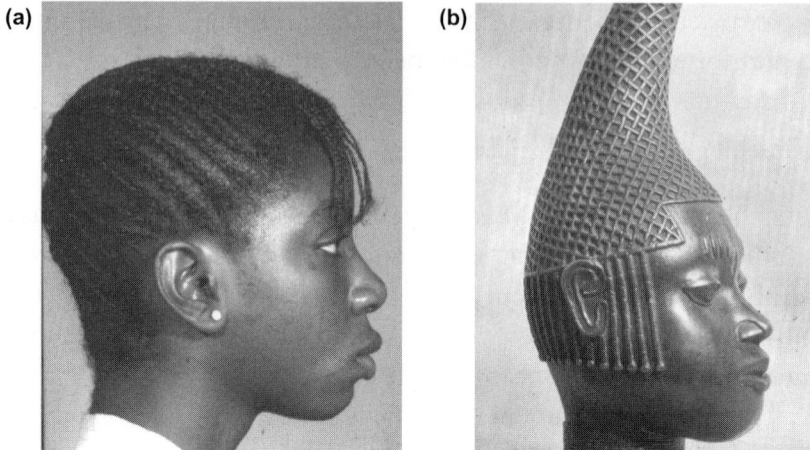

Figure 6.1   **(a)** and **(b)** British girl of Nigerian origin who wanted to look like her European school friends, compared with the ideal beauty of the Benin bronze.

stated, or when the patient is referred from a psychiatric unit specialising in gender reorientation, the aim of the treatment is obvious. However, occasionally the demand for a less prominent mandible or more prominent malar bones in an otherwise satisfactory face can be difficult to understand unless seen as part of this problem. Again, psychiatric assessment of the patient is essential.

Conclusions

Patients who seek surgery for dentofacial deformity frequently harbour emotional concerns and require careful psychological assessment, sound informative discussion and comprehensive information sheets. It is important to detect those patients with facial deformity and latent psychopathology who require specialist psychological assessment and support prior to treatment. Clinicians must also be aware that occasionally patients may reveal unexpected postoperative psychiatric disorders which require treatment. The body dysmorphic disorder patient must be identified early and treated appropriately. Surgery is rarely an appropriate option. Gender and ethnic dysphoria are allied idiopathic conditions where the patient appears determined to achieve an apparently irrational change in their features.

The importance of well established team care cannot be over-emphasised.

7

The Recording and Transfer of Orthognathic Planning Data

Introduction

Orthognathic surgery involves three-dimensional movements based on a series of non-surgical and surgical procedures. This is particularly evident in osteotomies which change the occlusal level.

The main planning concerns are:

- prediction of the tooth-bone-soft tissue changes,
- operative reproducibility of the treatment plan, and
- postoperative dentoskeletal stability.

Confounding factors are:

a) planning data transfer inadequacies,
b) the adaptation of the TMJ complex,
c) diversity of surgical skills, and
d) relapse forces.

The definitive preoperative planning process has the following stages:

- clinical estimated measurements,
- impressions,

- occlusal record (squash bite),
- face bow registration,
- face bow transfer to the articulator and mounting of the maxillary model,
- mounting of the mandibular model,
- maxillary model surgery,
- intermediate occlusal wafer fabrication,
- mandibular model surgery, and
- final occlusal wafer fabrication.

These ten processes all require care but are subject to inaccuracies which render fine degrees of planned measurement inappropriate.

With a single jaw mandibular osteotomy, precise model surgery planning using a facebow and anatomical articulator is not required. However, all maxillary and bimaxillary procedures require an accurate transfer of the jaw relationship to the articulator, for surgical planning.

The Planning Process

1. *Clinical Measurements*

There are inherent difficulties in accurately recording the clinical data. For instance patients may camouflage an occlusal cant by tilting the head and many Class II division 1 patients posture their mandible forwards. There are also important occlusal changes due to the effects of gravity in the conscious patient compared to the loss of muscle tone in the anaesthetised patient.

2. *Impression Procedure*

a) The impression procedure is more demanding than for standard impressions for dental appliances. Apart from the jaw deformity, malocclusion and postural camouflage, the presence of orthodontic brackets create a challenge for the inexperienced. It is important that the orthdodontic archwire is passive in the brackets at the time of taking the impressions.

b) The impressions must be taken as near to the surgery as possible. Soft red wax may be applied on the gingival side of the orthodontic brackets to avoid splitting adherent alginate. The application or flow of wax onto the occlusal side of the bracket can obliterate the occlusion. Two full upper and lower impressions which detail all the teeth are taken using irreversible hydrocolloid impression material (Claudius Ash. UK). It is essential to include the terminal cusps of the most posterior molars as failure to record these could lead to unplanned prematurities in occlusal contact at the time of surgery. The impressions are cast in Crystacal R Class III stone plaster (Newark Works, Bowbridge Lane, Newark, Nottinghamshire) and based in plaster (British Gypsum). One set of models is anatomically trimmed for model surgery (Figure 7.1a) and the second angle trimmed as study models (Figure 7.1b).

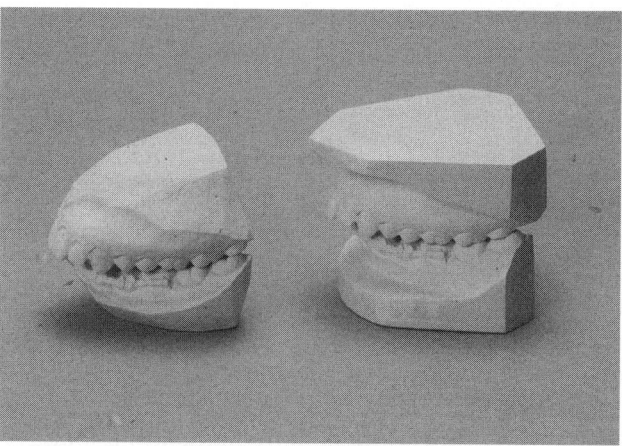

Figure 7.1   (a) Upper and lower models after removing non-anatomical parts, ready to articulate. (b) Standard angle trimmed study models.

3. *Recording the Occlusal Relationship*

The dental occlusion is dynamic with a three-dimensional envelope of movement which will change with altered patterns of neuromuscular function such as, postural habits, gravity, the level of consciousness and even psychiatric factors. It is crucial to recognise that preoperative planning is conventionally done on a conscious upright patient using centric occlusal records (CO), i.e maximal intercuspation in the X axis, despite the osteotomy taking place with the mandible in an anaesthetised supine centric relation position (CR), i.e the occlusal retruded position in the Y-axis (Figures 7.2a and 7.2b).

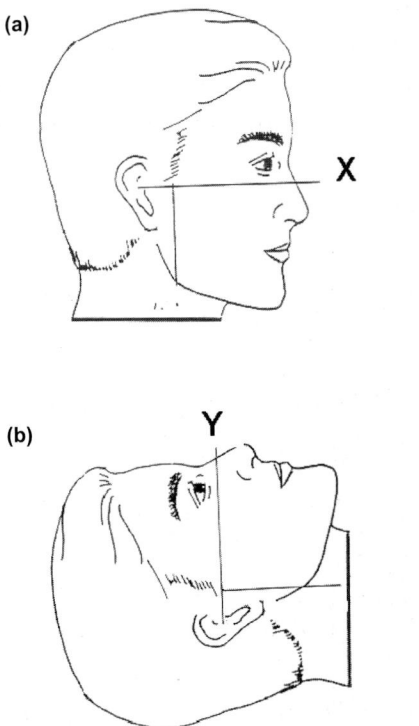

Figure 7.2 **(a)** and **(b)** Osteotomies are planned in the upright X-axis but carried out in a supine anaesthetised Y-axis.

A significant difference between the conscious CO and supine anaesthetised CR will produce unexpected discrepancies between the planned and postoperative occlusion, for instance when the osteotomised maxilla is temporarily fixed to the unoperated mandible and rotated upwards and forwards into its planned position for plate fixation. The anaesthetised mandibular CR will give rise to a loss of maxillary advancement which is seen when the patient wakes and sits up with the mandible recoiling forwards.

This may not be apparent in the bimaxillary procedure as the osteotomised mandible is then related to the previously fixed maxilla.

Conversely with a Class III mandibular setback there will be a loss of push back with the conscious upright recoil (Figures 7.3a and 7.3b). This is beneficial in a Class II division 1 mandibular advancement and helps to compensate for any distal relapse.

To avoid these potential problems the osteotomy should be planned from the CR occlusal registration, taken in a relaxed supine patient. Any minor residual CO-CR discrepancies are usually compensated for by proprioceptive adaptation within the envelope of movement of the condyle-disc-fossa relationship.

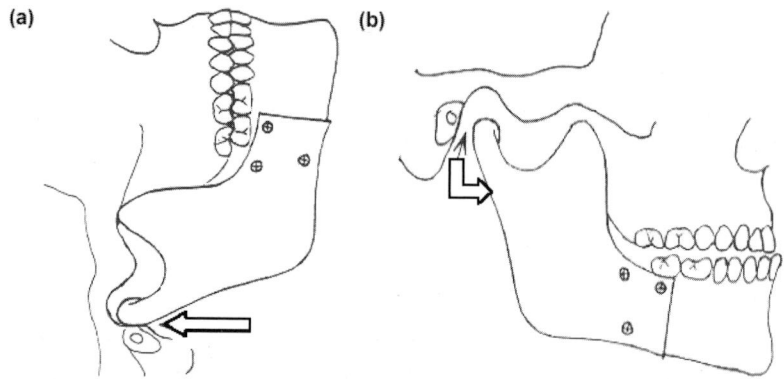

Figure 7.3   (a) Fixation in supine and (b) occlusion when upright.

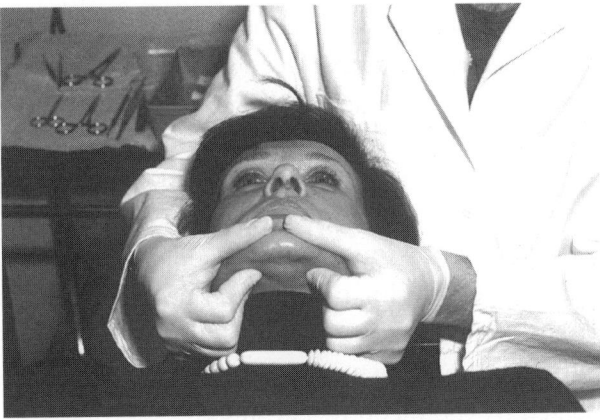

Figure 7.4   The centric jaw relation recording in supine conscious posture using bilateral manipulation technique.

The Registration of Supine Centric Relation

Centric relation is recorded using the bilateral manipulation technique, with the patient in a relaxed supine position and the operator seated behind and with the patient's head between the two arms. The operator supports the patient's mandible bilaterally by placing the fingers of each hand below the lower border of the mandible on each side and the thumbs in the depression of the labiomental fold (Figure 7.4). This technique emphasises the "posterior" placement of the condyles in the fossae. With the softened wax occlusal wafer in place the mandible is then guided into the centric relation position.

Appreciation of this plasticity of the condyle-disc-fossa relationship is essential in orthognathic surgery planning.

4. *Facebow Recording*

a)   The facebow is designed to record the relationship of the maxilla to the terminal hinge axis of the patient's mandibular condyles and a Frankfort-like plane. When transferred to the articulator this becomes the relationship of the maxillary cast to the condylar assemblies of an articulator. Although this axis can vary with posture, when standardised, the facebow/articulator transfer method has proved to be reproducible for orthognathic planning.

a) The Denar (and similar systems) is clinically reliable except where there is gross facial asymmetry. It has a reference point of 43 mm above the lateral incisor edge which defines the anterior point on an arbitary plane within the maxilla (Figure 7.5). The posterior reference point is the bony margin of the external auditory meatus, conveniently located by the facebow earplugs.

Although careful facebow registration shows a high degree of accuracy in the vertical plane there is a wider variation in the horizontal plane which together with the eight other variables in the transfer process, may invalidate

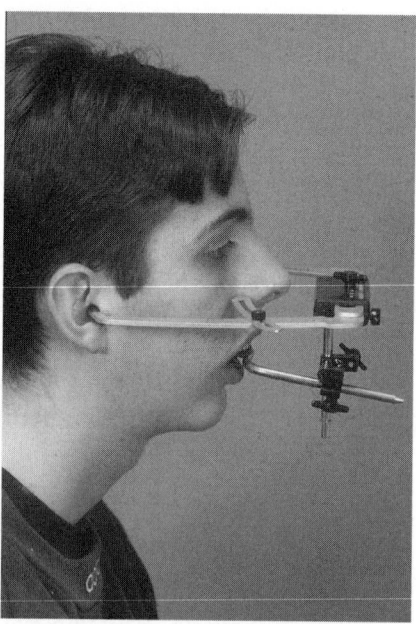

Figure 7.5 Clinical picture of Denar Slidematic facebow with ear plugs for hinge axis point and an anterior reference point 43 mm above central incisor.

the use of small planning movements. Furthermore small variations cannot be controlled surgically nor perceived by the eye. For this reason forward and backward movements of the maxilla are most reliably planned in 3 mm units which also simplifies clinical decision making when translated into minor 3 mm, moderate 6 mm and major 9 mm moves. Similarly vertical movements are more accurately estimated as 2, 4 or 6 mm. impactions again representing minor, intermediate and major defects. The exception to this "3-unit rule" is the cleft palate case with a major iatrogenic disturbance to facial growth.

b) The facebow registration procedure: Facebow ear pieces are placed into the external auditory meati and manipulated until the subject feels equal pressure in both ears. The anterior reference pointer is adjusted to the pre-determined reference mark 43 mm above the incisal edge of the right maxillary lateral incisor and the transfer jig screws are tightened (Figure 7.5).

The facebow bite fork registration can be taken using a silicon based material which gives definition of the occlusal surfaces (Figure 7.6a) and can be easily trimmed with a scalpel should the material inadvertently encapsulate the orthodontic brackets.

Prior to mounting the upper and lower models, silicon moulds of the master casts/models can be prepared (Figure 7.6b). This enables copies of the models to be prepared should damage occur during the construction of the splints and for one to be kept in the patient's study model box for record purposes.

5. Facebow Transfer to the Articulator and the Mounting of the Casts

Only the Denar transfer jig and bite fork need to be sent to the laboratory, the facebow does not have to leave the clinic. Unless the

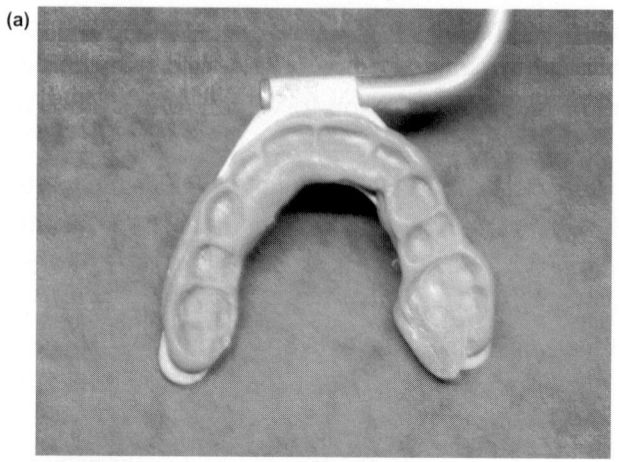

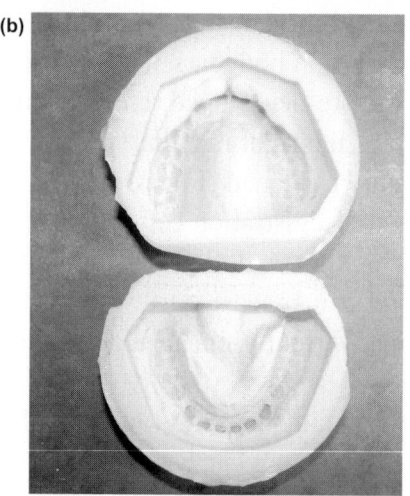

Figure 7.6   **(a)** Silicon bite fork registration. **(b)** Silicon mould of master models for duplication and record keeping.

procedure is carried out very carefully errors can be introduced when seating the cast into the bite fork indentation and during the subsequent mounting

Using a small amount of dental plaster mixed with an anti-expansion solution (Alan Pharmaceuticals Ltd., London) the maxillary model is mounted on the articulator (Figure 7.7a).

(a)

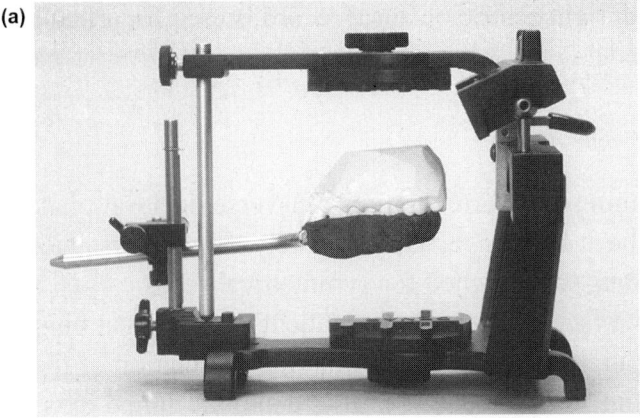

(b)

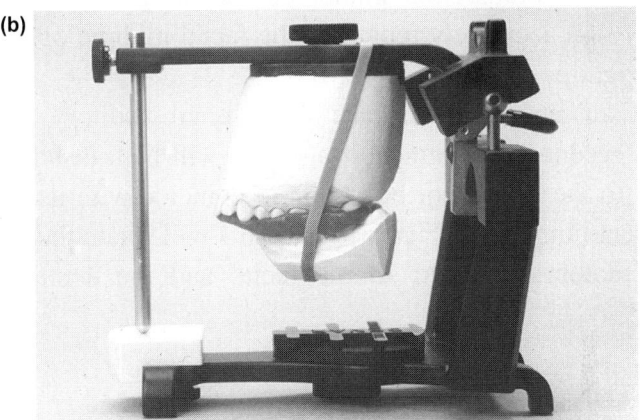

Figure 7.7 (a) The Denar facebow transfer jig assembled in an articulator with upper cast ready to be mounted. (b) Lower cast ready to be mounted in the Denar articulator.

This is followed by mounting the mandibular cast using the supine centric relation record (Figure 7.7b). The models are mounted in two stages; firstly using plaster mixed with anti-expansion solution as described, to eliminate any potential distortion. When set, the models together with their respective assembly plates are removed from the articulator and "anatomically" shaped with white plaster vacuum mixed in plain water.

The upright centric occlusal record is used for articulation of the study models.

Facial Asymmetry

The planning and correction of transverse occlusal plane asymmetry can be a challenge. Unfortunately articulators, facebows and cephalostats are designed for symmetrical faces.

With a facebow record, the patient's anatomical hinge axis (the external auditory meati) determine the orientation of the maxillary cast within the articulator. If this anatomic hinge axis is at right angles to the mid-sagittal plane, the resulting articulator model assembly will accurately represent the facial midline of the patient in an upright position (Figure 7.8).

With an asymmetrical face or external auditory meati, the patient's eccentric anatomical hinge axis will be transferred by the facebow to the articulator but made to coincide with its horizontal mechanical hinge axis (Figure 7.9a). This will rotate the maxilla in the articulator space and so the facial and the dental midlines

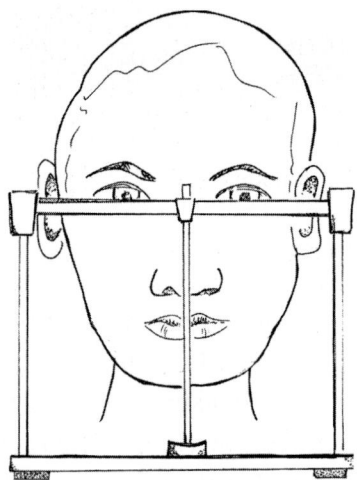

Figure 7.8 Symmetrical ears give symmetrical alignment with facebow recording.

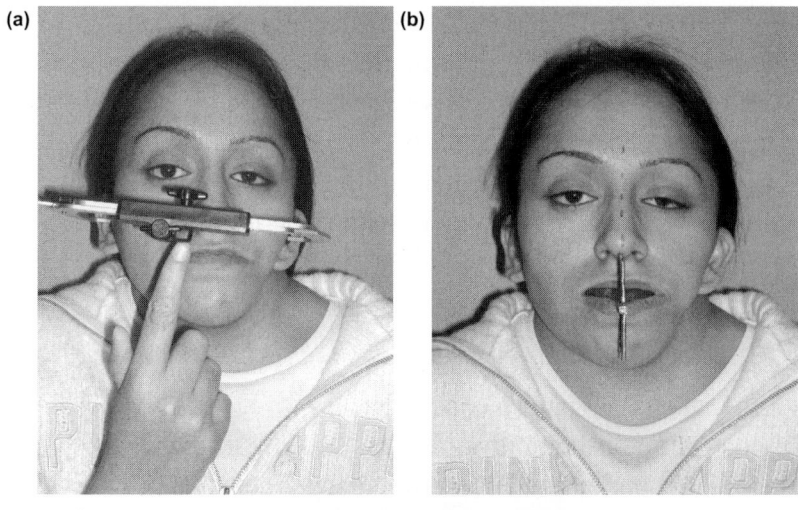

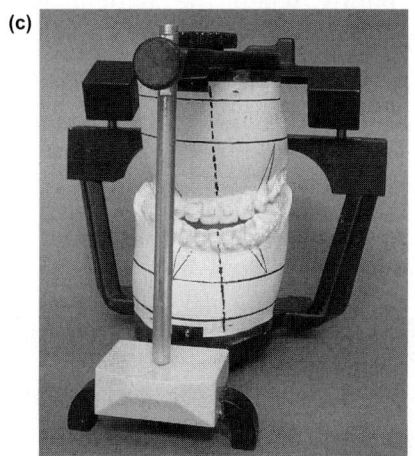

Figure 7.9 (a) Asymmetrical ears would give asymmetrical recording when using a standard facebow transfer. (b) The midline jig records the true facial midline. (c) The ear asymmetry is reflected in the mounted models as a pseudo cant when using the facebow record.

will not coincide with the articulator incisal pin. When due to asymmetrical external auditory meati, a pseudocant will suggest the need to correct a facial midline discrepancy, which does not exist (Figures 7.9b and 7.9c). For this reason it is very important that the patient's facial midline is recorded clinically and independently of the facebow with a facial midline jig, and transferred to the articulated models for the preoperative work-up. Figure 7.9c shows how the inferiorly placed left ear has been recorded as a pseudocant with the true midline traced obliquely to the left. Planning is done supporting the articulator in space to render the midline vertical.

The anatomical structures used to determine the vertical facial midline are:

(i)   from the centre of the glabella to the centre of the chin, unless the chin is deviated to one side;
(ii)   the centre of the philtrum unless it is deformed; and
(iii) a right angle to the interpupillary line at a point midway between the pupils when the patient is looking directly forward (Figures 7.10a and 7.10b).

The Transfer of the Facebow Record of Maxillary Asymmetry

The facebow record is taken with the midline mark on the facebow bite fork matching the patient's facial midline, not the dental midline.

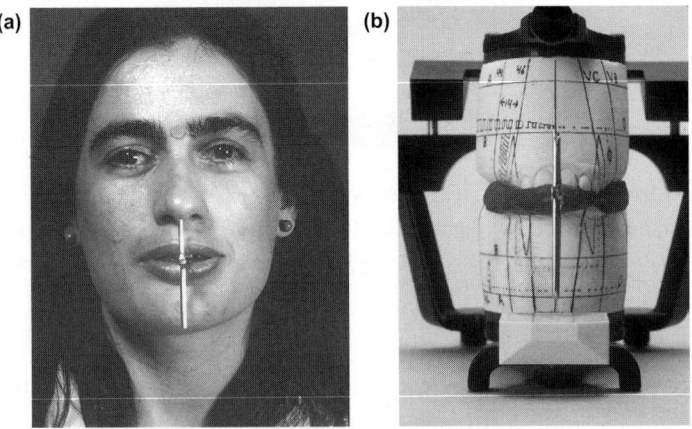

(a)   (b)

Figure 7.10   **(a)** Clinical picture of a midline jig in use with facial midline marker. **(b)** Jig transfer of midline to articulated models.

With asymmetry a facial midline indicator (FMI) jig is used which has a U shaped nickel silver wire tray, to take composition, silicon or wax, similar to a facebow bite fork. Its extraoral extension has two parallel vertical bars to register the long axis of the face. Each bar has notches on the upper and lower ends to help to align them to the facial midline (Figures 7.11a–7.11d). Wax or composition is softened and applied to the U shaped part of the jig. While soft, the jig is placed in the mouth and the patient asked to close slowly into centric occlusion

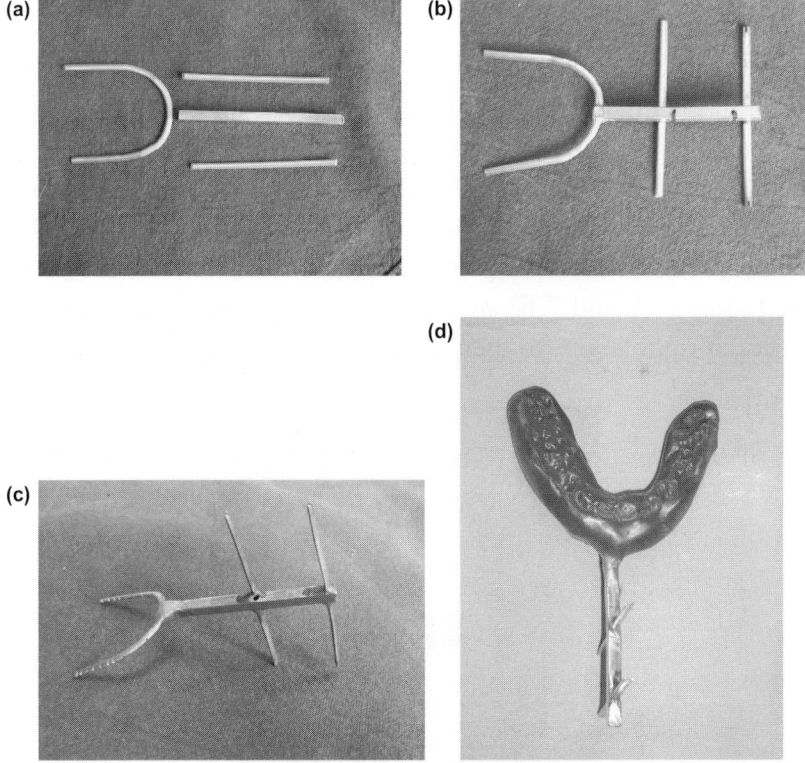

Figure 7.11 Midline jig: **(a)** Components: 4 mm nickel silver (NS) tube and 3 mm oval wire. **(b)** 3 mm oval NS wire is bent into a U shape and soldered on the end of the 4 mm NS tube, and two 3 mm NS wires with V cut are ready to be soldered on the tube at right angle to the U shape bite fork. **(c)** Midline jig with all components soldered together **(d)** with wax squash bite.

while the operator adjusts the vertical bars so that they match exactly the patients facial midline (Figure 7.10a). Heavy body silicon can also be used. When the material has set the jig is removed from the mouth and chilled.

The dental casts are mounted in the articulator using the face-bow record. The jig is then located by the impression of the cast teeth. Using the notches on the parallel vertical bars two reference points are marked on the surfaces of upper and lower mounting assembly plaster work. A third reference point is then taken from the facebow bite fork midline mark and the facial midline is drawn, using these three reference points, from the upper mounting plate A line to the lower mounting plate A line (Figures 7.10 and 7.12). This line represents the patient's true facial midline and the long axis of the face. This jig is an invaluable device, which facilitates the correction of the maxillary midline and occlusal cant with accuracy. Figure 7.10 shows a true occlusal cant with a symmetrical face. The maxillary model shows the planned bone removal to level the occlusion. Figures 7.9 and 7.12 are both pseudocants where the occlusal plane is at right angles to the midline jig alignment.

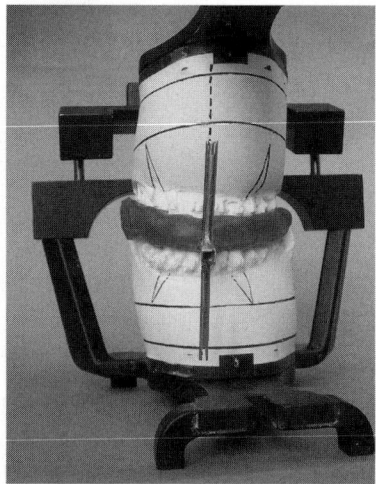

Figure 7.12   The midline jig is transferred to the articulator for midline cast marking.

6. *Model Surgery*

Bimaxillary surgery is usually sequenced with the maxilla mobilised and repositioned first although some surgeons correct the mandible at the outset. Regardless of which jaw, it is imperative that it is planned accurately because once fixed, it becomes the basis for repositioning the other jaw. For example a false asymmetrical maxilla will show itself by asymmetry of the mandible.

The following are important.

a) Midline dental discrepancies or an occlusal cant are corrected to the facial midline as drawn on the articulated models from the midline jig and not the articulator pin (Figure 7.9c).
b) The angular relationship of the occlusal to the Frankfort horizontal plane;

$(8^0 \pm 4^0)$ is also important in treatment planning.
Changes in the occlusal plane angle are used to

i) close an anterior open bite and
ii) retrocline maxillary incisal inclination.

In both cases the amount of occlusal plane alteration be carefully estimated clinically and radiolographically and then carried out on the articulated models.

c) Model Surgery Technique (Figures 7.13a to 7.13e)

- The preoperative relationships of the maxillary and mandibular models are recorded by horizontal lines (A, B and O) and vertical lines.
- The A lines are within half a centimetre of their mounting plates and the B line is at the estimated apices of the canines (Figure 7.13a).
- The O line (Figure 7.13b) is drawn to represent the site of the estimated osteotomy cut. The vertical lines are drawn through

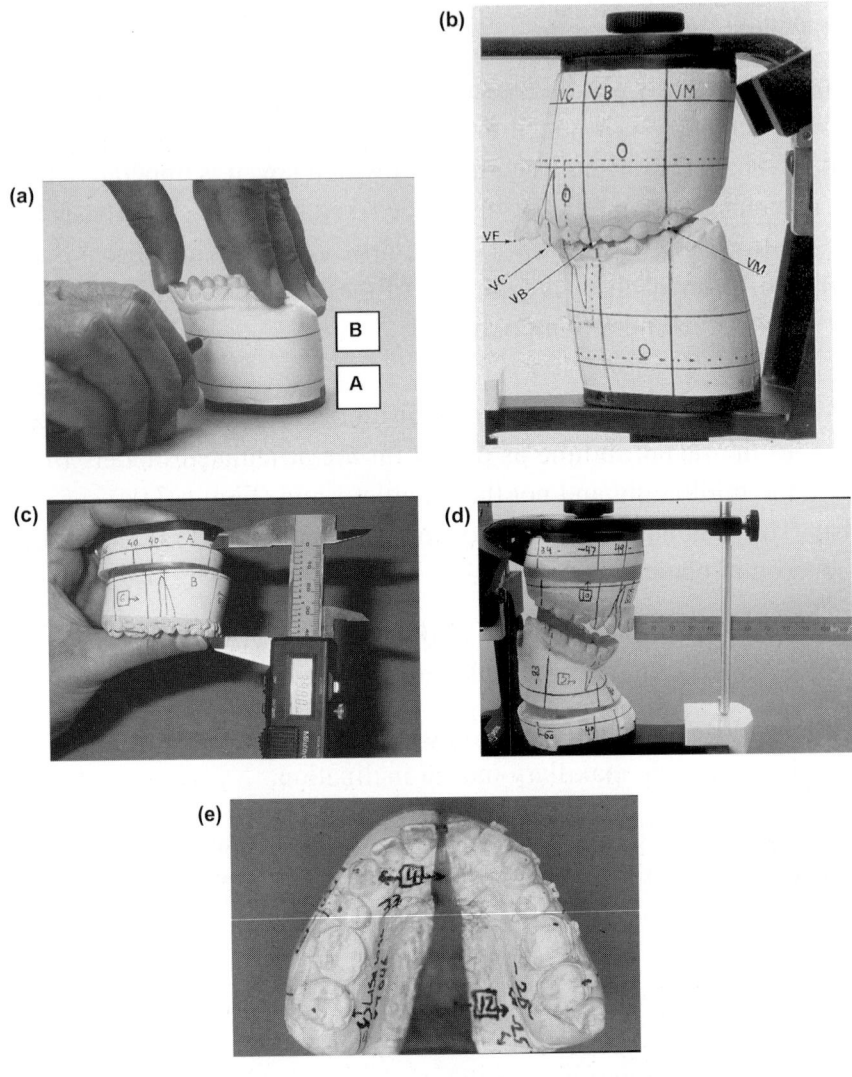

Figure 7.13 **(a)** Horizontal reference lines A and B are drawn with a fine tipped felt pen. **(b)** Models mounted in the preoperative position on the Denar articulator, using the Slidematic facebow and centric relation records, The anatomically-orientated models in preoperative positions showing the cusp reference points (as pointed out with arrows) used for pre- and postoperative measurements. VM = Mesial buccal cusp of a molar tooth; VB = buccal cusp of a premolar; VC = canine cusp; and VF = interincisor midline at the crown tip, unless the teeth or the maxilla are asymmetrically rotated in which case the most anterior

the following reference points: VM, molar buccal cusp tip; VB, buccal cusp tip of the second bicuspid; VC, canine cusp tip; and VF, interincisal edge or marker of the facial midline. The distance from each cusp reference point to its A line and the transpalatal intercanine and intermolar distances are measured with a Vernier calliper and metal ruler or Ericsson model platform and recorded on the models (Figures 7.13c to 7.13e).

- The model is cut at the O osteotomy line with a hand or electric saw, and where an impaction is to be carried out, the required amount of plaster is removed with the saw or electric sander to achieve the planned jaw movements. The segments are assembled in the postoperative position using red ribbon wax, which allows easy manipulation into the required position. When the final position is achieved the red soft wax is replaced with sticky wax. If any adjustments are necessary the wax can be softened and the maxillary or mandibular segments repositioned.

- The relative postoperative positions of the jaw segments are measured as the distances between the references points and the actual movements are indicated in boxes with direction arrows.

- It is advisable to complete the whole model surgery procedure, check the final occlusion and see if any adjustment is required in the maxillary position before making any occlusal wafer.

- For the intermediate wafer fabrication the postoperative mandibular model can be replaced with the preoperative

---

point at the incisor edge is used, where it coincides with the facial midline. Note: A and B base lines, O = simulated osteotomy line and the vertical reference lines. **(c)** The vertical maxillary movements measured with a digital Vernier calliper from the A line to the cusp tips of maxillary teeth. **(d)** The modified articulator anterior pin with a slot for the steel rule is used to confirm anteroposterior jaw movements. **(e)** Occlusal view of a patient cast showing 4 mm intercanine and 12 mm intermolar maxillary expansion.

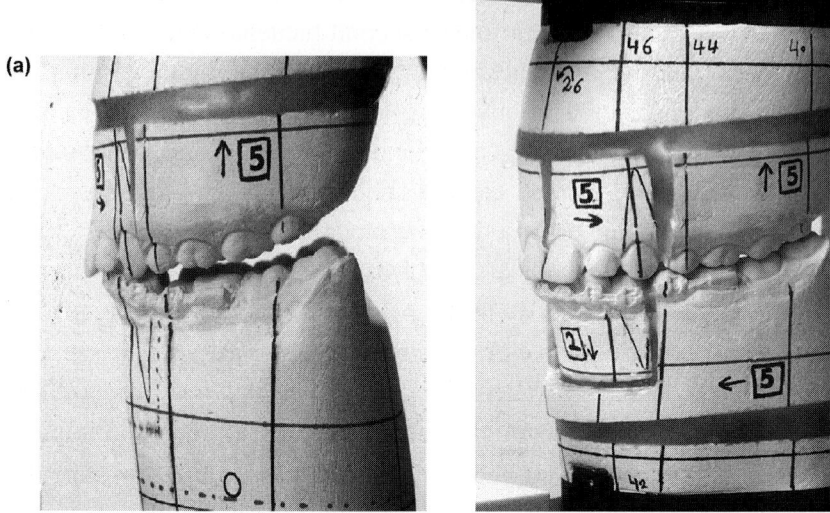

Figure 7.14 Models in **(a)** intermediate and **(b)** final position after the model surgery and before making intermediate and final occlusal wafers.

mandibular model mounted with the supine CR wax occlusal record (Figures 7.14a and 7.14b).

The Ericsson Table for Model Surgery (Great Lakes Orthodontics)

This is a precise tool for carrying out the model surgery. The registration bite and transfer jig are used for the articulation of the upper then lower models as described previously. Once the plaster has set both mountings are allowed to dry completely overnight in a drying oven.

* The Ericsson system consists of a highly polished smooth granite platform (Figure 7.15a) with an electronic calliper mount inserted into the base at 90 degrees to the surface platform and a model block (Figure 7.15b). The models mounted on the model block can be measured in three planes. The calliper's tip in addition to measuring can also be used to scribe lines onto the plaster models.

- The plaster model with its articulator ring is mounted on the rectangular model block in an identical manner to that on the anatomical articulator. The surface of the model block is therefore equivalent to the mounting surface of the articulator arm and is the reference plane for measuring vertical impaction changes (Y) (Figure 7.15b).
- With the model block on its posterior side on the granite table measurements are recorded from the platform surface to the dental midline and cusp reference points to simulate "horizontal — anteroposterior (X) movements.
- Transverse measurements (Z). are recorded with the block on its lateral side (Figures 7.15c and 7.15d).
- The measurements are taken as described in the previous technique, from the tip of the mesio-buccal cusps of the maxillary right and left first molars, the tips of the maxillary right and left canines, and the incisal edges of the maxillary central incisors to the appropriate mounting block surface .
- All measurements are recorded on a model surgery planning grid, drawn on a blank paper or lab-card and are repeated to ensure accuracy.
- The facial midline has already been drawn on the model when mounted on the articulator. The simulated O osteotomy line is drawn parallel to the granite base on the plaster mounting (Figure 7.15e).

When undertaking model surgery it is important to ensure that the clinically planned movements are in agreement with the reference points and measurements applied during the model surgery procedure.

- Planned vertical impaction movements can be first measured from the O line opposite the first molar cusps and incisor reference points and scribed on the plaster model mounting. (Figures 7.15f and 7.15g). Using a band saw, the mounting is cut along the O line. Plaster corresponding to the amount of maxillary

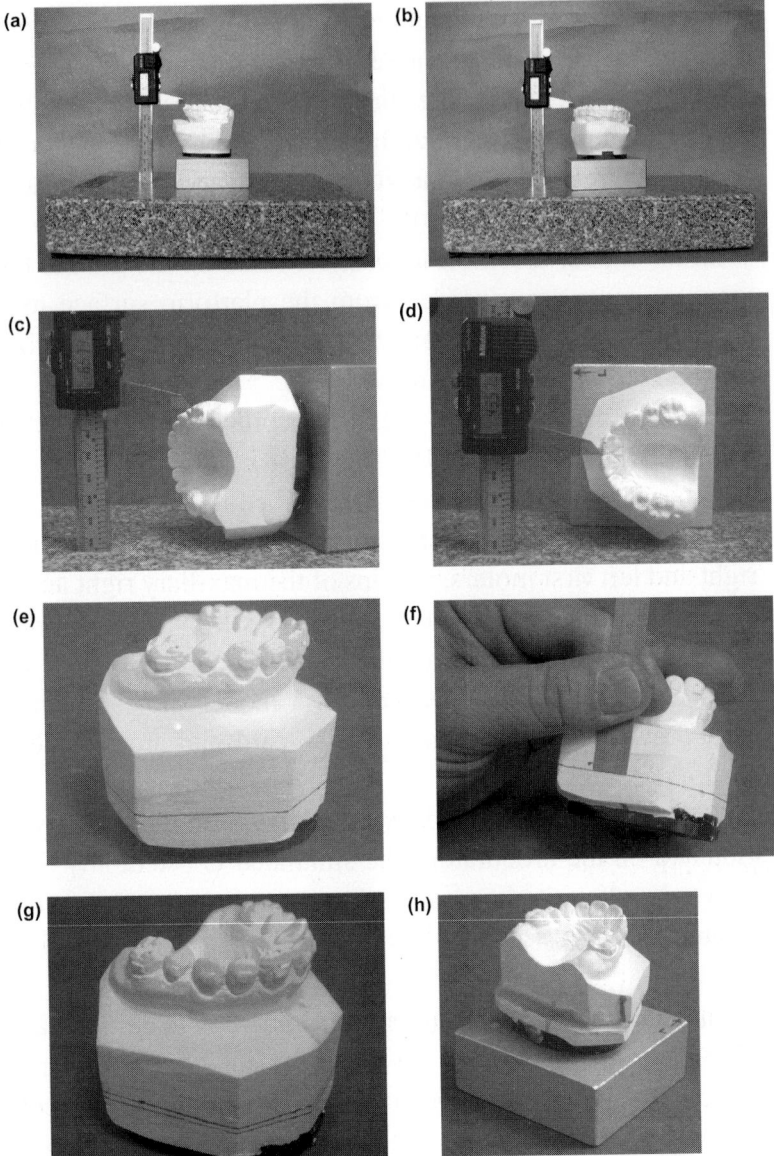

Figure 7.15   (**a**) Ericsson model platform with caliper and mounted casts. (**b**) Model with mounting ring on block. (**c**) and (**d**) Electronic caliper assembly showing identification of incisor and bicuspid reference points. To be measured against platform plane. (**e**) O osteotomy line for sectioning the model. (**f**) and (**g**) Measuring planned impaction to be removed from plaster base. (**h**) Assembled model after "surgery".

impaction is removed from the model plaster mounting using a model trimmer. The total amount of plaster removed will be slightly greater that that required. This is taken up by flowing a thin layer of warmed carding wax between the cut model and the mounting base to relocate the two elements (Figure 7.15h).

- Planned anteroposterior or rotational movements of the maxilla are checked against the marked centre line and cusp reference points.
- Transverse or segmental surgery requires additional cuts to the plaster model but the same principal is applied.
- The recombined cut maxilla is then replaced on the model block and Ericcson table and the measurements are confirmed using the electronic calliper.
- Warming the interpositional wax by flaming, allows fine adjustments to be made to to ensure the new planned postsurgical measurements to correspond to those recorded on the planning grid. The model is then sealed to the mount using either sticky wax or a glue gun, and rechecked.
- Fabrication of the intermediate and final wafers is as described below.

7. Occlusal Wafers

Osteotomy wafers locate the dental arches in any preplanned relationship and eliminate unreliable intraoperative guesswork.

Wafers are used for the following purposes.

a) To reposition the mobilised maxilla relative to the intact mandible (or *vice versa*). This intermediate wafer has a horizontal inaccuracy of about 2 mm of the planned position due to the discrepancy between the distalised centre of mandibular rotation in the supine anaesthetised patient and the mandibular rotation in the conscious upright patient. Overcorrection of the maxilla is therefore essential in a single jaw maxillary osteotomy to ensure the planned advancement. This maxillary discrepancy is masked in a bimaxillary procedure when the mandible is placed in a Class I incisor relationship to the maxilla regardless of its position.

b) To achieve the planned intermediate and final occlusion.

c) For postoperative proprioceptive guidance. After rigid fixation of the mandible the wafer may be wired to the maxilla or mandible to provide postoperative proprioceptive guidance for up to two weeks, with or without the help of elastics. However this causes discomfort to the patient and appears to have no proven value except to reassure the surgeon.

d) To stabilise the segments in the planned position when the dental arch is segmented and mobilised whilst an orthodontic supplemental arch wire or arch bar is secured into place. Without an occlusal wafer, this can be difficult and will give poor results. Without the supplemental arch wire the planned occlusal relationship may be unstable.

e) The wafer is invaluable when the postoperative occlusion is not sufficiently stable after the release of intraoperative IMF in cases requiring substantial postoperative orthodontics or with poorly contoured crowns or bridges which need to be replaced.

Wafer Fabrication (Figures 7.16a to 7.16d)

Wafers may be fabricated from cold cured (autopolymerising) or quick cure methylmethacrylate. A poorly designed inaccurate wafer will spoil the most skilful surgical technique. It is common practice to construct both the intermediate and the final wafers as thin as possible. The justification has been that thick wafers introduce discrepancies in the final occlusion.

As stated the condylar recoil from the distalised anaesthetised centric relation to active conscious centric occlusion can reduce the

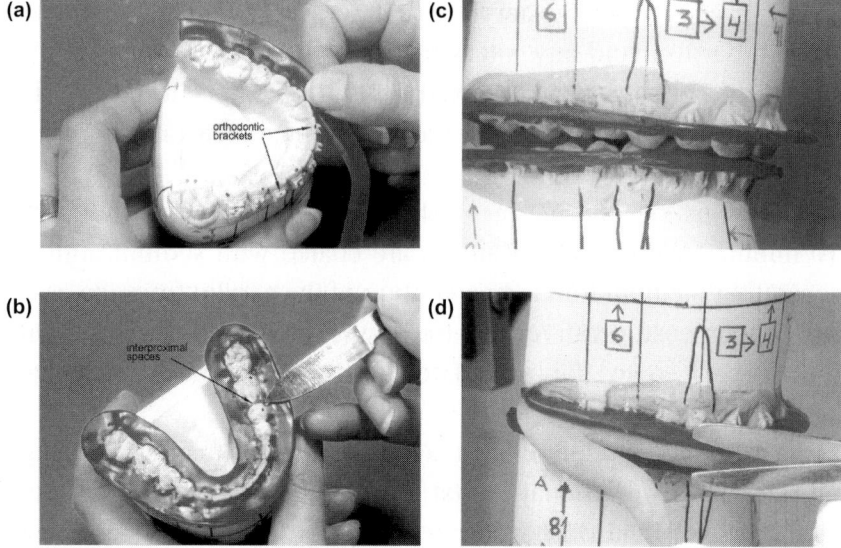

Figure 7.16 (a), **(b)**, **(c)** and **(d)** After the model surgery, the maxillary and mandibular models with the mounting assembly are removed from the articulator for wafer fabrication — see text.

setback in Class III corrections. This is anticipated by overcorrection of the planned posterior position of the mandible by at least 2mm.

Similarly, the inevitable degree of postoperative distal relapse in the Class II mandibular advancement justifies a forward overcorrection to an incisor edge to edge final occlusion.

The Construction Technique Using Quick Cure Acrylic

After the model surgery, the maxillary and mandibular models with the mounting assembly are removed from the articulator. All the undercuts along the palatal, lingual and buccal aspects of the dental arches are relieved by applying a strip of soft red beading wax (Utility Wax, Kem-Dent, Associated Dental Products Ltd, UK).

The occlusal margins of the orthodontic brackets are the limit of the coronal extension of the wafer. It is advisable to have about

1 mm space between the acrylic wafer and the orthodontics brackets or arch bar to avoid any interference at the time of insertion. The Interproximal spaces are blocked out with the wax to ensure that the wafer does not extend into these unwanted areas and impair fit during the surgery.

The tips of the plaster teeth are soaked in the water for 10 minutes and the dental arches are coated with sodium alginate separating medium for easy separation of the acrylic from the casts. The upper postoperative and the lower preoperative models are placed back onto the articulator to fabricate the intermediate occlusal wafer.

A quick cure high impact acrylic is mixed using 70% high impact polymer (Austenal Dental Products Ltd., The Crystal Centre, Harrow, UK), and 30% rapid repair polymer with its monomer. When the mix is at the dough stage, a U-shaped role is placed over the occlusal surface of the mandibular arch. The acrylic dough is moulded and directed towards the buccal and lingual surfaces of the teeth with a spatula, ensuring full coverage of the occlusal surfaces.

The upper arm of the articulator is closed down firmly until its incisal pin touches the incisal table. The acrylic material is thus sandwiched between the maxillary and mandibular dental arches indexing the occlusal surfaces of the teeth. While still soft, the excess acrylic is trimmed with a pair of scissors. At the initial polymerisation stage, the articulator is carefully opened and closed, to ensure that the wafer could be removed from both the upper and lower models when processed. This will also eliminate acrylic contraction around the incisal tips and minimise any damage to the teeth at wafer removal, when fully polymerised and hard.

After removal of the excess acrylic and ensuring that the dental arches are fully covered, the articulator with the models and wafer is secured with a rubber band and placed in the hydro-flask for 10 minutes for curing. Once processed, the upper arm of the articulator is unlocked and removed gently before removing the wafer. It is then trimmed and polished, avoiding frictional heat, which may

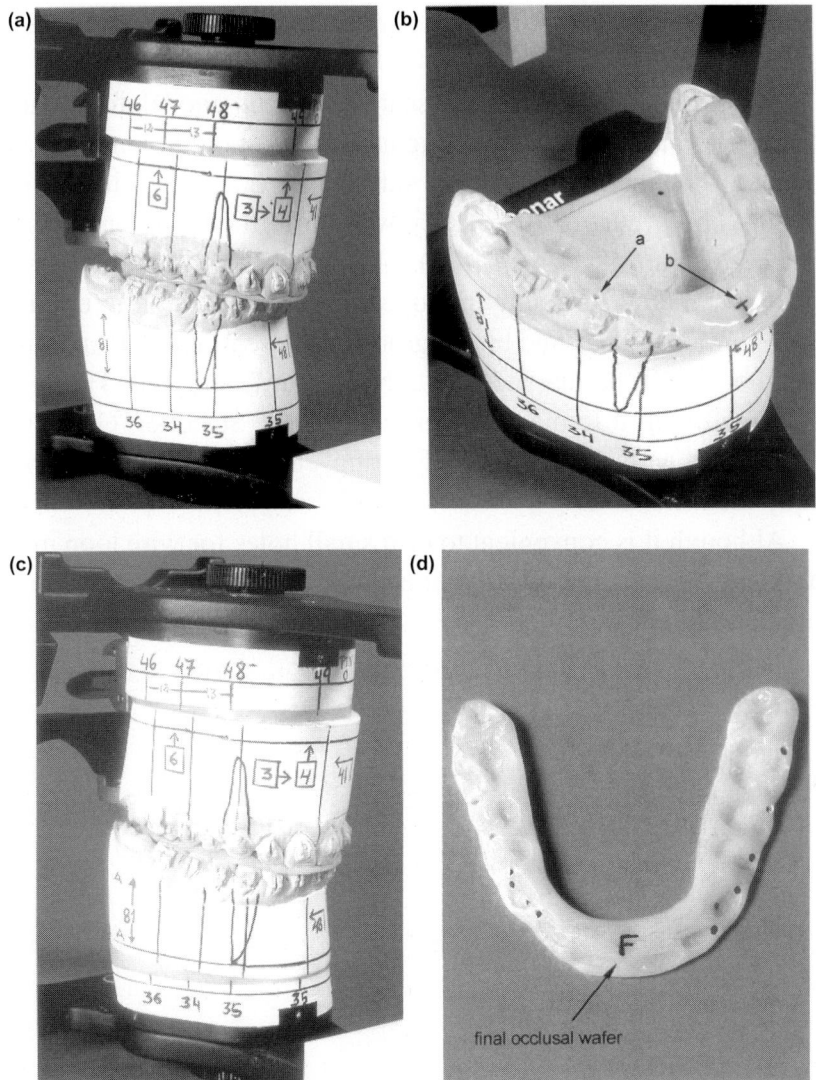

Figure 7.17   **(a)** The buccal and lingual aspect of the wafers should blend into the tooth morphology. **(b)** On buccal aspects of the wafer small holes are drilled using a round bur No. 5 to pass wires through to suspend the wafer to orthodontic brackets or arch bars. **(c)** Final occlusal wafer is tried in on the models. **(d)** For identification letter (I) for intermediate and (F) for final is engraved and a groove representing the midline can also be marked with No. 2 bur. These letters can be reinforced with lumocolor permanent pen (Staedtler, Germany).

warp the acrylic. The process is repeated with both postsurgical models for the final wafer.

The completed wafers are seated on each model for a final check. The buccal, labial and lingual aspects should blend into the tooth morphology. On the buccal sides, small holes are drilled using a round No. 5 bur for suspensory wires to orthodontic brackets or arch bar (Figures 7.17a to 7.17d).

It is essential for ready intraoperative identification to engrave I or F with a No. 5 round bur. A groove representing the facial midline should also be marked with a No. 2 flat fissure bur. These are reinforced with a Lumocolor permanent pen (Staedtler, Germany) and can be embedded with self-curing clear resin, thus ensuring ready identification.

Although it is convenient to drill small holes for wire loop maxillary suspension, embedded ball end clasps are occasionally a useful alternative.

8

Fixation Techniques

Introduction

The most commonly used fixation methods for orthognathic surgery are the following.

External Fixation.

- Fixed orthodontic appliances, with occlusal wafers.
- Fixed orthodontic appliances with supplementary arch wires and tubes.
- Arch bars — either prefabricated flexible, wrought wire, or cast cobalt chromium.
- Cortical screws and intermaxillary fixation.
- Eyelet wires.
- Cast metal splints.

Internal Fixation.

- Miniature titanium bone plates and cortical screws.
- Bicortical screws.
- Bioresorbable fixation plates and screws.

Most surgeons find orthodontic fixed appliance archwires with or without the addition of hooks are the most versatile and reliable method for intra- and postoperative fixation, especially when used with carefully constructed occlusal wafers. Where there has been no recent orthodontic treatment, a cortical screw placed in the buccal alveolus in each quadrant or some form of arch bar is essential for intraoperative fixation. Eyelet wires are a simple substitute but are less convenient to work with. Cast metal splints have become less popular because of the clinical and laboratory complexity and are usually confined to the unstable components of a cleft case.

With the use of miniature titanium plates and screws, wire osteosynthesis is almost outdated except where plate systems are not available. However precise temporary intermaxillary fixation (IMF) is very important to secure the mobilised segments of the maxilla and the mandible whilst applying the internal fixation plates and screws.

Bicortical bone screws or buccal plates in mandibular procedures have totally revolutionised postoperative rehabilitation by dispensing with prolonged intermaxillary fixation. Whatever the method of fixation, it should be decided upon early so that there is adequate time for fixation appliances to be carefully designed, made and if appropriate, tried for accuracy of fit. If the arch bars are the method of choice, theatre time may be saved by fixation on the teeth preoperatively under local anaesthesia, with or without intravenous sedation.

The material and design of the fixation appliance must be capable of maintaining the bone fragments in the planned position until union has occurred. This is particularly important in a cleft osteotomy.

Fixed Orthodontic Appliances

Most patients require presurgical fixed appliance orthodontic treatment, these may be modified for intermaxillary fixation and segmental stabilisation with the help of rectangular wire attachments and hooks (Figure 8.1).

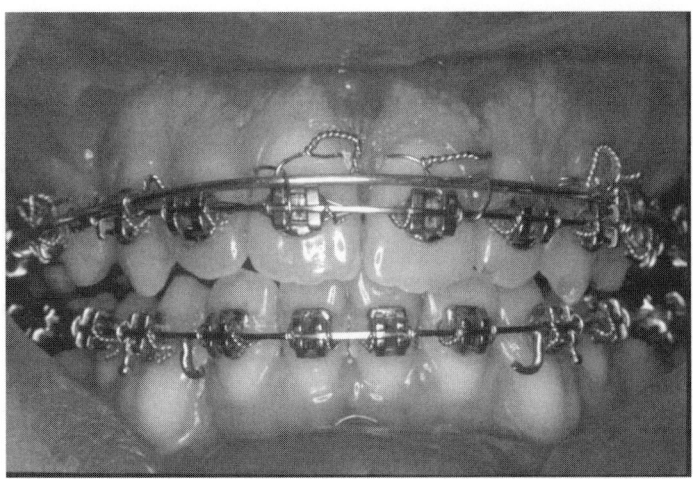

Figure 8.1 Orthodontic brackets, wires and hooks for fixation. Note the 1 mm maxillary supplemental arch wire to augment the internal fixation used to localise a divided dentoalveolar segment.

The attachment must fit well and be cemented securely to avoid dislodgement during surgery and intermaxillary fixation. The heavy rectangular wire in Edgewise brackets gives good stabilisation for fixation, and if required can be improved with the addition of crimpable steel hooks or soldered brass wires. Unfortunately it can be tedious when the hooks ensnare swabs. With segmental surgery, intra- and postoperative dentoalveolar stabilisation is essential to avoid any rotation around the internal plate fixation. Although this can be an archwire shaped on the sectioned and repositioned model used for surgical planning and which can be fitted intraoperatively by an orthodontist, it is more convenient to:

- section the arch wire at operation to facilitate the osteotomy,
- localise the segments with a wafer, and then
- stabilise them by ligation to a heavy 1 mm supplemental arch wire inserted into tubes fitted on the molar bands (Figure 8.1). On the upper molars these can be the headgear tubes but in the lower arch bands with double tubes are required.

Advantages

- Orthodontic fixation does not require laboratory facilities.
- With a rectangular arch wire every type of movement can be controlled.
- It is invaluable for intraoperative immobilisation whilst applying the plates and screws for "rigid fixation".

Disadvantages

- Direct bonded attachments are occasionally lost because the cementation fails.
- It is advisable to remove any lingual attachments which may have been present during the orthodontic treatment.

Cortical Screws

These may be specifically designed for IMF and are inserted through a stab wound into the dense basal bone between the canine and first premolars. Either wire or postoperative elastics may be applied to immobilise the occlusion.

This technique is only applicable when both arches are intact.

Arch Bars

Prefabricated Flexible

A prefabricated form (Erich — Dentaurum, Pforzheim, FRG) is made of semi-rigid stainless steel (Figure 8.2). It can be easily contoured to the arch form and ligated with stainless steel wires passed around the arch bar and the necks of the adjacent teeth. Cleats for intermaxillary fixation are also an integral part of the design. Stainless steel wire (0.5 mm) which has been prestretched by 10% is used to ligate the arch bar to the teeth, starting in the midline and working backwards.

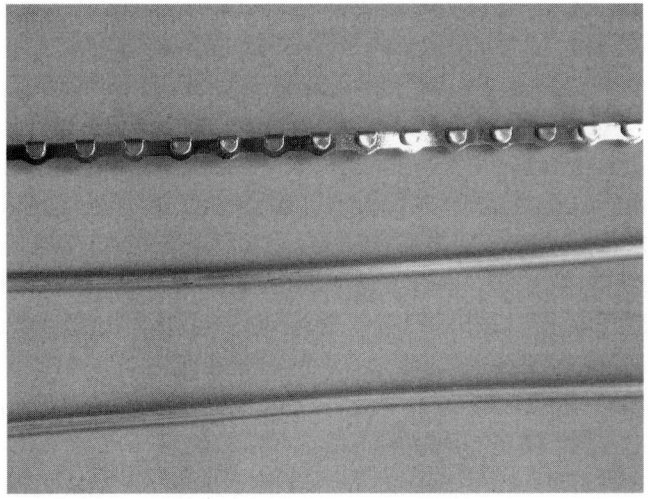

Figure 8.2 Prefabricated Erich arch bar and wrought wire used for making custom-made arch bars.

Advantages

- These are useful where orthodontic treatment has not been used.
- No technical assistance is required for this type of fixation, and the bars can be easily adapted into the desired shape.
- Arch bars can be placed before the operation, under local anaesthesia supplemented with intravenous sedation. This reduces the time spent in the operating room.
- The occlusion can always be checked and at the end of the fixation period the arch bars can easily be removed without an anaesthetic.

Disadvantages

- An adequate number of suitable teeth are required to get rigid and reliable fixation.
- They may not be suitable in osteotomies where there are many crowns and bridges.

Wrought Wire Arch Bar

These arch bars are a very satisfactory method of fixation, especially in segmental procedures.

Casts of the patient's teeth are obtained. If any segmental movement of the jaws is involved, the segments are sectioned and reassembled in the required position. The arch bar is constructed from nickel silver 1/8 inch (3.00 mm × 1.5 mm diameter) oval or 2 mm half-round wire and is shaped to fit as close as possible to the tooth surfaces and into the interdental spaces (Figures 8.3a and 8.3b).

The extreme ends of the bar are bent to fit around the distal aspect of the last tooth on each side. Cleats (hooks), tubes and locking plate attachments, if required, can be soldered to the bar. The bar is trimmed and polished in the usual way. Notches or grooves are made to stop ligature wires slipping. These arch bars are ligated to the teeth with 0.5 mm stainless steel wire which has been prestretched by 10% of its original length. If no segmental movement is involved, the arch bars can be wired to the dental arch preoperatively.

(a) (b)

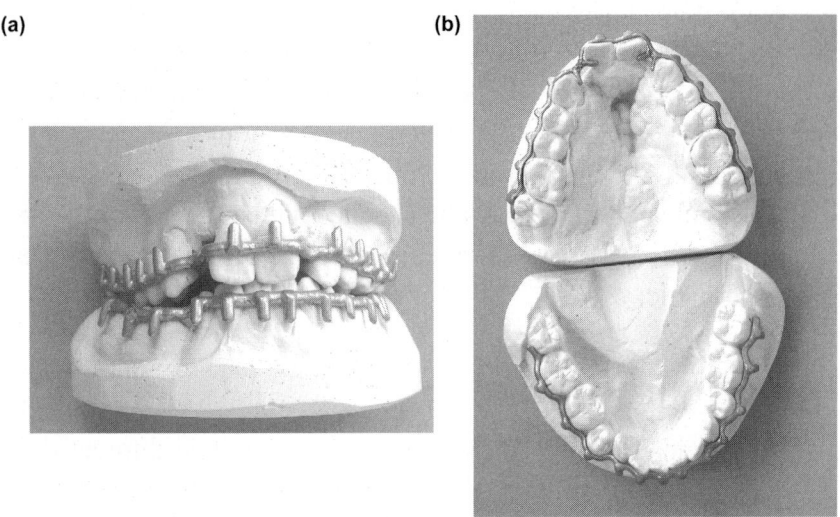

Figure 8.3 (a) and (b) Custom-made wrought arch bars with soldered cleats.

Advantages

- This method of fixation requires no casting facilities.
- There is no occlusal coverage and interference.
- They can be easily removed without too much discomfort to the patient.

Disadvantages

- This method may permit rotational movement in segmental surgical procedures without additional internal rigid fixation.

Cast Cobalt Chromium

If properly designed and manufactured, this type of arch bar has many advantages, whilst at the same time avoiding any interference with the occlusion. Cobalt chromium is the metal of choice because of its high tensile strength and so arch bars of this material are reliable and not bulky.

The casts are mounted on an articulator, sectioned and positioned in the planned position. Although it is advisable to prepare the wax pattern as close to the cervical margins of the teeth as possible, it is essential to avoid any contact with the gingival margin in the interdental area so as to leave space to pass and tie the 0.5 mm wire ligatures. The wax pattern also must not be formed close to the incisal edges to avoid interference with the postoperative occlusion. An arch bar made too close to the occlusal surface will be displaced gingivally when tightening the ligature wires. Intermaxillary fixation is achieved with two cleats placed on the buccal and labial segments on each bar. Each cleat should be opposite the one on the opposing arch. This can be precisely designed as capstan cleats (Figure 8.4) which are very helpful in stabilising the repositioned mobilised jaws in the planned position. Grooves must be provided to accommodate the interdental ligatures. The arch bar is cast using the "lift off" technique, and in segmental cases it is cast in the postoperative position.

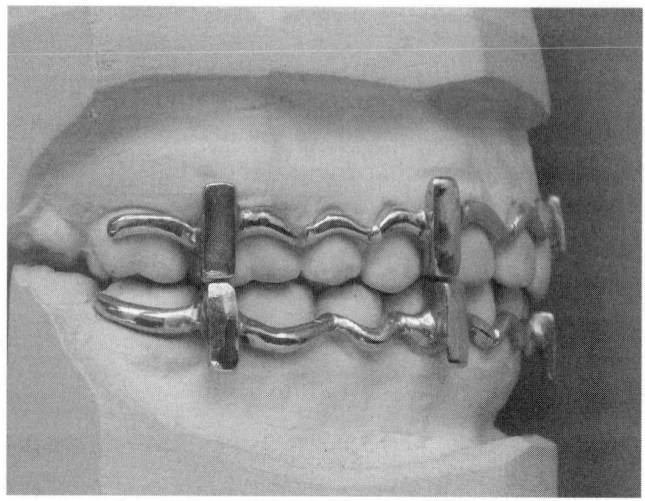

Figure 8.4   Cast chrome cobalt arch bars with matching cleats to confirm accurate localisation.

Advantages

• These arch bars provide reliable and precise fixation without any occlusal interference and with minimum discomfort to the patient.
• The facilities and skills for their construction are usually readily available in maxillofacial laboratories.

Disadvantages

• Casting facilities and skilled technical help are required. In common with any other arch bar they need to be ligated to the teeth with 0.5 mm soft stainless steel wires.

Ligating Arch Bars

A simple 0.5 mm wire ligature around the tooth and arch bar is unsatisfactory and the addition of a loop around the bar creating a figure of eight between tooth and bar produces stable anchorage (Figure 8.5).

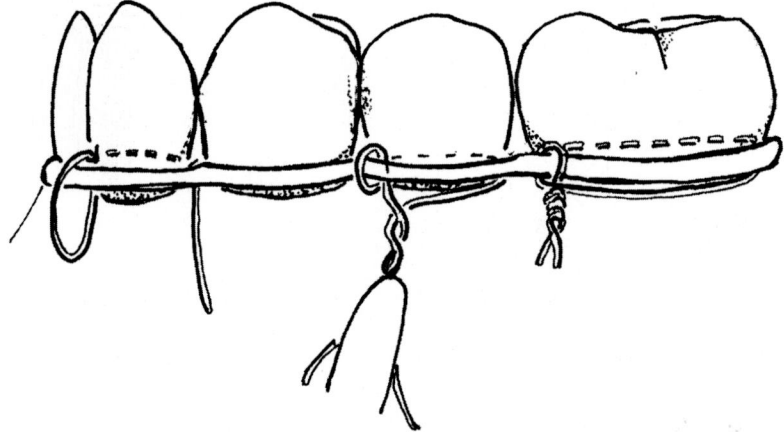

Figure 8.5   Ligation of custom-made arch bar with 0.5 mm stretched stainless steel wire.

Eyelet Wires

Are used primarily in the immobilisation of jaw fractures because of the simplicity of their fabrication and application. However, they are valuable for intraoperative immobilisation with rigid fixation.

Wire of 0.5 mm is preferable to 0.35 mm as it is sturdier and easier to pass through tight contact points and gingiva without getting lost. Three metres of wire can be stretched 10% between heavy artery forceps and then cut into lengths of approximately 12 cm. Each is grasped at both ends by heavy forceps and the centre placed against a headless nail (2 mm diameter) fixed in a suitable surface, or a bur shank in a vice. The wire is firmly bent around the nail and then twisted twice to produce the eye. The eyelet wire is then removed and the ends are cut at 45^0 and trimmed (Figure 8.6).

Advantages

- The wires can be easily prepared and applied preoperatively with no technical support or dental casts (models).

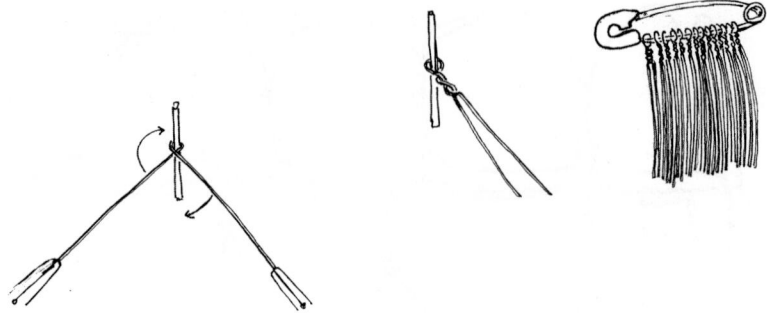

Figure 8.6   Making eyelet wires from 0.5 mm stretched stainless steel wire.

- They are ideal for temporary intermaxillary fixation when rigid fixation, i.e. plates and screws are being used.

Disadvantages

- This is a time-consuming procedure where an adequate number of suitably shaped teeth are essential.
- The use of eyelet wires on crowns and bridgework intraoperatively, can produce embarrassing displacement.
- Even when used with a wafer they will not stabilise small segments.

Occlusal Wafers (See Chapter 7, Figures 7.16–7.17)

As a final step in the presurgical planning, occlusal wafers are fabricated on the articulator mounted casts to establish the intermediate and postoperative positions. After surgery, the occlusal wafer can also provide a solid interdigitation of the teeth, especially in cases of mandibular advancement where the goal is a "3-point landing". It is therefore possible to defer any final orthodontic refinement of the occlusion or the replacement of crowns and bridgework until comfortable bone union has taken place.

When the dental arch is sectioned and the segments repositioned, the wafer establishes the planned position whilst securing the osteotomy site with screws and or bone plates. However the occlusal wafer alone will not prevent rotation of the dento-alveolar segments, which must be secured with an orthodontic archwire, an arch bar or a sectional splint despite the internal rigid fixation.

Internal Fixation

Transosseous Wiring

This is a simple traditional method of holding bone fragments together. For the mandible with its rigid cortical plates, 0.5 mm stretched, soft stainless steel wire is satisfactory. However, a finer 0.35 mm wire is essential for maxillary osteotomies to avoid pulling through the thin bone margins of the drill holes. Although the bone plate has superceded transosseous wiring there are occasions when wires can be an invaluable salvage technique.

Miniature Bone Plates and Cortical Screws

Titanium bone plates and screws,[1] are an excellent means of internal fixation. The introduction of L- and Y-shape plates should eliminate apical damage when screwing into the maxillary alveolar segment. The screw holes must be prepared with a slow, well-cooled matching drill, or a tapering tungsten carbide fissure bur (No. 101). High speeds and heavy hand pressure amplify eccentric rotation and produce a large, charred useless hole, especially in the thin maxillary wall. There are broader salvage screws available to rescue such situations. Plates provide greater security against relapse especially in cleft cases. In non-cleft osteotomies, the use of buccal plates in the maxilla and mandible or 9–13 mm bicortical screws for sagittal split osteotomies have made postoperative intermaxillary fixation unnecessary. This has dramatically simplified postoperative nursing

---

[1] Gebruder Martin GmbH & Co. KG, Tuttlingen, Germany; Leibinger (QS Leibinger, Muhllheim-Stetten, Germany), Albert Waeschle, Germany.

and patient rehabilitation. Unfortunately, some plates when superficially placed submucosally give rise to irritation or become infected and have to be removed. However, when inserted with slow, gentle carefully cooled drilling of the bone, long-term incorporation is the rule rather than the exception.

Bioresorbable Fixation Plates and Screws

Resorbable fixation systems[2] may have the potential for avoiding the possibility of a secondary procedure to remove plates. These are mainly produced from two alpha hydroxyl acids; polylactic and polyglycolic acids which resorb approximately in a year to lactic acid, carbon dioxide and water. Some may take up to 3 years. The ideal bioresorbable system should facilitate fixation with sufficient initial strength to stabilise bone segments and allow uneventful bone healing. It should be biocompatible and degrade predictably and completely after osteosynthesis has restored adequate intrinsic bone strength. They must be easy to use and cost effective.

At the moment most of designs are not suitable for the mandible to return to early masticatory function, as they can lose their strength within six weeks.

Cast Metal Cap Splints (See Figures 8.7a and 8.7b)

In procedures for gross facial deformity where prolonged fixation is required, metal cap splints still prove to be more reliable than any other method. Many variations exist. For repositioning of dentoalveolar fragments, the splint can be made

i)   in separate parts and joined together with precision locks and connecting bars;

---

[2] Gebruder Martin GmbH & Co. KG, Tuttlingen, Germany; Albert Waeschle, Germany. Inion Ltd, Tampere, Finland.

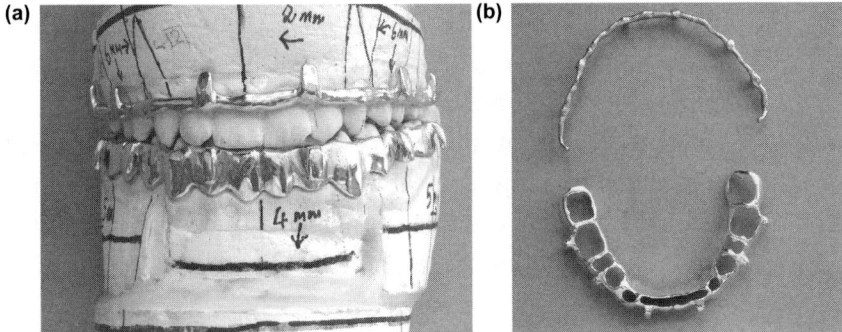

Figure 8.7 (a) and **(b)** A combination of a custom-made arch bar and open occlusal metal splint.

ii) as a one-piece open cast splint can be constructed on the surgical planning cast and fitted both as a template and fixation at the operation; or
iii) the splints can be secured to the mandible with circumferential wires during the operative procedure.

Advantages

- Teeth which are subjected to traction over long periods of time tend to migrate and extrude if not locked into a single unit by a rigid appliance.
- Important when few teeth are widely distributed.
- Excellent immobilisation can be achieved for a long period without causing discomfort or damage to the periodontal structures.
- The laboratory preparation of segments with locking plates and connecting bars in a planned position can reduce time spent in the operating theatre.

Disadvantages

- Splints require accurate impression techniques.
- Requires a skilled technician and maxillofacial laboratory facilities.

- Require adequate time for their construction, although this should not be an important factor when orthognathic operations can be planned weeks beforehand.
- Due to the thickness of metal between the occlusal surfaces of the teeth there is a slight error of occlusion after cap splints have been used. This resolves spontaneously or rarely requires postoperative orthodontic treatment.

The Design

They should fit as closely as possible against the gingival margins. To reduce the construction time and ensure uniform strength, everything that can be cast, such as hooks and rings, should be included in the wax pattern rather than be formed and soldered on at a later stage. The wax pattern should be smooth to reduce finishing time to a minimum. Given good organisation, the most complicated upper and lower splints can be produced in 6 hours. The use of cleats (hooks) tends to be the most popular method for intermaxillary fixation. Where accurate movements and positioning of the jaws is required, precisely matching capstan cleats can give superior results. The most useful design is the open cap splint where its open occlusal surfaces allow the escape of excess cement. This facilitates full seating and enables an accurate occlusion to be visualised at operation.

Splints should be cemented preoperatively and scrupulous care taken to remove residual cement from the occlusal surfaces, gingival margins, under cleats and from within locking plate recesses and screw holes.

Lines must be marked on the splints preoperatively to correspond to the facial midline. This can be of crucial importance in the operating theatre in establishing the desired fixation of two mobilised jaws in a bimaxillary procedure.

Also, where necessary, grooves for circumferential wires are incorporated into the design. The locking plates must be marked to indicate their position on the splint by engraving with small matching cuts on the top and soldered base of the locking plate.

Splint Attachments (See Figures 8.8a and 8.8b)

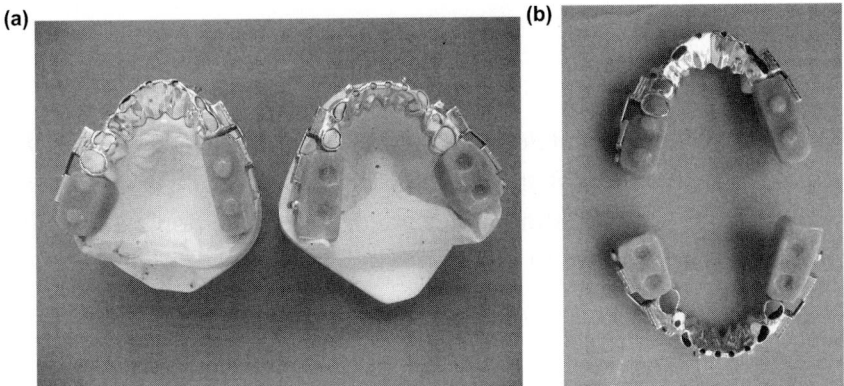

Figure 8.8 (a) and (b) Metal splints with posterior bite blocks for edentulous areas.

Locking Plates (See Figures 8.9a and 8.9b)

These are made of nickel silver. They can be purchased prefabricated and are in two sizes: a small, single screw type and a double screw, larger size with either 6 or 8 BA (British Association) screw sizes. They may also be specially fabricated in the laboratory from 1–5 mm

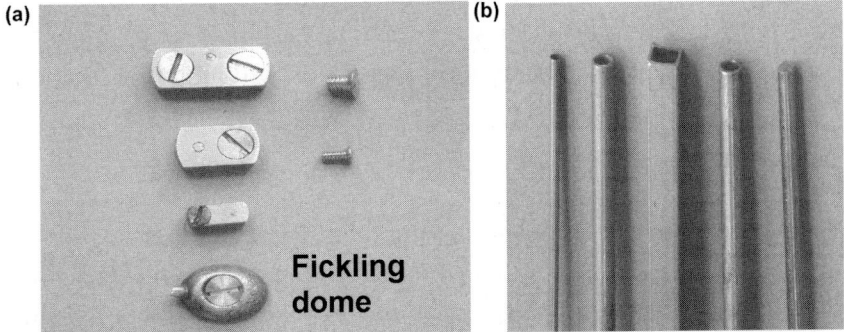

Figure 8.9 (a) Locking plates and screws for metal splint attachments. (b) Tubes and rods for splint attachments.

thick strips of nickel silver. All locking plates provide a base for additional intra and extraoral attachments such as connecting bars.

Fickling Domes

This type of locking plate is cast in silver at the same time as the splint. A recess is built in the splint for the Fickling dome at the wax-up stage. After casting, holes are drilled in the dome and splint recess and then tapped to accept a screw of an appropriate size.

Screws

These are also constructed from nickel silver and are available in the following sizes: 4 BA, 6 BA, 8 BA and 10 BA, the highest number being the smallest size. Screws are normally supplied with countersunk heads. The most common choice is a 6 BA but smaller screws may be necessary if crown size is small.

Connecting Bars

These are used where the splints are made in sections and are joined together after surgery. The most suitable size of rod has an oval section (3 × 2 mm). This size is rigid enough to give excellent stability and yet at the same time is sufficiently malleable to be shaped into almost any desired form. They may also be cast in silver for any special need. Projecting bars are rarely used now with internal fixation.

Replacing Teeth

Where upper incisor teeth are missing the patient's appearance can be markedly improved during the fixation period by adding an acrylic tooth bearing flange to the splint by means of a pin and tube system.

9

Surgical and Osteodistraction Procedures

This chapter provides basic preoperative, intraoperative and post-operative instructions for surgical procedures and a section on Distraction Osteogenesis. At first sight these may appear adequate for the correction of all deformities. However, in practice most cases have a complexity requiring the integration of several procedures, as described in Chapter 10.

General Preoperative Considerations

Informed consent is essential. Patients should be given an accurate although reassuring description of the immediate post-operative period. The possibility of prolonged neurapraxia of the mental or infraorbital nerves must be stressed and recorded. They should be given details of postoperative regimens for feeding and oral hygiene and also be asked to bring to hospital a child's small soft and medium toothbrush. All this is best done as a handout.

The patient must be fit, with a normal haemoglobin concentration. A chest film is probably only necessary where a rib graft is required as a base line should there be any postoperative problem. The nasal airway must be bilaterally patent. Enlarged tonsils may create postoperative oropharyngeal obstruction when swollen, especially with maxillary osteotomies.

Emotionally unstable patients are usually unsuitable for surgery and find intermaxillary fixation intolerable. However this is rarely a problem with rigid fixation.

Preoperative Investigations

1. Haemoglobin, full blood count and blood film.
2. Urinalysis.
3. Blood group and transfusion antibody screening.
4. For major procedures especially when a bone graft is taken, cross-matching blood should be arranged at the last preoperative visit.
5. Sickling test, hepatitis B surface antigen (HBsAg) and HIV screening where appropriate.
6. Chest radiograph, if indicated by the medical history or procedure.

Blood Replacement

Loss of blood can be significantly reduced with hypotensive anaesthesia and antifibrinolytic medication. Mandibular procedures rarely require transfusion, however it is good practice to group the patient's blood and screen for transfusion antibodies but hold the serum for emergency cross-matching. With the increased concern about cross-infection, autologous blood is now being used in some centres for elective surgery.

Antibiotics

Preoperatively

Microbiologists advocate minimal regimes for non-infected surgery. The following **alternatives** are reasonable choices.

- Amoxicillin 1G intravenously at induction followed by 500 mg intravenously 3 hours postoperatively is recommended.

However there is anecdotal evidence that continuing the antibiotic orally 500 mg 8-hourly for the traditional 3 days reduces the low incidence of postoperative infection at the sagittal split site. But this may be prevented by using mandibular vacuum drains after the osteotomy rather than more antibiotics.

- Metronidazole can be given as a 1g rectal suppository pre- and postoperatively. This is more convenient than a 500 mg slow intravenous infusion, to be followed by 400 mg orally 12-hourly for 2–3 days.
- Clindamycin 300 mg intravenously at induction and 150 mg iv. 3 hours postoperatively. This can be extended to 300 mg 6-hourly orally for 2–3 days.

Antibiotics are not required more than 3 days postoperatively unless there is evidence of wound infection or a persistent pyrexia.

Antioedema

Preoperatively

Dexamethasone 8 mg is given intravenously with the anaesthetic induction agents and repeated 12 hours later.

Postoperatively

Dexamethasone 8 mg is given i.v. or i.m. 12-hourly on postoperative day 1, followed by 4–5 mg 12-hourly on day 2.

Operating Considerations

1. The patient must be anaesthetised via a nasal endotracheal tube centrally secured across the forehead. A simple low profile connector between the endotracheal and anaesthetic tubing is essential. A 12 FG nasogastric tube for postoperative aspiration

should also be passed prior to the operation. Some anaesthetists will also pass a fine-bore feeding tube at the same time.

2. Clean the face and mouth with an aqueous antiseptic such as chlorhexidine or povidone-iodine.

3. Drape so that the orbital margins may be exposed for orientation. Cover the nasal tube and eyes with an adhesive drape (Steridrape — 3M, US; Opsite — Smith and Nephew, UK) (Figure 9.1).

4. If a bone graft is being taken, strip the patient, clean the hip or chest twice with iodine detergent and square drape the area with towels; cover and seal the site with a Steridrape or Opsite.

5. Check bipolar diathermy is in place. The anaesthetic machine is best placed with a long hose at the lower end of the table on the opposite side to the graft site. If used, the compressed air cylinder can also be conveniently placed at the foot end of the table so that the air drill hose may pass upwards along the long axis of the patient to the head end. This is avoided by the use of an electric drill.

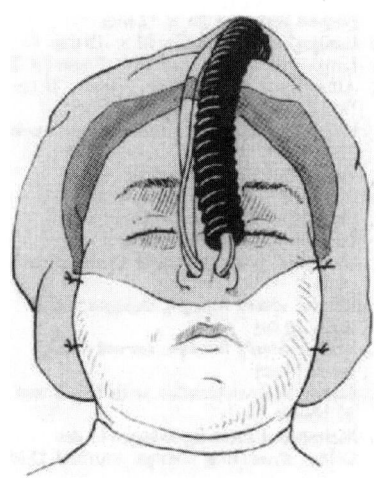

Figure 9.1

6. Tilt the feet down and the head up. Lubricate the lips initially and repeatedly with 1% hydrocortisone ointment.

Instruments

The following list gives the basic osteotomy instrumentation. Most of the instruments are shown in Figures 9.2a–9.2d.

1. Ward's cheek retractor
2. Prognathism channel retractors (×2)
3. Chin holding retractor
4. Cairn's malleable retractor 17 mm
5. Cairn's malleable retractor 11 mm
6. Lac's tongue depressor — child
7. Lac's tongue depressor — adult
8. Kilner cheek retractors — insulated (×2)
9. Forked retractor 70 × 12 mm
10. Langenbeck retractors 44 × 13 mm (×2)
11. Langenbeck retractors 23 × 7 mm (×2)
12. Allis tissue forceps, 4 in 5 teeth, 15 cm (×2)
13. Halstead Mosquito artery forceps, curved 12.5 cm (×10)

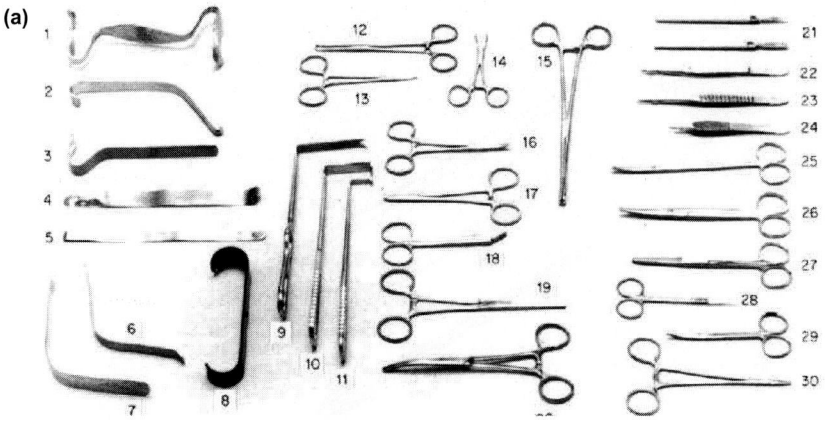

Figure 9.2   (a)

(b)

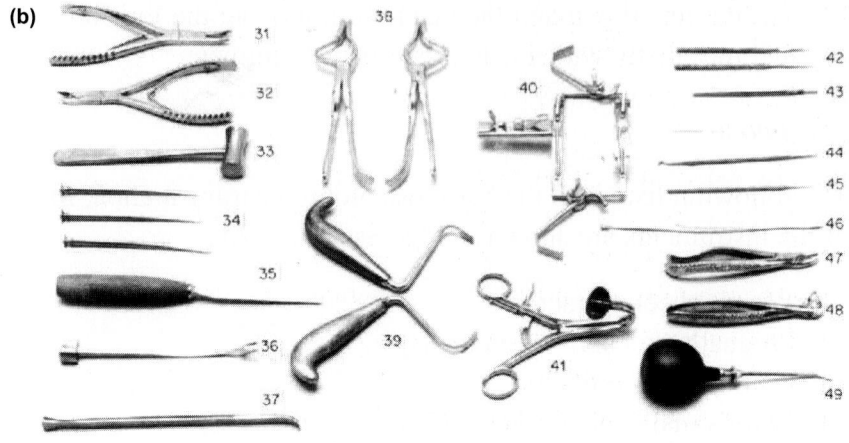

(c)

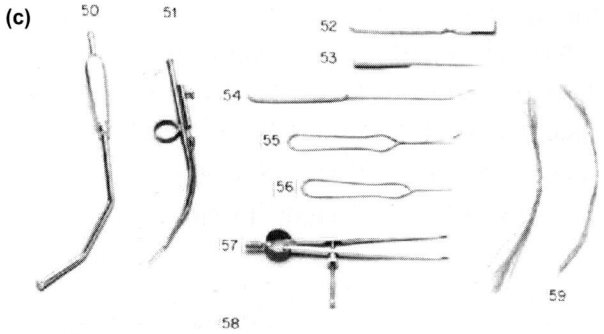

(d)

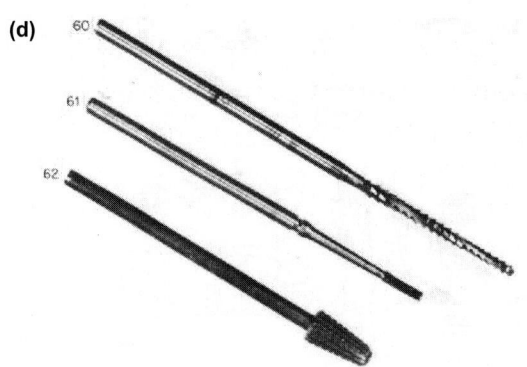

Figure 9.2   (b), (c), (d)

14. Bachaus towel clips (×10)
15. Rampley spongeholders 24 cm (×3)
16. Dunhill artery forceps 13 cm (×10)
17. Lawson Tait artery forceps (×2)
18. Universal wire and plate shears 12 cm (×2)
19. Kocher artery forceps, straight 1 in 2 teeth 18 cm
20. Kocher artery forceps, curved 1 in 2 teeth 18 cm
21. Barron scalpel handles with No. 5 and 10 blades (×2)
22. McIndoe dissecting forceps 15 cm
23. Gillies dissecting forceps, toothed 15 cm
24. Adson dissecting forceps, toothed
25. McIndoe scissors T/C edge 18 cm
26. Mayo scissors T/C 17 cm
27. Blunt-ended scissors 15 cm
28. Iris scissors T/C 12 cm
29. Strabismus scissors T/C 11.5 cm marked with black tape
30. Crilewood needleholders T/C jaws 15 cm (×2)
31. Luer Jansen bone rongeur 19 cm
32. McIndoe bone cutting forceps 19 cm
33. Small mallet
34. French osteotomes 5 mm, 7 mm and 11 mm
35. Osteotomes ½" (13 mm) with round handle (×2)
36. Obwegeser nasal septal chisel
37. Pterygoid chisel
38. Rowes disimpaction forceps — right and left
39. Tessier maxillary mobilisers — right and left
40. Dingham mouth gag. Frame with cheek retractor, 3 blades S, M, L (not shown)
41. Featherstone or other self retaining mouth gag
42. Kilner skin hooks 15 cm (×2)
43. Mapping pen (with nib)
44. Mitchell trimmer
45. Dental probe No. 6
46. Howarth's nasal raspatories (periosteal elevators) (×2)

47. Dental extraction forceps 76 N
48. Dental extraction forceps 74 N
49. Chip syringes (×2)
50. Yankauer suction tube
51. Self-clearing suction tube
52. Farabeouf rougine curved 11mm
53. Flat screwdriver
54. Obwegeser mandibular awl
55. Kelsey Fry bone awl — curved
56. Kelsey Fry bone awl — straight
57. Caliper
58. Ruler
59. 0.50mm and 0.35mm stainless steel tie wires (×25)
60. Long shanked Lindemann surgical bur (Meissinger)
61. Tungsten carbide surgical bur (Ash)
62. Cone shaped acrylic bur

There are an infinite number of refinements such as a coronoid stripper and coronoid forceps, and many types of periosteal elevator.

Not shown are: surgical handpieces for drills and oscillating and sagittal saws or arm miniature titanium bone plating set with transfacial trocar, canullae and retractor.

Note: To ensure a harmonious operation, check the radiographs, study models with the patient the day before and the instruments, especially burs, drills and wafers *preoperatively*. A pre-admission checklist can be invaluable.

Postoperative Care

Immediate

The patient is nursed at 45° for comfort and access. A nasopharyngeal airway is left *in situ* overnight, with *strict* instructions to staff to suck out the nasopharynx every 30 minutes with a fine catheter passed through the tube. Ideally it should be humidified to prevent crusting. Some anaesthetists prefer to leave the endotracheal tube *in situ* overnight. However, it is doubtful whether suction of blood and mucus from the entire length of the tube to maintain the airway can always be guaranteed. Oxygen (40%) in air is usually administered by face mask at approximately 5 litres/min.

Hourly aspiration of accumulated blood, oral and gastric secretions, and bile from the stomach help to eliminate vomiting. As most patients are fit prior to the procedure, dedicated nursing supervision with half-hourly observations is required rather than intensive care.

Analgesics

Pain experience is variable and surprisingly often absent. However repeated moderate doses of a subcutaneous or intravenous opiate, such as morphine 10 mg p.r.n. × 4 doses each 24 hours (more useful than 10 mg 4-hourly), with an antiemetic such as metoclopromide 10 mg, should be prescribed. Control is better and the analgesic dose lower when morphine is given 1 mg/ml by a Patient Controlled Administration "pump" system. This may be administered as morphine 50 mg in 50 ml normal saline into a drip or by a separate cannula.

The infiltration of the long-acting local analgesic 0.5% (5 mg/ml) bupivacaine hydrochloride (Marcain) with adrenaline (1:200 000) is said to reduce postoperative pain experience in addition to its intraoperative analgesic and vasoconstrictor effects. It is interesting to note that this reduced pain experience extends beyond the possible action of the drug. Up to 2 mg/kg may be used in any operative procedure.

First Postoperative Day

Check in particular:

1. Airway and chest clinically and if not clear, radiographically. All patients benefit from chest physiotherapy.

2. Fluid balance, i.e. blood and fluid replacement should approximate to blood and fluid loss. Note the urinary output and ensure the patient's bladder has been emptied, especially as transient retention may follow narcotic analgesics. Remember the loss via gastric aspiration, vomiting and the drains. Two litres of compound sodium lactate intravenous infusion (Hartmann's solution) should suffice in addition to blood replacement.

3. Occlusion and elastic fixation if used.

4. Cutaneous sensation and facial motor function.

5. Drug regimen. Antibiotics should be given intravenously or rectally, and analgesics and antiemetics intravenously. However, many patients will tolerate soluble analgesics orally or by nasogastric tube on a regular as required basis. A rectal non-steroidal anti-inflammatory analgesic, such as flurbiprofen 150 mg 12-hourly, is also useful to avoid continuous opiate analgesia.

6. Nutrition. During the first 24 hours continue the Hartmann's solution, 2 litres i.v., but try 100 ml/h water by mouth, then tea or orange juice, etc. as soon as the patient can tolerate feeding, using a syringe and quill, feeding cup or straw. If this is not possible use a fine-bore (Clinifeed — Roussel, UK) nasogastric tube which should be passed preoperatively to permit feeding until the patient can accept fluid and calories by mouth. If a fine-bore tube is not available, the standard Ryle's tube (12 or 14 FG) may be used. (See also Chapter 9 for postoperative feeding regimen.)

7. Oral hygiene with Chlorhexidine 0.2% solution is commenced.

Second Postoperative Day

Repeat the above but change from intravenous to an oral or nasogastric regimen, increasing the feed to a full diet.

Note: Oral fluids may be difficult for some patients up to 3 days after major procedures, especially those involving the chin, producing difficult lip control.

Discharge from hospital is determined by the nature of the procedure, the individual, and the care available at home. Most patients can be discharged on the second or third postoperative day, and on discharge should have adequate simple analgesics and instructions on oral hygiene, especially the use of a small tooth brush with chlorhexidine gluconate gel or mouthwash. Advice on a blended diet and the provision of a diet sheet is also important.

Follow-Up

The occlusion may be checked weekly or fortnightly. It is reassuring for the surgeon to assist maximal intercuspation with the final wafer and elastics. However wafers are uncomfortable and difficult to keep clean and are probably unnecessary. Soluble sutures should be left or removed when they are accessible and are a source of irritation. Patients require reassurance that impaired labial or infraorbital sensation will return to normal within 6 months and that excess soft tissue will also remodel and disappear over this period.

The Operative Procedures

The Obwegeser Sagittal Split Osteotomy

Indications

This versatile operation may be used for placing the mandible backwards or forwards, but should not be used for an anterior open bite without a simultaneous maxillary impaction to reduce the posterior upper facial height.

Technique

The operation for a backward correction will be described first.

1. The jaws must be supported as widely apart as possible by a self-retaining gag which gives better access than a prop (Figure 9.3a).

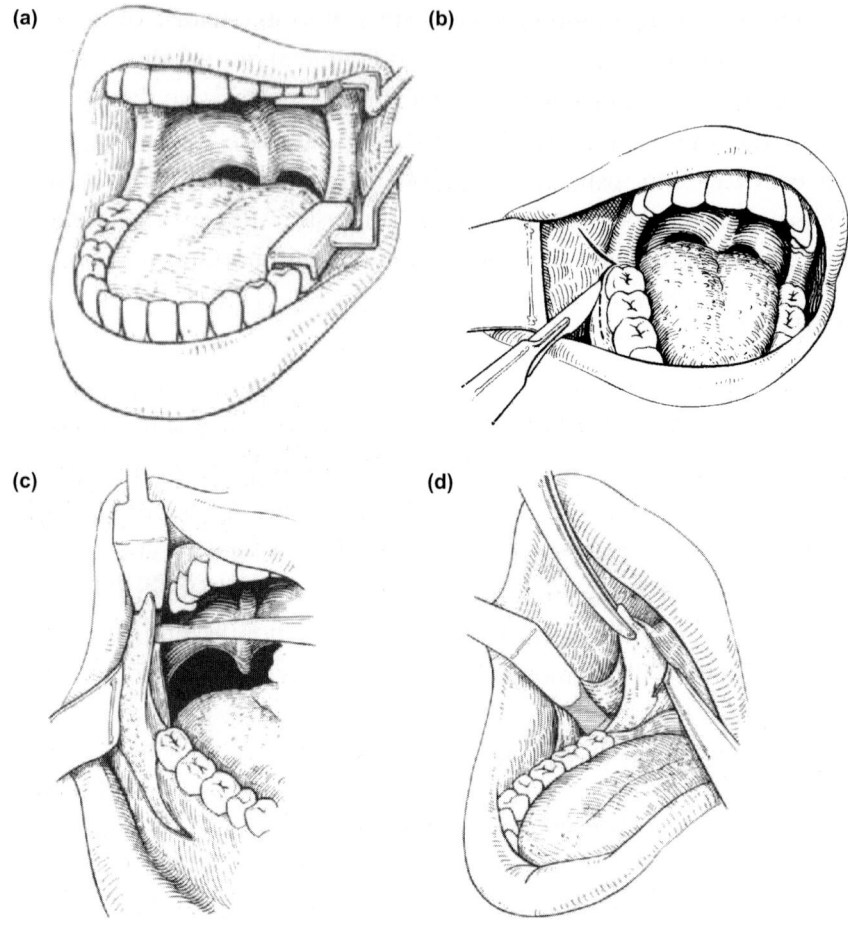

Figure 9.3   **(a), (b), (c), (d)**

2. The tissues on the lingual and buccal aspect of the ascending ramus and adjacent body of the mandible are infiltrated generously with a vasoconstrictor containing local anaesthetic, e.g. 0.5% bupivacaine with 1:200 000 adrenaline.

3. The incision is a buccally based triangular flap with the apex at the back of the last standing molar (Figure 9.3b). The anterior limb should leave a generous skirt of alveolar mucoperosteum

attached to the gingival margin of the first molar to assist suturing (Figure 9.3c).

4. The buccal periosteum is widely elevated, exposing the outer surface of the body and ramus of the mandible. This can be facilitated by using the forefinger, stretching and incising the periosteal layer to produce a buccal space which helps retraction of the tissues with a channel retractor and also provides good operative access for the insertion of bone plates. Techniques recommending limited exposure are difficult to understand (Figure 9.3d).

   Raise the lingual flap, with a Howarth periostal elevator, detaching the mucoperiosteum downwards and forwards from the anterior aspect of the ascending ramus to the distolingual aspect of the last molar. The inferior extent of the periosteal reflection needs to be no deeper than the mylohyoid ridge.

5. Dissect up the anterior aspect of the ramus, detaching the temporalis tendon with the sharp end of the Howarth elevator or a forked coronoid stripper. By inserting the Obwegeser coronoid retractor half way up and applying strong traction, the exposed tendon can be gradually stripped off with the elevator so that the retractor may be eventually seated comfortably on the coronoid tip. This degree of elevation greatly helps the access to the lingual aspect of the ramus (Figure 9.3c). The application of a heavy pair of curved Kocher's or coronoid forceps to the coronoid will now dispense with the forked retractor and provide a comfortable and secure alternative for the assistant.

6. Carefully raise the lingual periosteum to the level of the sigmoid notch and follow its margin until the condylar neck is reached; then smoothly detach the tissues downwards until the lingula is reached. Care will avoid troublesome venous bleeding, which usually ceases after the channel retractor (or a reversed bent Lacs retractor) is inserted with its tip passed behind the condylar neck.

7. The horizontal cut should be made as low as possible close to the lingula where the cortices are always separated by adequate cancellous bone. The higher the cut the less chance there is of splitting the ramus cleanly. Improved access is obtained by rotating the flat or channel retractor 45° to the vertical plane so that it lies parallel to the neurovascular bundle (Figure 9.3e).

8. The cut is made through the cortex of the bone with a long-shanked, medium-sized tapering fissure bur (Ash, Meissinger, Busch) and should be extended beyond the concave inner surface to the distal aspect of the ramus as the Hunsuck modification does not always work! With maxillary impactions parallel medial cuts allow a fillet of cortex to be removed. This allows the mandible to follow the maxillary vertical displacement (Figure 9.3f).

9. The buccal channel retractor is now placed vertically opposite the mid-point of the second molar with its tip below the lower border of the mandible (Figure 9.3g).

10. Access is remarkably improved by taking out the gag and all other instruments bringing the teeth into occlusion. A line of bur holes is made parallel to the external oblique ridge, which is continued onto the lateral surface of the mandible following the lateral bony prominence as it curves down on the buccal surface towards the lower border (Figure 9.3h).

11. This ensures an accurate line when they are joined together, and produces a natural continuous, lingual-buccal cortical cut. It is important to emphasise the cuts through the cortex proximally at the junction of the medial (lingual) and mid section and also antero-inferiorly through the thick cortex of the lower border to a depth of 2 mm.

    If the mandibular osteotomy is part of a bimaxillary procedure the cuts are done bilaterally, tonsil swabs inserted, and the maxillary osteotomy carried out and fixed with the intermediate wafer against the unchanged mandible.

12. The split is traditionally done with two ½ inch osteotomes which must have thick round handles enabling a firm twisting

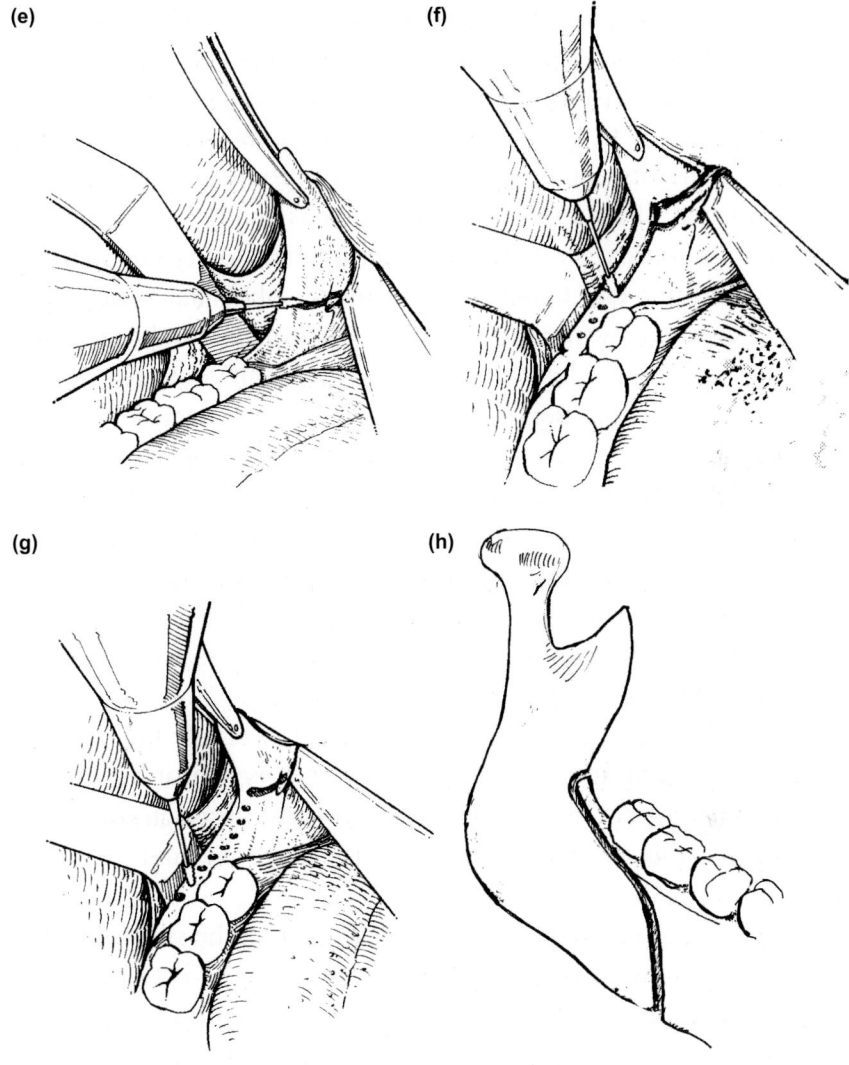

(e)   (f)   (g)   (h)

Figure 9.3   (e), (f), (g), (h)

action to be used without the glove slipping. However a more
controlled division can be achieved with a narrow 5 mm.
osteotome tapped first distally below the horizontal medial bur
line "feeling" the inner surface of the outer cortical plate. This

is repeated at least twice with an identical osteotome obliquely downwards and backwards through the buccal cut, and then downwards just within the line of the external oblique ridge which seems to be a natural plane of cleavage (Figure 9.3i). This bone dissecting manoeuvre may produce an instant and clean split. If not the ½ inch osteotome is gently tapped into the anterior cortical cut until firm, and rotated slowly but continually until the cancellous bone begins to split. The cortical split is generated by rotating anticlockwise on the right side and clockwise on the left. Slow separation permits the neurovascular bundle to be identified if exposed and dissected from the outer fragment where it may be adherent. If a single osteotome is used, it should then moved from the anterior buccal end of the cut to the superomedial end (Figure 9.3j). The two segments must be completely separated by inserting a finger into the depths of the osteotomy cut to vigorously detach all muscular and periosteal restraints. Where the mandible is narrow or the fragments refuse to separate on twisting, the fine 5 mm osteotome can be used as just described to divide the bone by gently tapping it through to the lower and posterior borders on the inner aspect of the buccal cortex. However such resistance suggests that the cortical bur cuts are inadequate and should be repeated.

13. The estimated setback has been measured on the study models. This amount of buccal plate is held firmly in Kocher or Dingman bone-holding forceps and cut off with a Lindemann fissure bur protecting the underlying inferior dental bundle with a flat retractor (Figure 9.3k). A horizontal fillet of bone may have to be trimmed with an acrylic bar from the upper margin of the inner cut on the ascending ramus to allow a good fit, especially in cases where the maxilla has been elevated — and the mandible has to rise to maintain the occlusion.

14. The forward correction requires the buccal cortical cut to be made at the mesial aspect of the second molar. After the split, no bone is removed.

(i)

(j)

(k)

(l)

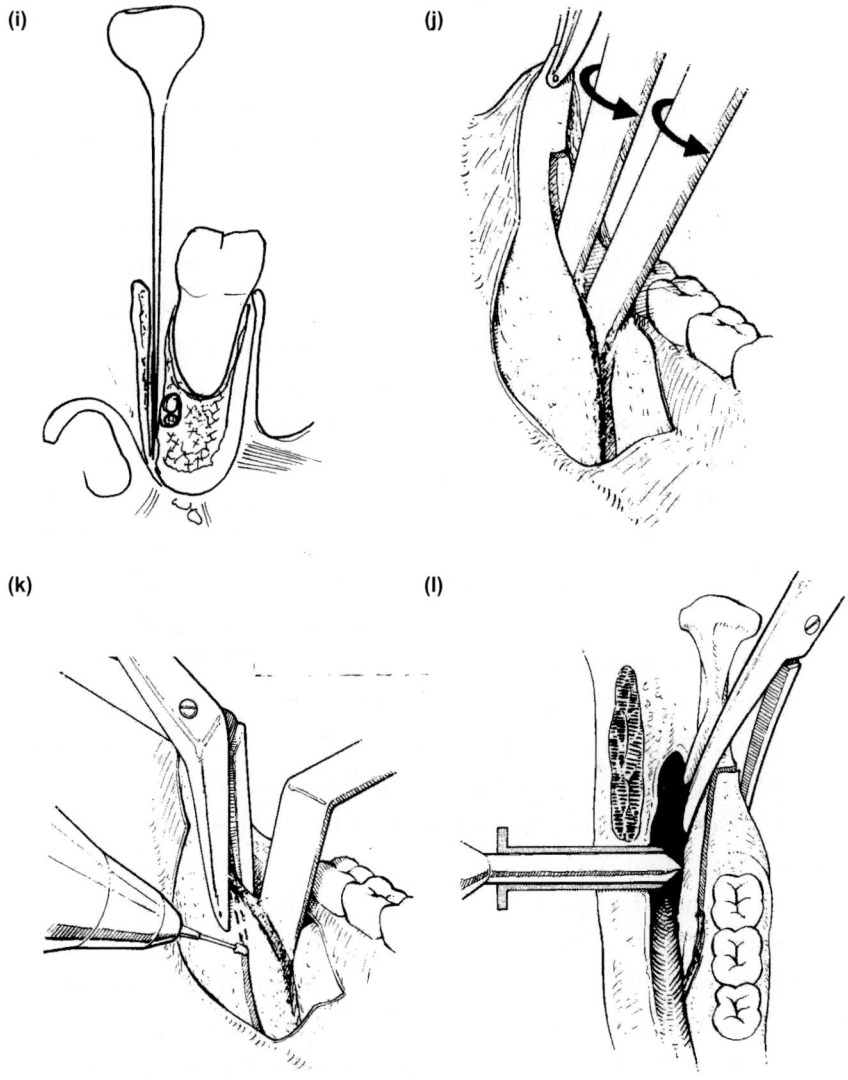

Figure 9.3 (i), (j), (k), (l)

15. Internal fixation requires accurate, firm intraoperative inter-maxillary fixation which is applied after the osteotomy cuts have been completed.
16. A transfacial trocar, cannula and retractor are essential for bicortical screws. A short stab wound (5 mm) is made through

the skin, a finger's breadth above the lower border of the mandible just anterior to the masseter muscle. Fine mosquito forceps are pushed through the tissues to enter the wound in the mouth, opened and closed, rotated through 90°, and opened again to create an entry for the canulla.

17. The trocar and cannular sleeve are then firmly pushed through to reach the buccal plate (Figure 9.3l). The trocar is removed and the cannula is attached to the extra and intraoral arms of the retractor. The design varies with the manufacturer. The cannula has a projection which helps to immobilise the buccal plate if a bone clamp is not used (Figure 9.3m).

18. The antero-posterior position of the proximal fragment (ascending ramus) is crucial Light self-retaining bone-holding or Allis forceps are used to grip the proximal fragment which is pushed back for mandibular advancements and pulled forwards for push backs. It should also be rotated downwards to lower the buccal plate just below the upper margin of the retromolar lingual cortical surface. This maintains the contour of the gonial angle which can be lost if the proximal fragment is inadvertently allowed to rotate forwards (Figure 9.3n).

   The two bone plates can then be stabilised by clamping them with an Allis until the screws have been inserted or with experience the tip of the cannula can so be used to hold them in place.

19. If there is sufficient bone beneath the neurovascular bundle the first screw hole may be drilled with the special long-shanked twist drill at this level. The drill should be applied gently as the shank is fragile and does not take kindly to torsion. A sense of give is felt when each plate is penetrated. The lingual side should be protected.

20. Screws 9–13 mm are usually adequate for bicortical fixation and are inserted with a screwholding screwdriver, which should be ready mounted to use the moment the hole is drilled. Two further screws are inserted above the bundle behind the last

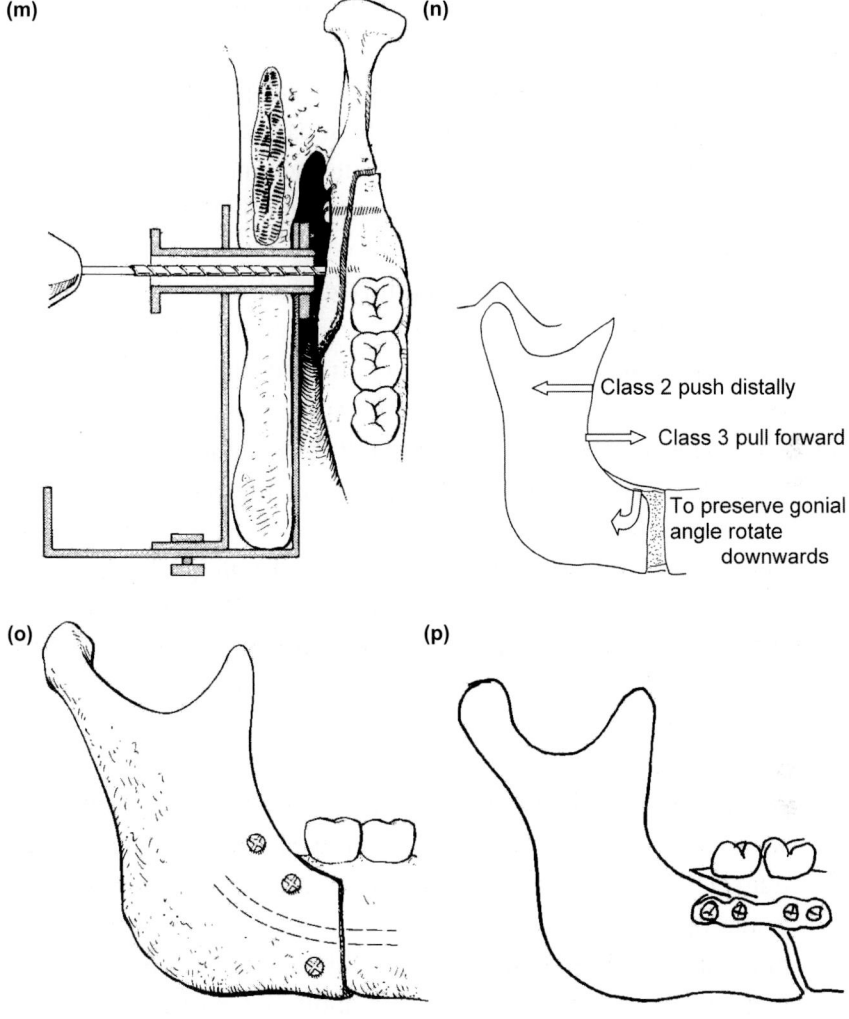

Figure 9.3   **(m), (n), (o), (p)**

standing molar (Figure 9.3o). When the opposite side is complete the intermaxillary fixation is released.

21. The stab wounds are closed with 6/0 prolene.
22. An alternative and simpler technique of intraosseous fixation is the application of a buccal titanium plate bridging the

osteotomy gap and fixed intraorally with 5 mm moncortical screws (Figure 9.3p).

23. Vacuum drains are inserted in the buccal pouches bilaterally, sutured to the skin and attached to separate bottles. There are those who do not use drains despite evidence that the subperiosteal sump gives rise to morbidity and infection without this standard practice.

24. The intra oral wounds are carefully closed with a 3/0 polyglycollate suture.

25. When all bleeding has been controlled the throat pack is removed and the pharynx carefully sucked out.

26. The wafer may be left suspended to the maxillary arch wire, but intermaxillary fixation with elastics is unnecessary and the patient is returned to the recovery area.

27. The use of the wafer and postoperative training elastics for 2 weeks is uncomfortable for the patient of no proven value except for providing comfort for the surgeon.

Additional Notes

- As varying degrees of relapse invariably take place, especially with large movements, the planning should be based on a relaxed supine centric relation squash bite, as close as possible to the operating position. In addition overcorrection should be built into the model surgery. This should be an edge to edge incisor relationship for forward mandibular movements and a class 2 div1 relationship for mandibular setbacks.

- With major facial deformities, such as a hemifacial microsomia, the neurovascular bundle often lies superficially adjacent to the buccal cortex and can be easily severed whilst carrying out the buccal cut. With such a mandible, an extraoral subsigmoid osteotomy is recommended for vertical lengthening or an inverted L osteotomy with a bone graft for forward movements.

- Despite careful intraoperative intermaxillary fixation and a perfect immediate postoperative occlusion, occlusal discrepancies can still mysteriously appear from 24 hours to 14 days later. The cause may be postoperative condylar recoil, intracapsular oedema or lack of muscle adaptation. This usually remits and the use of training elastics is probably unnecessary.
- If the preoperative arch co-ordination is imperfect and requires restorative or orthodontic correction, it is essential to construct a final wafer which will ensure that the midlines and incisor overjet are correct and the arch alignment is symmetrical. The underlying malocclusion can then be corrected as required.

The Subsigmoid (Subcondylar) Osteotomy

Indications

Although formerly a very popular operation and easier to perform than the sagittal split, the subsigmoid osteotomy is less versatile. It also requires elastic intermaxillary fixation unless secure plating is achieved. It can be carried out intraorally or through an external skin-crease incision, leaving a discrete scar.

The subsigmoid osteotomy is not an operation for lengthening the body of the mandible but it is useful where the mandible is narrow as in a congenital deformity, or atrophic in the older edentulous patient with unerupted wisdom teeth, when it can be used for setting back the body or lengthening or shortening the ascending ramus.

Extraoral Subsigmoid Osteotomy

Technique (Figure 9.4)

1. A 5 cm submandibular or retromandibular incision is marked with a pen and infiltrated with 4 ml local anaesthetic containing 1:80,000 adrenaline. This is made in a skin crease two fingers' breadth below the mandibular border to avoid the marginal

(mandibular) branch of the facial nerve. A lower crease requires a larger incision (Figure 9.4a). Note: Never mark an incision with the head rotated: this will produce unexpected changes in the surface anatomy.

2. The skin, fat and platysma are divided with a No.15 blade. The flap margins are undermined with MacIndoe scissors or the knife to increase the elasticity of the wound margins which are carefully retracted with cat's paw retractors.

3. The deep fascia is identified, picked up with fine-tooth dissecting forceps and divided widely beyond the ends of the flap incision with a knife or scissors. Deep veins, usually the posterior facial, can be identified, divided and tied with 3/0 polyglycollate.

4. Access through the submandibular incision requires the identification of the mandibular branch of the facial nerve which lies under the deep fascia just below the lower border of the mandible. As it passes upwards on to the face it crosses the facial artery and vein. This important motor nerve may be protected by identifying the facial artery and vein as they emerge between the submandibular salivary gland and lower border of the mandible. Use scissors or Spencer Wells forceps to separate the tissues, and divide and tie these vessels, then retract and suture the distal ends upwards over the lower border of the mandible. This will carry the marginal branch of the facial nerve with them.

5. The muscle and periosteum can now be incised along the lower border with a knife and stripped upwards to the sigmoid notch and coronoid process. The Obwegeser channel or Robertson ramus retractor may be hooked over the notch to expose the ramus (Figure 9.4b).

6. A small buccal prominence is a reasonably accurate landmark of the lingula area, so a cut downwards and behind this from the midpoint of the sigmoid notch to the beginning of the curve of the angle avoids the inferior dental neurovascular bundle. This

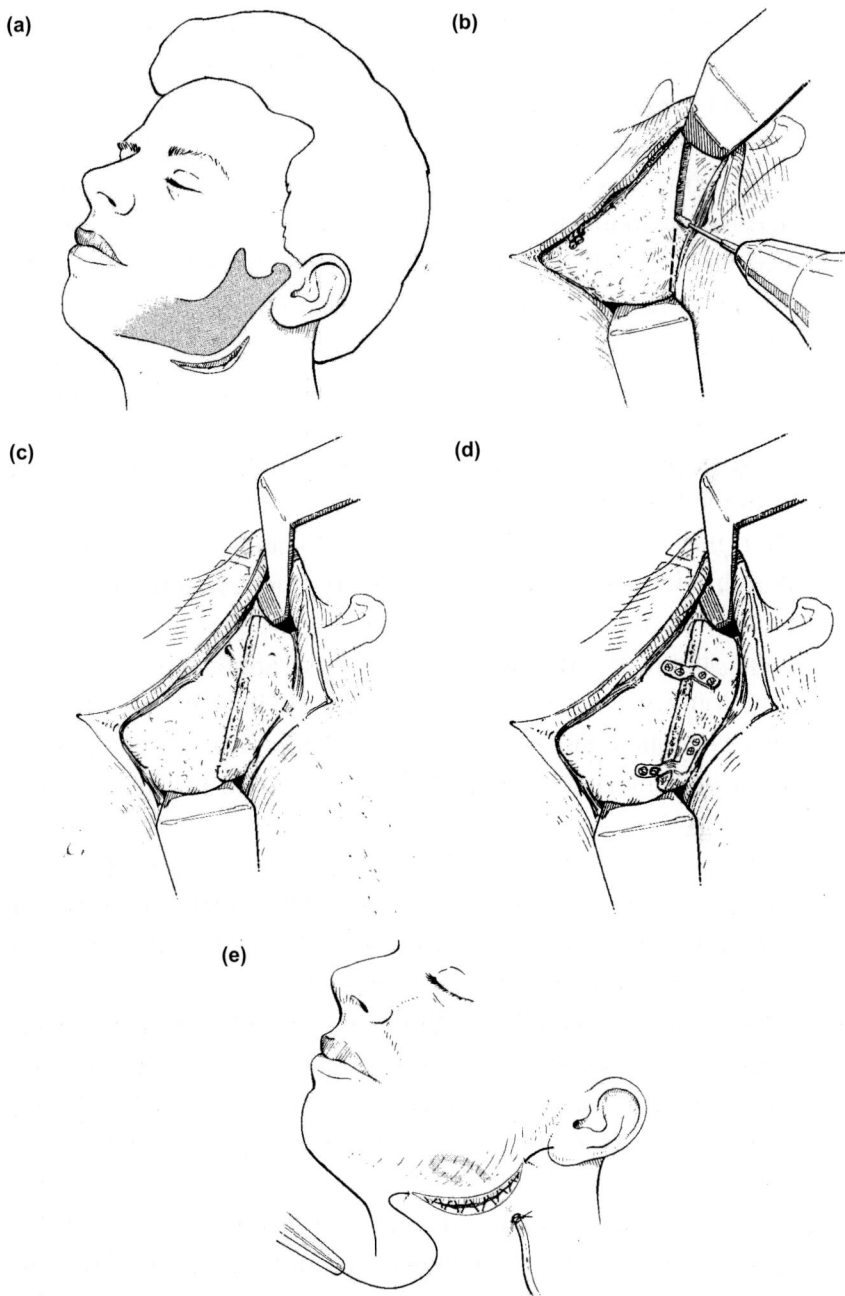

Figure 9.4 (a), (b), (c), (d), (e)

may be done with a fissure bur or reciprocating saw. A flat retractor should be placed on the medial aspect of the ramus to protect the soft tissues.

7. Once separated, the inner cortex of the narrow fragment and the outer cortex of the main segment may be bevelled with an acrylic bur to ensure good opposition.

8. For large distal displacements, i.e. greater than 0.7 cm, it is necessary to do a coronoidectomy to remove the restraining influence of the temporalis muscle (Figure 9.4c).

9. A saline-soaked tonsil swab is inserted in the wound and the procedure repeated on the opposite side.

10. With the appropriate wafer the intermaxillary wires are applied, with the teeth held in occlusion.

11. As rigid fixation is being used the cut should be as vertical as possible in order to leave a substantial posterior border. After putting on intermaxillary fixation the larger, i.e. distal, fragment should be trimmed to allow close approximation of the osteotomy margins. An L or T-shaped plate with six holes is then fashioned and screwed into the lateral aspects of the posterior and inferior borders of the mandible to bridge the bone cut firmly.

12. Vacuum drains are placed bilaterally overlying the bone surface and sutured firmly to the skin as soon as the introducer has been pulled through; ensure that at least 2 cm of non-perforated drain lies within the wound (Figure 9.4d).

13. The wound is closed by suturing the muscle and periosteum with 3/0 polyglycollate on a 22 mm half-round needle. The fascia/platysma layer and subcutaneous tissue are similarly closed, with the knots buried by suturing from deep to superficial. For a fine scar, the skin should be closed with a 3/0 continuous subcuticular monofilament [Prolene, Ethilon (Ethicon Ltd., Edinburgh, UK) or nylon] suture on a straight needle. This can also be done with a half-round non-cutting needle. Alternatively, wound closure may be achieved with 5/0 Prolene or Ethilon

interrupted sutures, or even adhesive Steri-strips (3M, US) if subcutaneous closure is satisfactory.
14. The throat pack is removed.

Intraoral Subcondylar Osteotomy

This is a relatively simple procedure and is a rapid way of treating minor displacements of the mandible, i.e. less than 7 mm, which may involve a backward or a rotational correction for asymmetry. Major movements should be accompanied by a coronoidectomy or even a horizontal ramus osteotomy because of the restraining influence of the temporalis muscle.

However neither have the great advantage of dispensing with intermaxillary fixation. The best application of the intraoral procedure is a means of salvaging a sagittal split that has not separated the condyle from the body of the mandible.

Technique

Buccal Ramus Approach (Figure 9.5).

Infiltrate the tissues on the buccal aspect of the ascending ramus with a vasoconstrictor (Figure 9.5a).

1. A buccal-based triangular incision is made with a No.15 blade with the apex behind the last molar tooth, the upper limb stopping at the external oblique ridge halfway up the ascending ramus (Figure 9.5b).
2. The flap is elevated subperiosteally as widely as possible, using the Howarth periosteal elevator and then the forefinger to stretch the periosteum and create a generous pouch. A J-shaped periosteal elevator is useful in freeing the muscular attachment at the posterior and inferior borders. The sigmoid notch, condylar neck and angle of the mandible should be readily palpated.

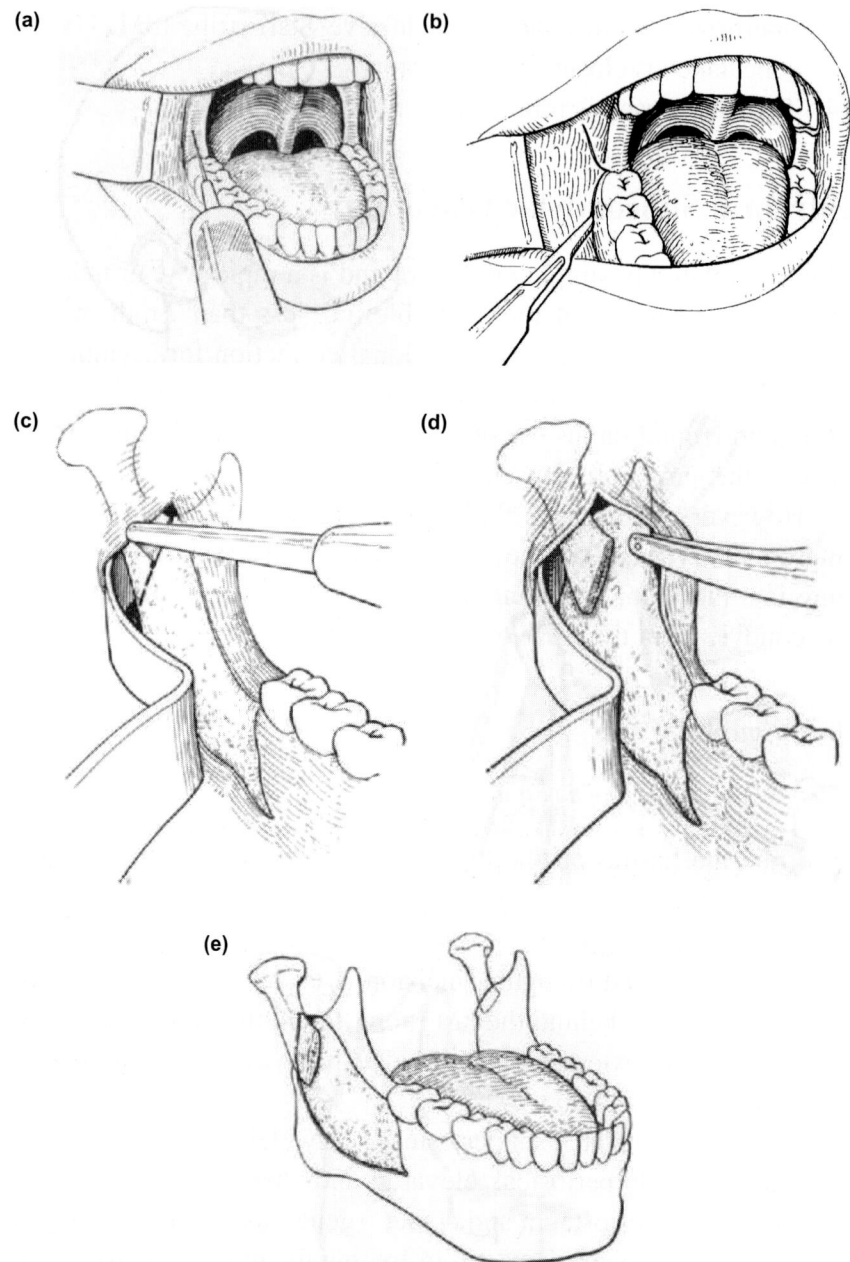

Figure 9.5   (a), (b), (c), (d), (e)

3. The Merrill or similar retractor is inserted so that the curved distal flange may be firmly placed behind the posterior border of the ascending ramus (Figure 9.5c).
4. The sigmoid notch may then be visualised and a 1.5 cm right-angled oscillating saw is used to cut downwards and backwards to 1 cm below the mid-point of the posterior border, i.e. where the condylar neck has narrowed and fused with the flat ascending ramus. It is essential to use a sharp-edged saw. Some operators prefer a blade which is 70° to the long axis of the saw.
5. Once separated, the condylar component is displaced buccally with the Howarth elevator. When both sides have been completed the mandible is displaced backwards between them (Figures 9.5d and 9.5e).
6. A vacuum drain is inserted into the wound prior to closure.
7. As this procedure does not lend itself to internal fixation elastic intermaxillary fixation is necessary.

Medial Ramus Approach (Figure 9.6)

This procedure is useful to salvage a failed sagittal split.
1. The basic exposure is almost exactly the same as for the sagittal split technique except that only minimal stripping is required on the buccal surface of the mandible. However, with the curved Kocher's forceps in place *above* the coronoid process and the ramus channel retractor inserted just above the level of the lingula and hooked behind the posterior border of the ascending ramus, an excellent view of the sigmoid notch and posterior border is achieved form the contralateral side of the patient (Figure 9.6a).
2. With a long-shanked fissure bur and oblique cut is made through the thick posterior ramus border as low as possible, passing forwards and upwards into the sigmoid notch (Figure 9.6b).

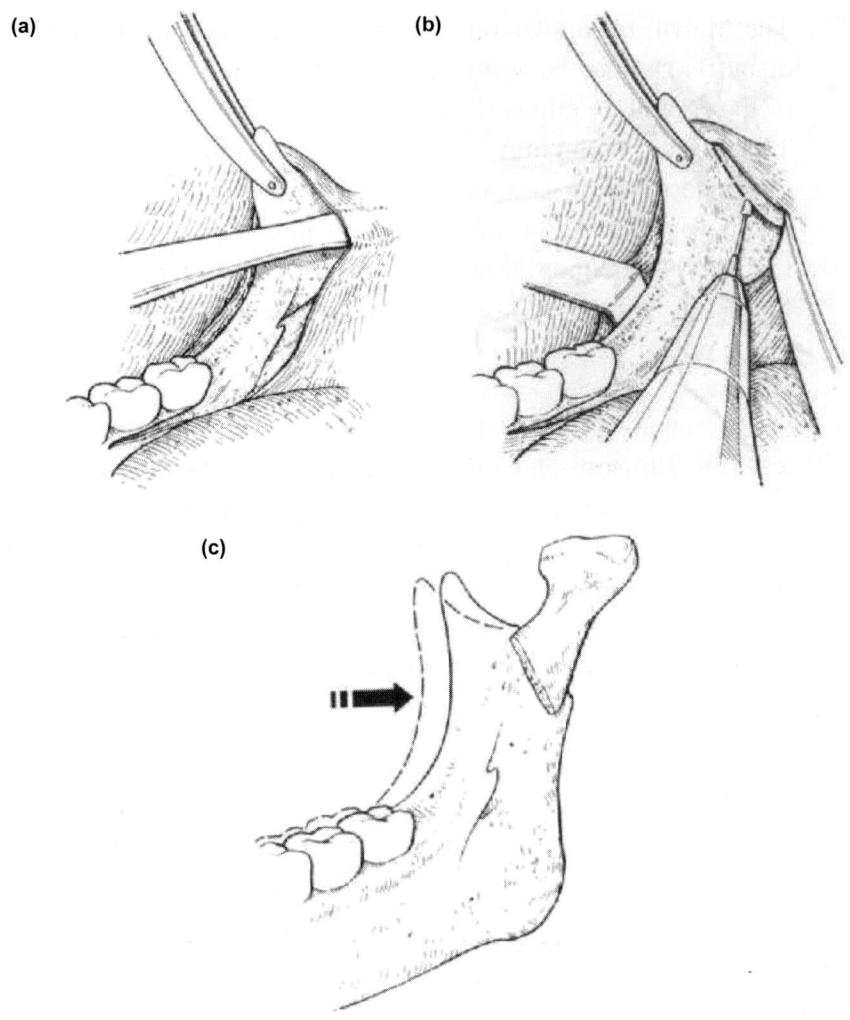

Figure 9.6   (a), (b), (c)

3. Separation of the osteotomy may be completed with a
    5 mm osteotome. The small condylar fragment is then
    manipulated medially with the channel retractor and a perio-
    steal elevator into the hollow medial surface of the ramus
    (Figure 9.6c).

4. This is repeated on the contralateral side and the mandible is placed into the planned occlusion.
5. The wounds are closed.
6. Again this procedure requires elastic intermaxillary fixation.

Note: Occasionally access is restricted where the medial aspect of the ramus is broad and concave, in which case an alternative osteotomy should be undertaken.

Body Osteotomies

This procedure is done intraorally, usually in the molar-premolar region. However, it shortens the alveolus and has not got the elegance or versatility of the sagittal split or subsigmoid procedures and requires more careful planning. For these reasons it is not considered here. The anterior mandibulotomy, in which the section is made anterior to the mental foramen, is a useful variant of this operation.

The Inverted L Osteotomy

Indications

This operation is valuable when there is a need to increase both the ramus height and body length at the same time, especially when the sagittal split osteotomy is not possible. Such cases are usually gross congenital mandibular hypoplasia or, occasionally, acquired hypoplasia following condylar fractures or when previous surgery has disturbed the bony anatomy. The operation differs in concept from the sagittal split procedure in that a bone graft is inserted to make up the deficiency.

Technique

1. The surgical approach is exactly the same as for the extraoral subsigmoid osteotomy (steps 1–6 and see Figure 9.4) except

that the bone cut is made from the anterior border of the ascending ramus, passing distally, to behind the estimated position of the lingula then downwards to the lower border anterior to the angle, i.e. to the antegonial notch (Figure 9.7a).

2. With bilateral deformities the approach is repeated on the opposite side.

3. The mandible is then temporarily fixed into occlusion. Where the maxilla is normal this presents no problems. However, if there is a deformity of the maxilla this must be corrected before the inverted L and fixed with bone plates.

    Mobilising the small mandible into the desired anterior position can be difficult and is facilitated by drilling a hole bilaterally in the lower border of the mandible just anterior to the osteotomy cut and passing a 0.5 mm traction wire to be attached to heavy forceps. When anterior traction is applied, explore the deep tissues medial to the mandible with a finger to find any restraining bands of periosteum, muscle or ligament. These must be vigorously divided with the finger to ensure stability.

4. With the proximal condylar fragment confirmed to be in the fossa, the gap created can be measured, and a template formed with sterile paper or card.

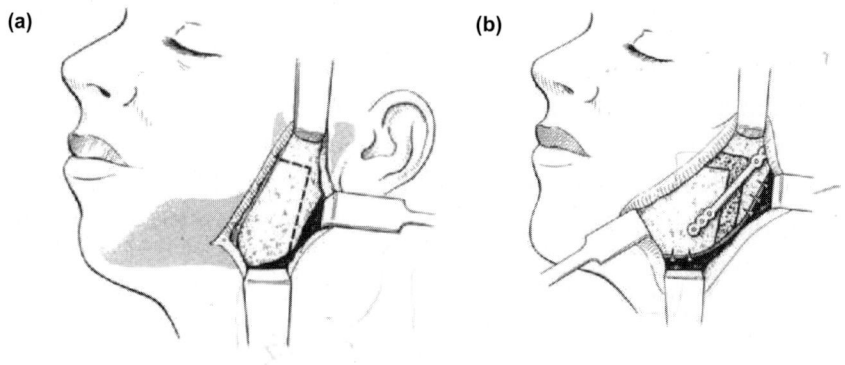

(a) (b)

Figure 9.7   (a), (b)

5. An interpositional graft is now obtained. The ideal source is cortico-cancellous bone from the iliac crest. A solid cancellous graft can be used but the incorporation of one cortex provides reassuring stability. Some surgeons use split rib for the gap. Two miniature bone plates provide excellent rigidity and form (Figure 9.7b).
6. A vacuum drain is inserted and the wound is closed in layers.
7. The intermaxillary fixation is released and the pack removed.

Note: Any mandible which requires lengthening with an inverted L osteotomy also requires an augmentation genioplasty.

The Lower Labial Segmental Osteotomy (Kole Subapical Osteotomy)

Indications

Although this operation may be used to move the dentoalveolar segment in almost any direction permitted by the angulation of the teeth, it should not be used as an alternative to presurgical orthodontics and is less useful and more difficult than the anterior mandibulotomy If carried out as a single procedure, intermaxillary fixation is not required. The alveolar segments can be secured with bone plates plus:

1. An arch bar, the best being a cast chrome cobalt bar designed on the surgical planning model.
2. An orthodontic arch wire fitted intraoperatively or more readily a heavy (1 mm) supplemental arch wire fitted into distal buccal tubes and ligated to the segment and the adjacent teeth. The segments are localised by a postoperative wafer and bone plates below, which are not enough without the dental control to prevent displacement.

3. Three-part cast German silver splints with locking plates and connecting bars (but this is labour intensive and requires a skilled technician).

Where preoperative extractions are not carried out, orthodontic tooth movement is required to ensure space to facilitate the surgical cut without root damage.

Technique

Downward and posterior movements (Figure 9.8)

1. A premolar is carefully extracted bilaterally to create space for a distal movement. For vertical movements without extractions it is imperative to confirm that there is sufficient bone between the roots of the teeth. The orthodontist can achieve increased separation with a fixed appliance.
2. Whichever incision is used (see below), extend the lips, dry the mucosa, and mark it out with a pen and Bonney's blue.
3. The procedure is done with a curved incision starting below the papilla distal to the site of the vertical bone cut (Figure 9.8a) at the reflection of the sulcus mucosa. The blade is then taken very superficially through the mucosa along the inner aspect of the lip anterior to the sulcus, returning in an arc of a circle to the equivalent point on the opposite side. Finger dissection with a gauze swab will reveal the three terminal branches of the mental nerve. These must be exposed by dissecting backwards to the foramen with scissors. The anterior labial section of the incision can now be deepened with a blade obliquely downwards to bone approximately halfway between the gingival margin and lower border of the mandible. This skirt of mucosa facilitates suturing and also provides a good seal if bone chips are being inserted.

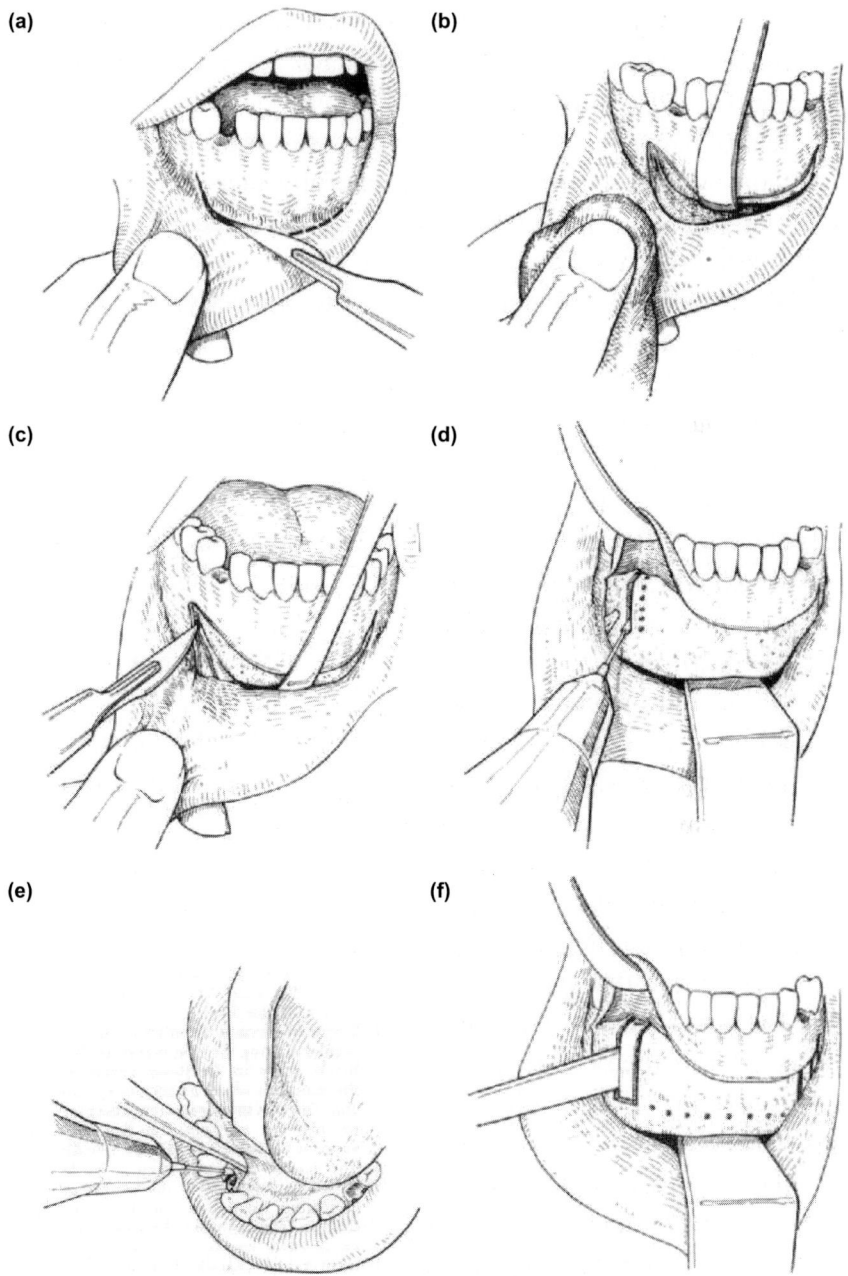

Figure 9.8   (a), (b), (c), (d), (e), (f)

4. The mucoperiosteum is then elevated distally revealing the mental nerve at its origin. At this stage, the periosteum above and behind the foramen may be elevated and incised without fear of damaging the nerve (Figure 9.8b). If the cone of periosteum around the nerve is now carefully incised with a sharp blade and the mental nerve dissected free, it becomes considerably more extensible and therefore easier to retract.

5. Using an elevator the anterior periosteum overlying the chin is then peeled firmly down to the lower border of the mandible where a Lack's or special chin (Awty, Obwegeser) retractor may be inserted to hold the flap and support the mandible (Figure 9.8c).

6. Incise along the gingival sulcus around the premolars and canines to facilitate elevation of the attached gingival flaps which will be widely undermined to form a bridge maintaining continuity of the gingiva.

7. The vertical bone cuts may be made with a narrow tungsten carbide fissure or an oscillating sagittal saw blade. If the first or second premolar has been extracted to enable the alveolar segment to be pushed backwards, the appropriate amount of bone is removed as a vertical strip (Figure 9.8d).

8. If no teeth are to be extracted the buccal cut can be made with a fine fissure bur through the outer cortex only. Then, after detaching the lingual mucoperiosteum, a cut is made vertically from above through the inner cortex. The Howarth periosteal elevator is held *in situ* to protect the mucosa (Figure 9.8e). The section is then completed between the teeth with a fine 3 mm osteotome (Figure 9.8f).

9. The horizontal cut may be completed with a bur or oscillating saw and must be placed well below the canine apices. It is useful to estimate the level of the canine apices from radiographs and the cortical contour and mark them with a bur hole on both sides. Where bone is removed for a setdown it is safer to make the upper cut first, marking it out with a series of bur holes (Figure 9.8g).

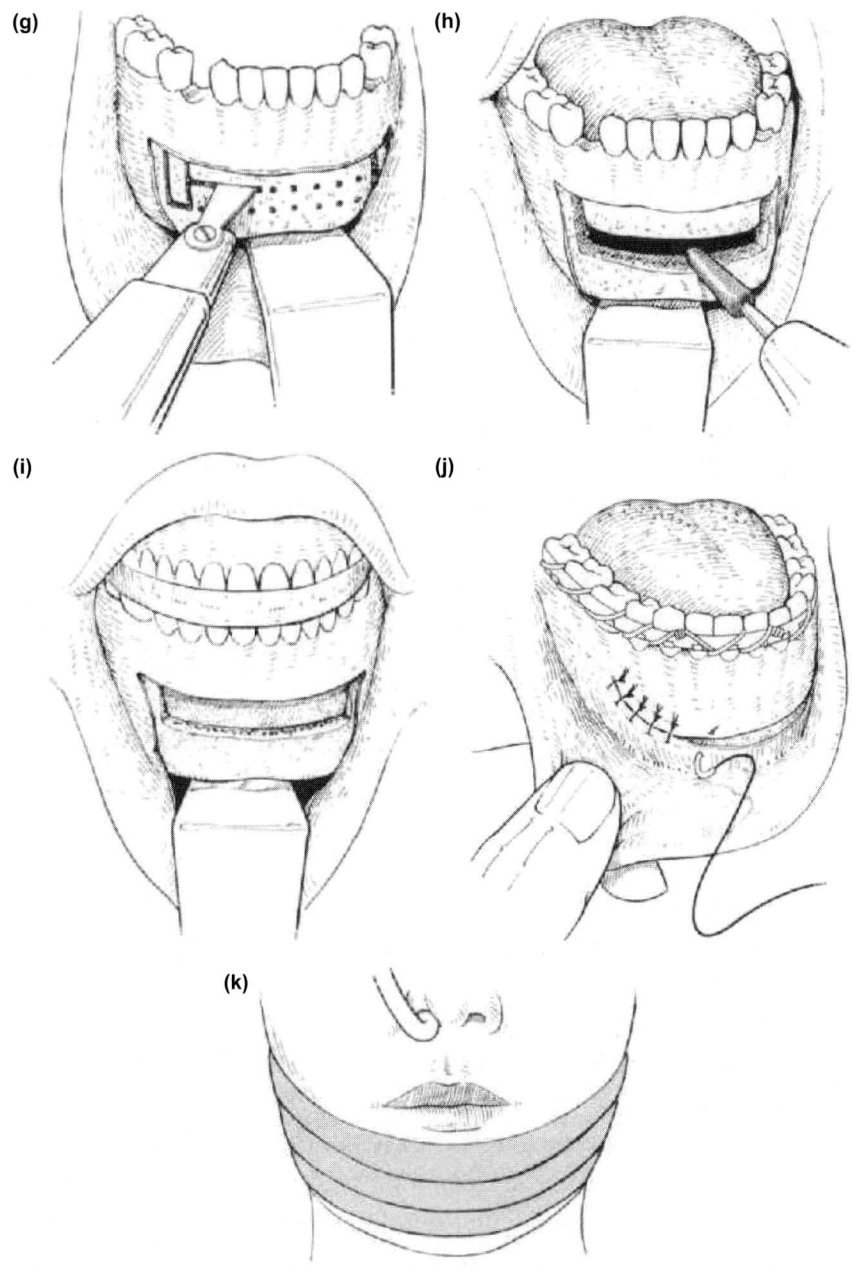

Figure 9.8 (g), (h), (i), (j), (k)

10. If there is insufficient room below the apices to remove adequate bone for the setdown, an anterior mandibulotomy must be performed. Furthermore in most situations this is a better procedure than the Kole. Save all fragments of bone in a blood-soaked swab to fill any residual dead space left after moving the segments.

11. Sometimes the mobilised segment which is pedicled on the genial muscles cannot be satisfactorily seated, in which case carefully trim off all cortical spurs, especially at the angular margins, with a well-cooled, narrow tapering acrylic bur (Figures 9.8h and 9.8i).

12. Accurate dentoalveolar localisation can be achieved by an acrylic wafer with an arch bar, heavy arch wire, or an open cast silver splint, all previously prepared on the lower model after model surgery. The splint is secured with circum-mandibular wires. The osteotomy is secured with bone plates.

13. The muscle and periosteum are closed with 3/0 polyglycollate and the mucosa is closed with a combination of simple and vertical mattress sutures (Figure 9.8j). A 2.5 cm elastic adhesive pressure dressing applied over the labiomental skin crease helps to reduce dead space and haematoma (Figure 9.8k).

Forward Movement

Occasionally a forward segmental movement is useful for correcting a Class II, division 1 deep overbite and overjet, where a sagittal split has been declined. This may be modified to include one or more of the premolars on the mobilised anterior segment, in which case the mental nerve is released from within the canal by removing the overlying cortex distally with a bur, by cutting two parallel grooves from the upper and lower edges of the mental foramen. The intervening bone can be carefully removed with a Mitchell's trimmer. The exposed neurovascular bundle is then retracted by an elastic or nylon tape held in a pair of mosquito forceps. Once the alveolar segment has been mobilised forwards and fixed by plates or a wafer and arch bars, the vertical gaps are packed with bone chips from the iliac crest and covered with a buccal mucosal flap rotated over the alveolar crest to be carefully sutured to the lingual mucosa with horizontal mattress sutures.

Upward Movement

The osteotomy is as previously described except that the space created at the subapical area by the upward movement is packed with cancellous bone chips.

The Anterior Mandibulotomy

Indications and Technique

This is anatomically a better operation than the Kole subapical procedure especially in patients with a short lower face, with little bone between the incisor apices and the lower border of the mandible and those with a deficient chin. In the former an adequate setdown cannot be achieved without damaging the apices or leaving a precariously thin strut of cortical bone. These problems can be overcome in two ways:

1. Take the vertical osteotomy cuts of the Kole down through the lower border to produce a three-part osteotomy of the mandible (Figure 9.9a). This enables a setdown which maintains or improves the lower facial height.
2. Combine the oblique advancement genioplasty cut with the two vertical segmental cuts, producing a four-part mandibuloto-genioplasty (Figure 9.9b). The anterior incisor segment is then set down and fixed as planned and will displace the genioplasty segment downwards and also allow advancement. These are not only simple solutions to anatomical difficulty but also increase the anterior inferior dentoalveolar height and improve the lower facial proportion. However, as the mandible has been completely divided bilaterally, dentoalveolar localisation is

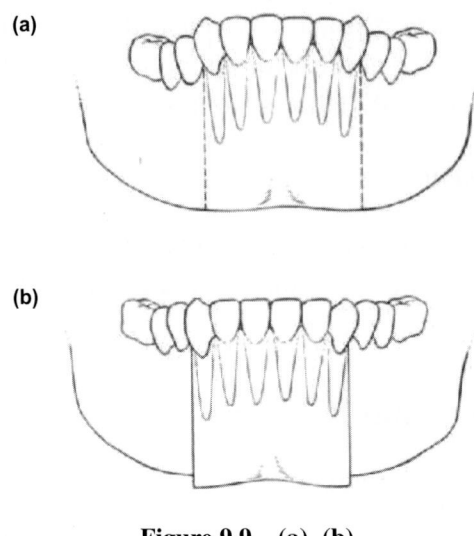

(a)

(b)

Figure 9.9   (a), (b)

done with a deep wafer, an arch bar or supplemental archwire in distal tubes and the lower level by bone plates.

Note: Do ensure that the osteotomy cuts at the lower border feel and look smooth prior to closure.

Genioplasty or Mentoplasty

Indications

Augmentation or reduction of the chin may be done for an isolated deficiency or combined with other osteotomies. This is discussed in detail in Chapter 10.

Augmentation is most easily achieved with a sliding genioplasty (Figure 9.10a). A short lower face with a reduced lower anterior dentoalveolar height can also be simultaneously corrected with an interpositional bone or alloplast sandwich filling. If, however, an incisor setdown is also required to flatten the lower occlusal plane, the anterior mandibulotomy (see above), which is a combination of a segmental osteotomy and genioplasty, should be used (Figure 9.10a).

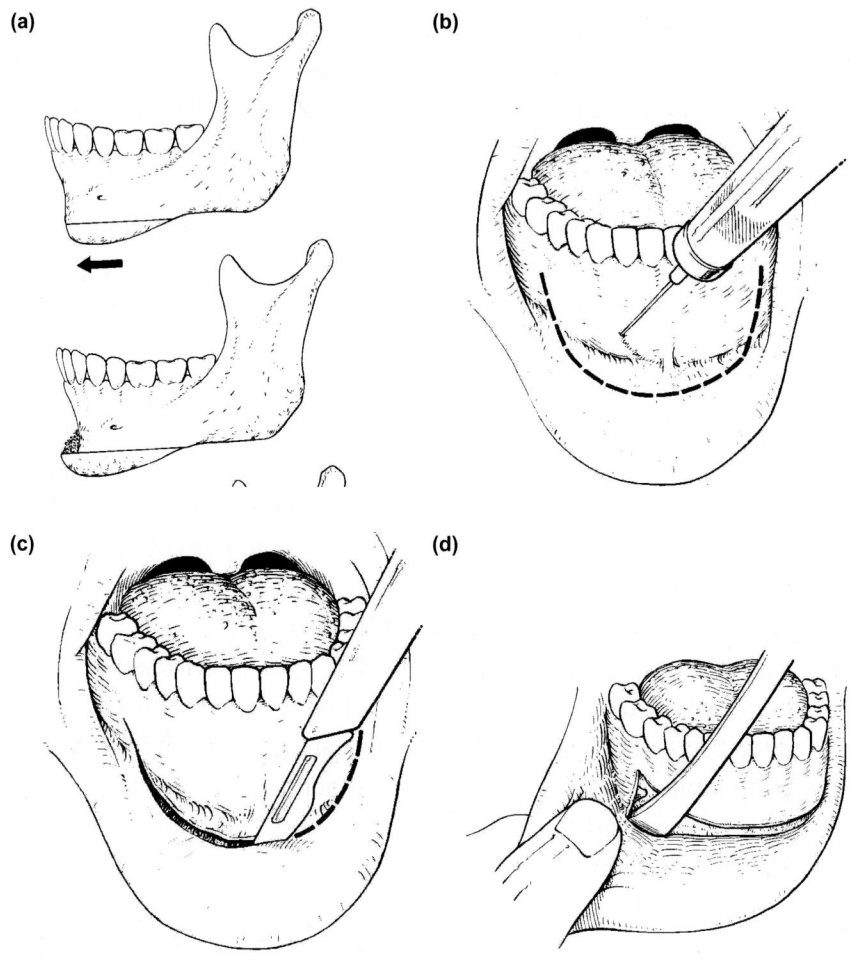

Figure 9.10   (a), (b), (c), (d)

The Augmentation Genioplasty

Technique

1. Mark a U-shaped incision with Bonney's blue from 46 to 36. Start just below the attached gingiva and cross the sulcus on to the labial mucosa anterior to the canine teeth (Figure 9.10b).

2. Infiltrate the sulcus with local anaesthetic containing 1:200 000 adrenaline. The incision is made very superficially from the first molar in the unattached mucosa. This is widened anteriorly by bringing the incision out on to the inner aspect of the lip. As the knife reaches the medial aspect of the canine area the tissues may be incised down to bone but is again brought to the surface at the opposite canine. It is imperative to leave a generous skirt of unattached mucosa on the gingival side to facilitate suturing (Figure 9.10c).

3. A dry gauze swab used to displace the tissues of the divided superficial incision will reduce bleeding and also bring the three branches of the mental nerve into view. These should be further exposed by dissecting backwards with fine scissors to the mental foramen. Then incise through the periosteum with a knife in a forward arc from behind, above and in front of the nerves as they emerge from the foramen.

4. The soft tissues may then be reflected with a periosteal elevator inferiorly to deglove the mandible (Figure 9.10d). This must be done firmly and will be facilitated by carefully incising the periosteum around the origin of the mental nerves. The soft tissues can then be retracted from the lower border of the mandible with a Lack's or genioplasty retractor (Awty, Obwegeser) (Figure 9.10e).

5. It is important that the chin periosteum and overlying fascia are now vigorously stretched with the finger, incising widely any tight bands, to make a pocket to accommodate the increased bony prominence. A damp swab should be inserted in this pocket to confirm that the overlying skin looks untethered.

6. When cutting the bone the mental nerves must be retracted with an elastic or nylon tape and also protected with a Howarth periosteal elevator or miniature Langenbeck retractor. The bone cut should commence at the lower border below the second premolar and come obliquely forwards and upwards on both sides. As usual, the choice lies between a tungsten carbide fissure bur or an oscillating sagittal saw, but must be carried through to divide the lingual cortex. The separation is done with a fine

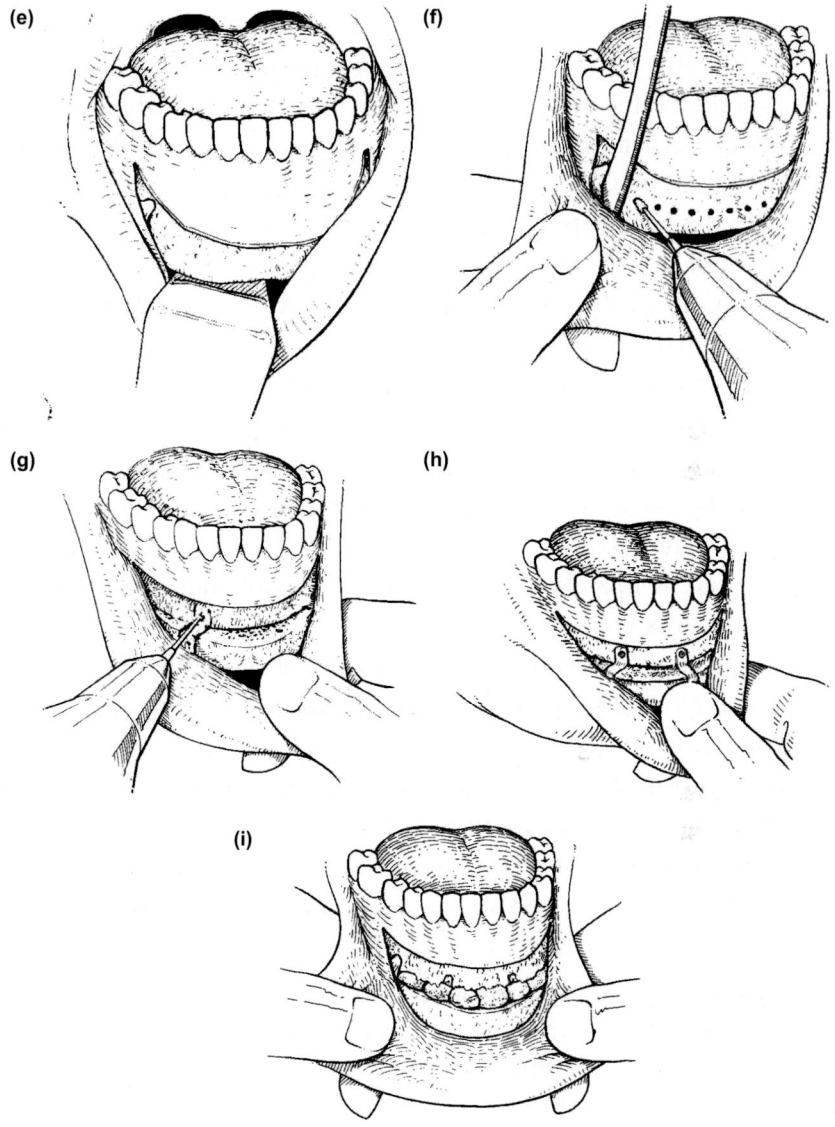

Figure 9.10   (e), (f), (g), (h), (i)

osteotome. It may be possible to cut two fine horizontal slices of bone which help to elongate and correct a severe retrogenia (Figure 9.10f). Leave the bone pedicled on the vascular digastric muscle behind improves the healing process. There is an approximate 15% loss of contour using this technique; this may rise to 30% if the muscle pedicle is divided.

7. A bone shelf is now created by attaching the anteriorly displaced lower border to the buccal cortex above with plates (Figures 9.10g and 9.10h). Two plates are fashioned into a three-part step with the horizontal "tread" representing a generously estimated forward move. The plates are screwed into place on the facial cortex above the section with two 5 mm screws avoiding the apices. The chin fragment is then firmly brought forward with bone holding forceps and secured with screws to the plate. Cancellous bone chips removed from the iliac crest through a short incision (the Flint Technique), fill dead space, enhance contour and promote union with large advancements (Figure 9.10i).

     An interpositional graft of bone or hydroxyapatite can be inserted at this stage to increase the lower facial height with severe deficiencies.

8. By placing the original incision well out on the labial surface, sound closure may be achieved in two layers, i.e. muscle then mucosa (Figure 9.10j).

9. An elastic adhesive pressure dressing is applied to the face to lift and compress the soft tissues overlying the enhanced chin. This prevents subsequent lip sag due to separation of the divided mentalis muscle.

The Reduction Genioplasty

In cases of progenia a simple technique is to deglove the chin and sculpt off the excess bone with fissure and acrylic burs. However, it is necessary to retain the concavity at the junction of the alveolus and basal bone, for the overlying labiomental fold is aesthetically important.

With the "deep mandible" (vertical chin excess) due to a markedly increased lower anterior dentoalveolar height, an intermediate wedge of bone is removed after completing the standard genioplasty oblique section (see Vertical Maxillary Excess,) but this has to be a significant

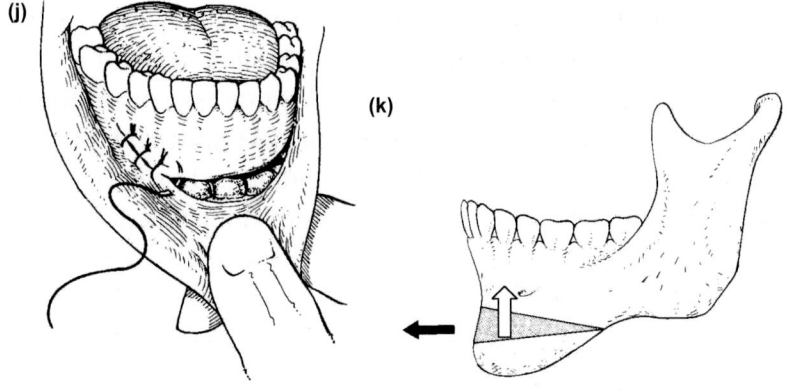

Figure 9.10   (j), (k)

wedge to make a difference externally (Figures 9.10j and 9.10k). Try not to apicect the canines. As for all genioplasty procedures, make sure the osteotomy cuts at the lower border look and feel smooth before wound closure.

Maxillary Osteotomies

The anterior segmental osteotomies, as described by Wassmund and modified by Wunderer, and the posterior segmental osteotomy of Schuchardt are rarely used compared to the more versatile Le Fort I.

Anterior dentoalveolar osteotomy (Wassmund/Wunderer)

Indications

Reduction of the overjet or localised anterior open bite. This is a simple operation but rarely achieves more than orthodontics.

Limitations

Where the upper lip is short or the dentoalveolar exposure is excessive this procedure will leave an unacceptable amount of upper incisor showing. In such cases a Le Fort I osteotomy with a vertical impaction sbould be the basis of the prescription. Also, if the maxillary first premolars have already been extracted for orthodontic reasons with forward movement of the buccal segment teeth, further extractions would leave only canines and molars. In such cases a Le Fort I osteotomy with distal movement is recommended to preserve a functional buccal occlusion.

Technique (Figure 9.11)

1. Local anaesthetic with a vasoconstrictor is infiltrated buccally and palatally on both sides (Figure 9.11a).
2. Either a first of second premolar is extracted and the gingival attachment incised from the first molar to the lateral incisor.
3. An inverted L incision is made above the apex of the tooth to be extracted, i.e. site of vertical bone cut. The gingiva is not incised but remains as a soft tissue bridge, after being carefully elevated from the alveolus from above downwards (Figure 9.11b).
4. A mucoperiosteal flap is raised forwards with the Howarth periosteal elevator, exposing the canine apex, and then extended into the pyriform fossa margin (Figure 9.11c).
5. The periosteal elevator is carefully turned through 100° and inserted submucosally along the lateral wall of the nose to protect the nasal mucosa (Figure 9.11d).
6. Bone is cut with a tapering fissure bur from the pyriform fossa margin distally, parallel to and slightly above the nasal floor, then vertically downwards into the socket of the extracted tooth, i.e. a vertical fillet is outlined. The buccal gingiva is protected by the periosteal elevator (Figures 9.11e and 9.11f).
7. The palatal mucosa may be elevated and tunnelled, but this is unnecessary. A transpalatal incision planned to rest on uncut bone provides better access. This may cross from canine to

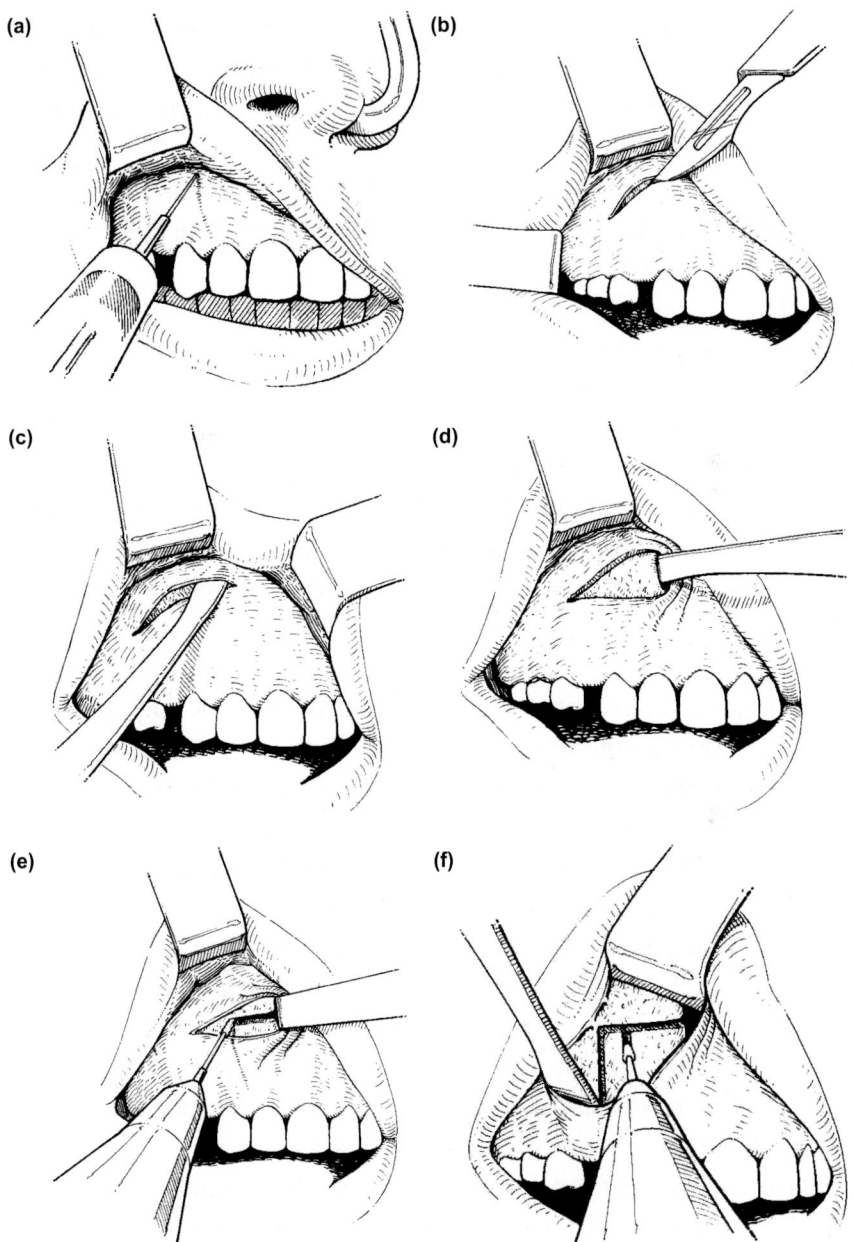

Figure 9.11   (a), (b), (c), (d), (e), (f)

canine and then be reflected backwards to expose the palatal bone. The greater palatine vessels should be tied or oversewn with polyglycollate to arrest bleeding from the posterior flap (Figures 9.11g and 9.11h).

8. The predetermined strip of palatal bone is then removed under direct vision, together with any remaining buccal plate (Figure 9.11i).

9. The buccal cuts are then made on the contralateral side.

10. Using a notched nasal septum chisel the septum is separated from the anterior fragment. This is done through a short vertical incision overlying the anterior nasal spine retracting the margins with miniature Langenbeck retractors (cat's paw) (Figure 9.11j).

11. The alveolar segment is now mobilised and repositioned. Judicious trimming with an acrylic bur, avoiding exposure of root surface, is often required to seat the segment.

12. Modifications:

   a) The intercanine width of the arch may be expanded by dividing the anterior segment in the midline through the anterior vertical incision. Start with a fine fissure bur but complete the interdental division with a narrow osteotome. This should be done before the final mobilisation (Figures 9.11k and 9.11l).

   b) Elevation of the anterior segment without distal movement can be achieved by omitting the premolar extractions and removing only the overlying cortical bone. If using burs, the buccal and palatal alveolar cortices are cut and a thin 3 mm osteotome is used for the interradicular separation. Some surgeons prefer an oscillating saw.

   c) The segment can only be elevated by careful submucosal trimming of the nasal septum and by cutting a V-shaped trough in the upper surface with a narrow cone-shaped acrylic bur or a large rosehead (Figure 9.11m).

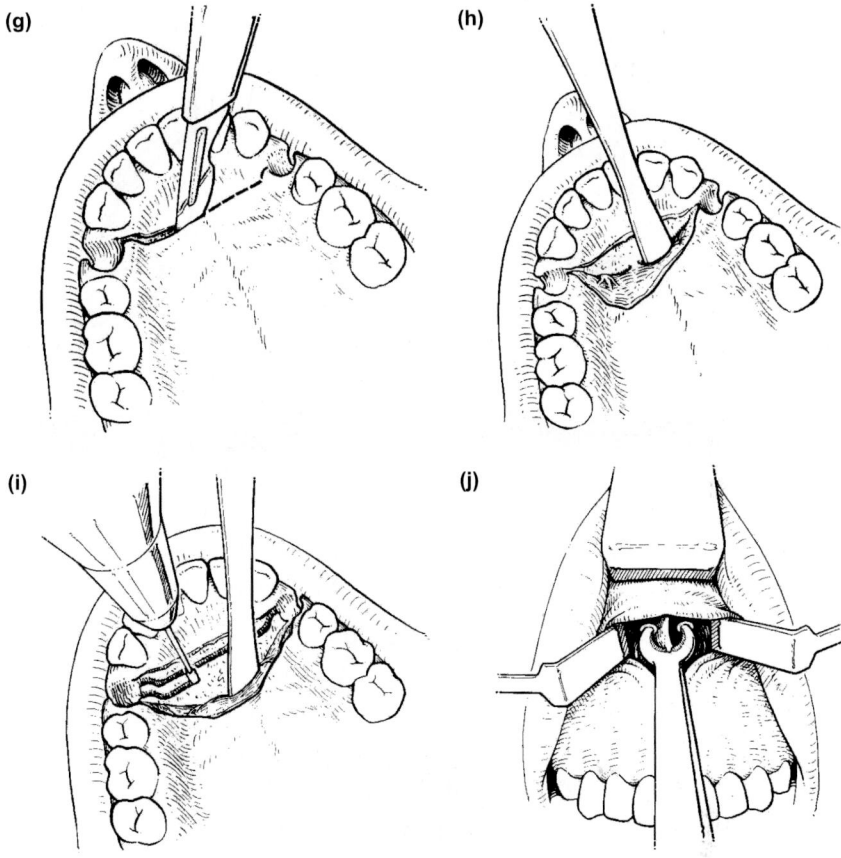

Figure 9.11   (g), (h), (i), (j)

13. The final position may be confirmed with a clear acrylic splint (wafer) covering the palatal, incisal and occlusal surfaces constructed on the surgical planning model.
14. L shaped bone plates are then bent to shape and fixed with screws.
15. The splint can be wired through a series of interdental holes to the teeth to provide definitive fixation, after the flaps have been sutured. Alternative means of fixation are using a wafer for

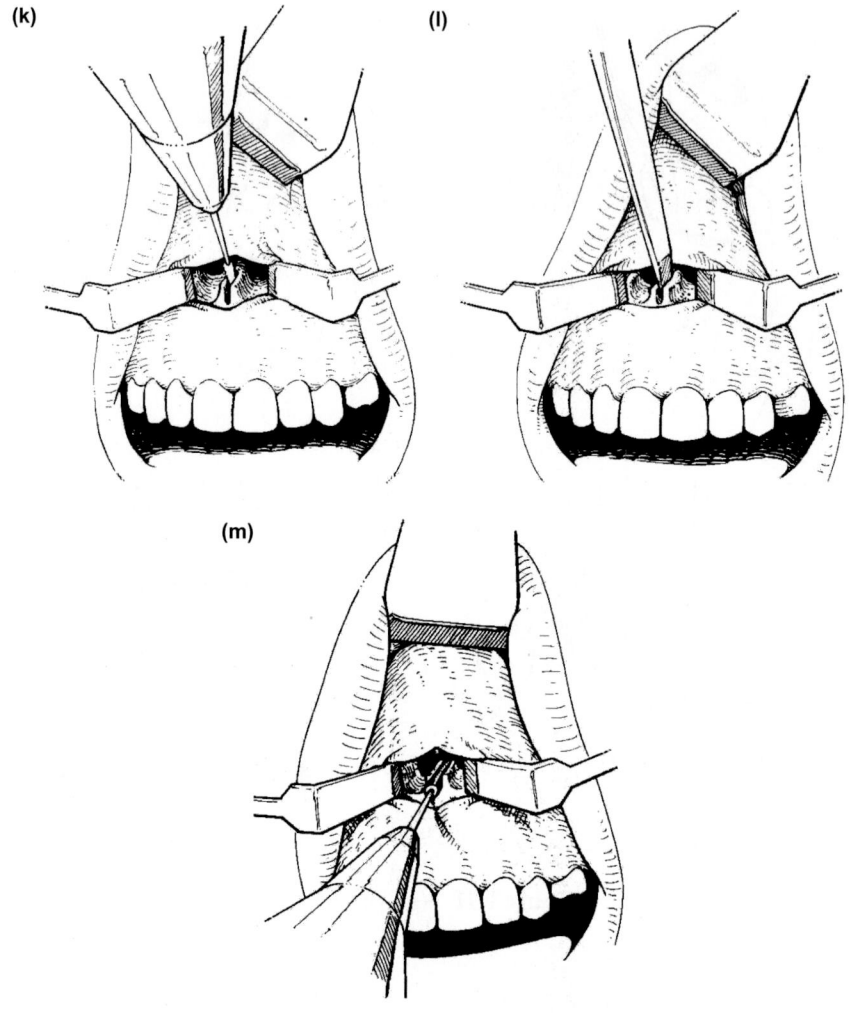

Figure 9.11   (k), (l), (m)

localisation and a wrought arch bar, or preformed orthodontic
arch wire and brackets (see Chapter 8).

16. A compression dressing of 2.5 cm elastic adhesive tape over the
lip helps reduce the swelling.

The Le Fort I Osteotomy

Indications

This is a versatile operation which can be adapted to move the whole maxillary dentoalveolar component in any direction; forwards, backwards, superiorly and inferiorly. Additional modifications can be added by segmental division from above after a down-fracture.

Remember that measured movements of the maxilla are not reflected completely by the overlying lip. The lip will be displaced only half the distance of most anterior movements. However the aesthetic outcome depends mostly on achieving a Class I incisor relationship. Approximately a quarter of an upward impaction will also be lost by elevation of the lip. Therefore, always overcorrect when planning the soft tissue changes.

Technique (Figure 9.12)

1. Infiltrate the entire buccal sulcus with local anaesthetic and a vaso-constrictor (Figure 9.12a).
2. Incise firmly down to bone with a No. 15 blade from the distal aspect of the first molar around to the opposite side. The incision must leave a generous skirt of unattached mucosa on the alveolar side for suturing (Figure 9.12b).
3. Firm upward pressure with a swab will help reflect the soft tissues and periosteum as well as drying the bone surface (Figure 9.12c).
4. With a Howarth periosteal elevator carefully extend the periosteal reflection distally behind the tuberosity and then insert the curved end of a Lack's retractor behind the maxilla until it contacts the pterygoid buttress (Figures 9.12d and 9.12e).
5. Continue the reflection forwards and upwards to identify the inferior orbital foramen and neurovascular bundle, then to the margin of the pyriform fossa of the nose. Insert the Howarth's

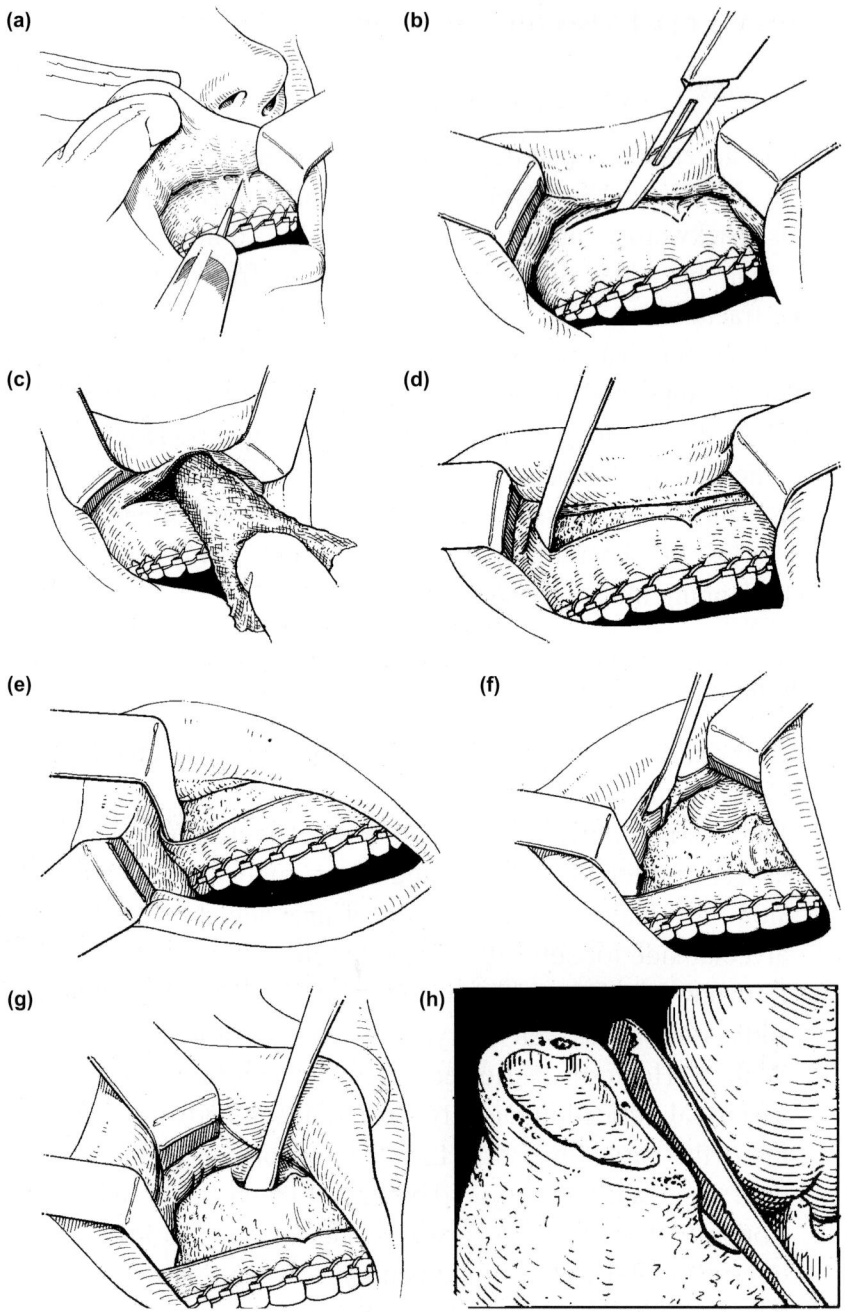

Figure 9.12   (a), (b), (c), (d), (e), (f), (g), (h)

elevator submucosally distally along the lateral nasal wall to the posterior end of the hard palate; this will protect the nasal lining (Figures 9.12f to 9.12h).

6. Bone is best cut with a reciprocating sagittal saw. A tapering fissure bur is also adequate but may produce a ragged margin (Figure 9.12i).

7. The osteotomy cut is extended from the pterygomaxillary fissure behind, forwards to the margin of the pyriform fossa approximately 15 mm above the gingival margin to clear the tooth apices, especially the canine. The cut is deepened posteriorly to section the distal and medial wall of the antrum, and also anteriorly where the medial and lateral walls of the antrum meet to form the thick triangular bony canine buttress.

   A useful variation is to fashion a step-shaped osteotomy (Figure 9.12j). Start as high as possible at the pyriform fossa margin and make a horizontal cut distally, parallel to the intended direction of maxillary movement. On reaching the zygomatic buttress cut downwards, i.e. at right angles, for 5 mm, then again turn distally through to the pterygoid plates in the usual way. This technique has the advantages of allowing more precise measurements and movements and enables the use of a horizontal miniature bone plate overlying the vertical component of the step, and so avoiding the apices of the molar teeth.

8. If the maxilla is to be elevated, make two cuts the appropriate distance apart, e.g. 2–4–6 mm, and remove the intervening strip of bone.

9. The curved pterygoid osteotome is then inserted horizontally between tuberosity and pterygoid plates and angled so that the cutting edge is tapped anteromedially with a light mallet; it may be felt protruding under the palatal mucosa with a forefinger when through the bone suture (Figure 9.12j).

10. This procedure is repeated on the opposite side.

11. The nasal septum is divided with a notched septum chisel. The Obwegeser septum chisel has a well-designed cutting

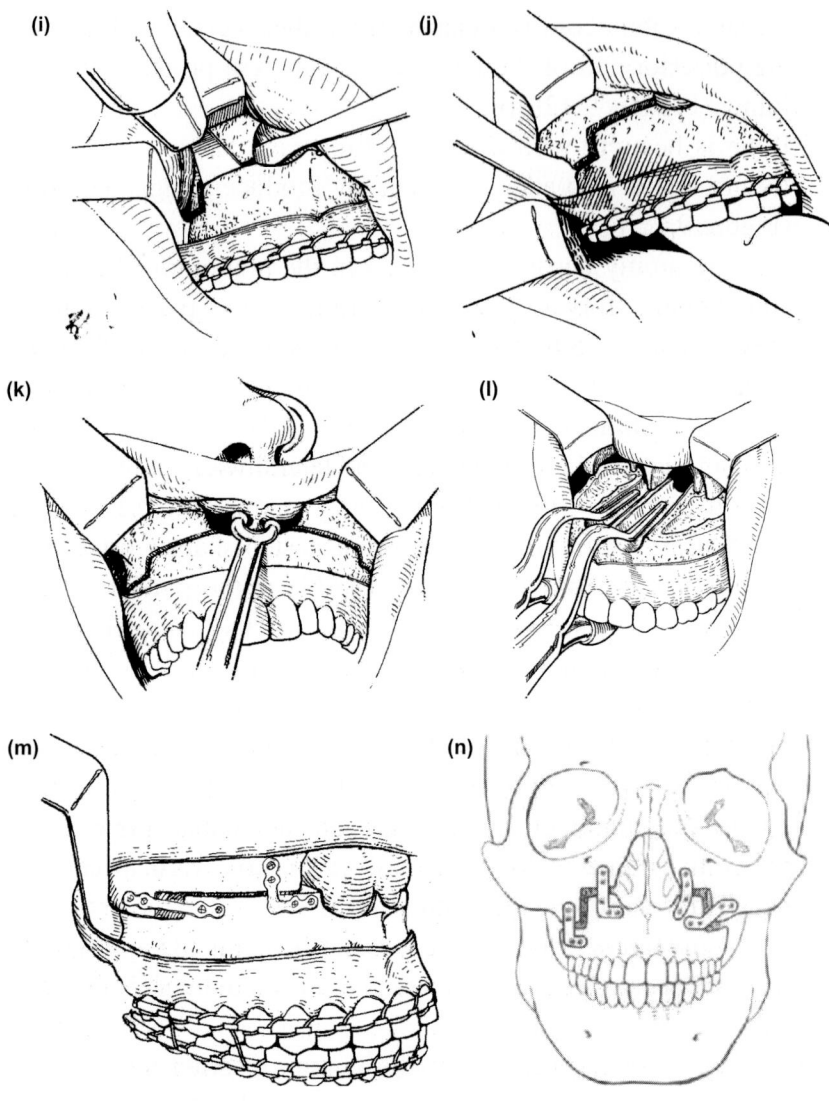

Figure 9.12   (i), (j), (k), (l), (m), (n)

protected end which prevents the chisel from straying away
from the base of the septum (Figure 9.12k). Some nasal septum chisels may perforate or sever the nasotracheal tube,
which produces a sudden burst of bloody bubbles. This may

be prevented by passing a protective finger to the back of the soft palate.

12. The maxilla may now be fractured downwards with firm digital pressure or Rowe's disimpaction forceps. Any restraining points are divided with bone shears, saw or bur. It is imperative that the tooth-bearing component is made completely mobile, leaving it loosely pedicled on the soft palate (Figure 9.12l). If the greater palatine neurovascular bundle, which can be seen or felt at the back, restricts forward movement, it can be divided with a forefinger. Upward displacement is usually prevented by the nasal septum at the back and the posterior wall of the antrum. Both need to be generously trimmed with bone rongeurs. Occasionally with upward or distal movements it is necessary to section the pterygoid buttress with an osteotome, and displace it backwards to enable repositioning of the maxilla satisfactorily.

13. At this stage the management will depend on the direction of the correction.

    Forward movements with an unoperated mandible. The dentoalveolar segment is placed in the planned occlusal position with temporary intermaxillary fixation. Malleable miniature bone plates are contoured and fitted across the posterior and anterior bony buttresses and screwed into place. An L-shaped plate will avoid the apices of the canine anteriorly, and a horizontal plate across the vertical cut of the posterior step osteotomy similarly preserves the molar roots (Figure 9.12m).

14. With large forward movements (e.g. >9 mm), improved stability may also be obtained by inserting cancellous bone blocks anteriorly between the inner aspect of the lower maxillary wall and outer aspect of the upper wall. These are secured by plates.

15. Always drill slowly with the appropriate drill or a tapering tungsten carbide fissure bur to ensure a firm bite by the screws. Rapid cutting, especially with a slightly eccentric rotation, will create a large, burnt hole. Use 5, 7 or 9 mm screws, depending

on the thickness of the maxillary wall. Rescue screws are invaluable to replace loose ones.

16. With bimaxillary osteotomies the maxillary dentoalveolar segment is positioned with an intermediate occlusal wafer designed to relate its postoperative position to the unchanged mandible. By putting on temporary intermaxillary function with 0.35 mm wires, the mandible can be used to rotate the maxilla up into a stable position whilst the bone plates are placed.

17. Although at this stage it may be possible to check the lip-incisor relationship and maxillary midline by carefully displacing the anaesthetic tube to release the nose this is not reliable compared to a precise planning process and an accurate wafer.

18. **Superior positioning** simply requires the removal of a bone strip of appropriate width. However, the septum must also be generously reduced and, if necessary, a V-shaped groove made on the superior surface of the downfractured palate. Remember that, with a nasotracheal tube in place, the nose and septum are artificially elevated after the palate has been separated; this may give a false impression of adequate clearance. Inadequate septal reduction will either displace the maxilla, producing an asymmetrical malocclusion, or distort the nose itself. If ignored, both will require surgical correction. With any significant elevation, remove the inferior tubinates to prevent nasal airway obstruction. This is easily done through the anterior nares with a pair of heavy straight scissors, or from below after incising and opening the nasal mucosa.

19. **Segmental division** can be carried out from above with a tungsten carbide fissure bur and fine osteotome or an oscillating sagittal saw. Care must be taken to preserve the mucosa of the hard palate beneath, which maintains the blood supply of the anterior segment. The buccal mucosa is protected by a Howarth periosteal elevator (Figures 9.12n and 9.12o).

20. **A transverse anterior** cut between the canine and first premolar is useful for levelling the occlusal plane in an anterior open-bite case with an exaggerated curve of Spee. As with all dentoalveolar

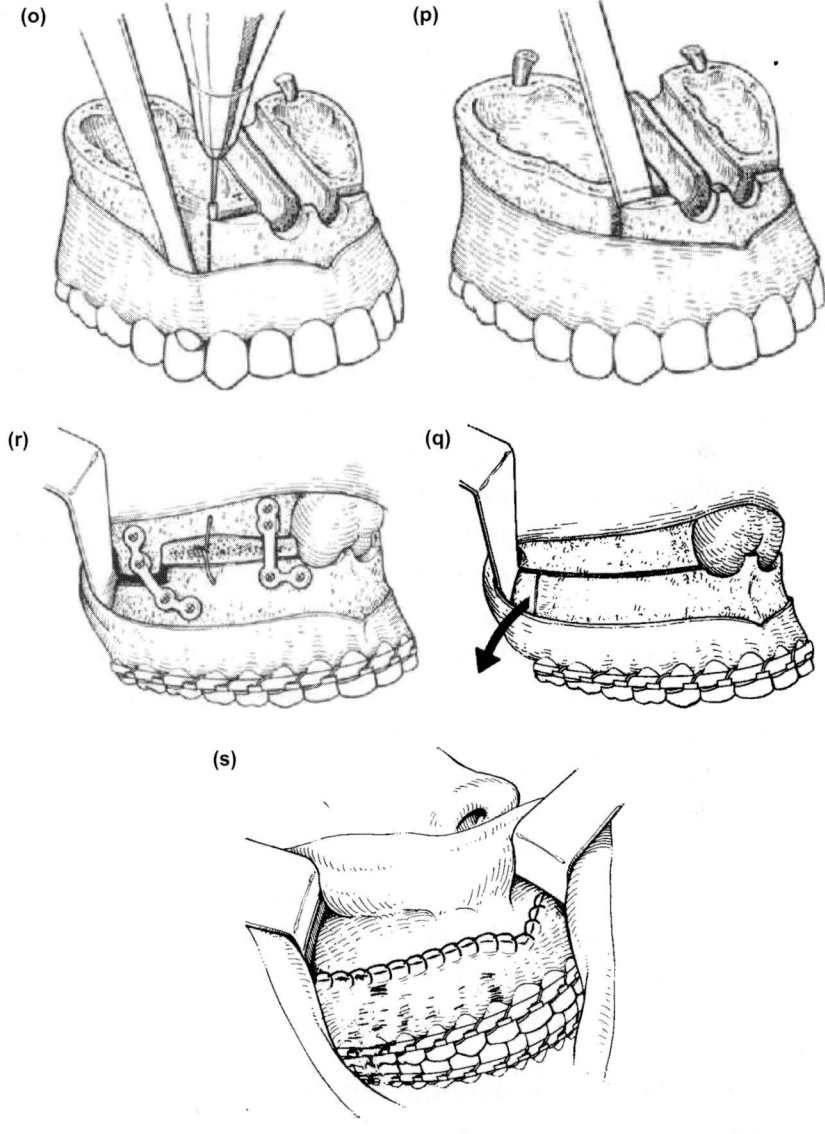

Figure 9.12 (o), (p), (q), (r), (s)

osteotomies, the buccal and palate cortex are cut with a fine bur, but even if a space has been created by orthodontics or an extraction, the alveolar section must be done with a fine osteotome to avoid damaging the roots of the adjacent teeth (Figure 9.12p).

21. **A complete midline** section will enable the arch to be expanded posteriorly. Again, the anterior interincisor division must be done with a fine osteotome. Careful elevation of the underlying palatal mucoperiosteum through the palatal section from above will allow the outward expansion. If a palatal tear occurs in the midline, lateral (Langenbeck) relieving incisions will facilitate closure with a 4/0 Prolene mattress sutures.

22. **All segmental procedures require dual fixation**. The segmental components are first related with a well fitting wafer and fixation is secured with bone plates (Figure 9.12q). In addition the dental arch is accurately secured with a supplemental 1 mm arch wire which has been prepared with the model surgery.

23. **The maxilla may be lowered** by placing contoured/bent split rib overlying the cut margins of the gap in the lateral maxillary wall. Place the cancellous surface outwards to contact the vascular soft tissues. Always overcorrect by 25%. This procedure will produce a downward and posterior rotation of the mandible requiring a sagittal split. Transosseous fixation with miniature bone plates gives adequate stability (Figure 9.12r). (See also The Short Face.)

24. **Posterior displacement** can be achieved by removing a triangular wedge of tuberosity sectioned through the third molar region. The tooth will, of course, be removed prior to this tuberositectomy. It is also necessary to divide the pterygoid buttresses at their midpoint with an osteotome and displace them backwards (Figure 9.12s).

25. The wounds are sutured; but no drains are required.

The Posterior Dentoalveolar Segmental Osteotomy of Schuchardt

Indications

With the development of the Le Fort I downfracture technique allowing segmental procedures under direct vision, this operation has become obsolete.

Le Fort II Osteotomy

Indications

Nasomaxillary hypoplasia, especially where there is a deficiency at the infraorbital margins giving the appearance of a pseudo-proptosis. The operation will accentuate a prominent nasal bridge, and so with a good nose a more suitable alternative operation is the Kufner modification of the Le Fort III osteotomy (see below).

The anatomical maxilla, together with the nasal bones and most of the septum, can be advanced and rotated downwards in the sagittal plane (Figure 9.13a). It is impossible to elevate the maxilla at the back with this operation and so the procedure is much less versatile than the Le Fort I osteotomy.

Technique

1. See the general preparation for bimaxillary procedures.
2. Prepare and drape the face, exposing the orbital margins and frontal area. Use a flexible armoured nasoendotracheal tube to give adaptable positioning of the anaesthetic hose. The nasal anaesthetic tube should be decontaminated with antiseptic and covered with an adhesive drape (Steridrape, Opsite) to allow the surgeon access to the frontal area.
3. Insert protective coneal shells and suture the eyelids. Also suture the towels to the margins of the operative area to prevent exposure of the adjacent non-sterile surface. Hair has a habit of crawling onto the operating surface and should be fixed by brushing it away from the face with undiluted scrub detergent on a sterile scrubbing brush before towelling.
4. Mark the blephoroplasty (subciliary) and frontal incisions with a pen then infiltrate with a local anaesthetic-adrenaline (1.200,000) mixture (Figure 9.13b). A transconjunctival incision may be used as a more aesthetic approach by those who

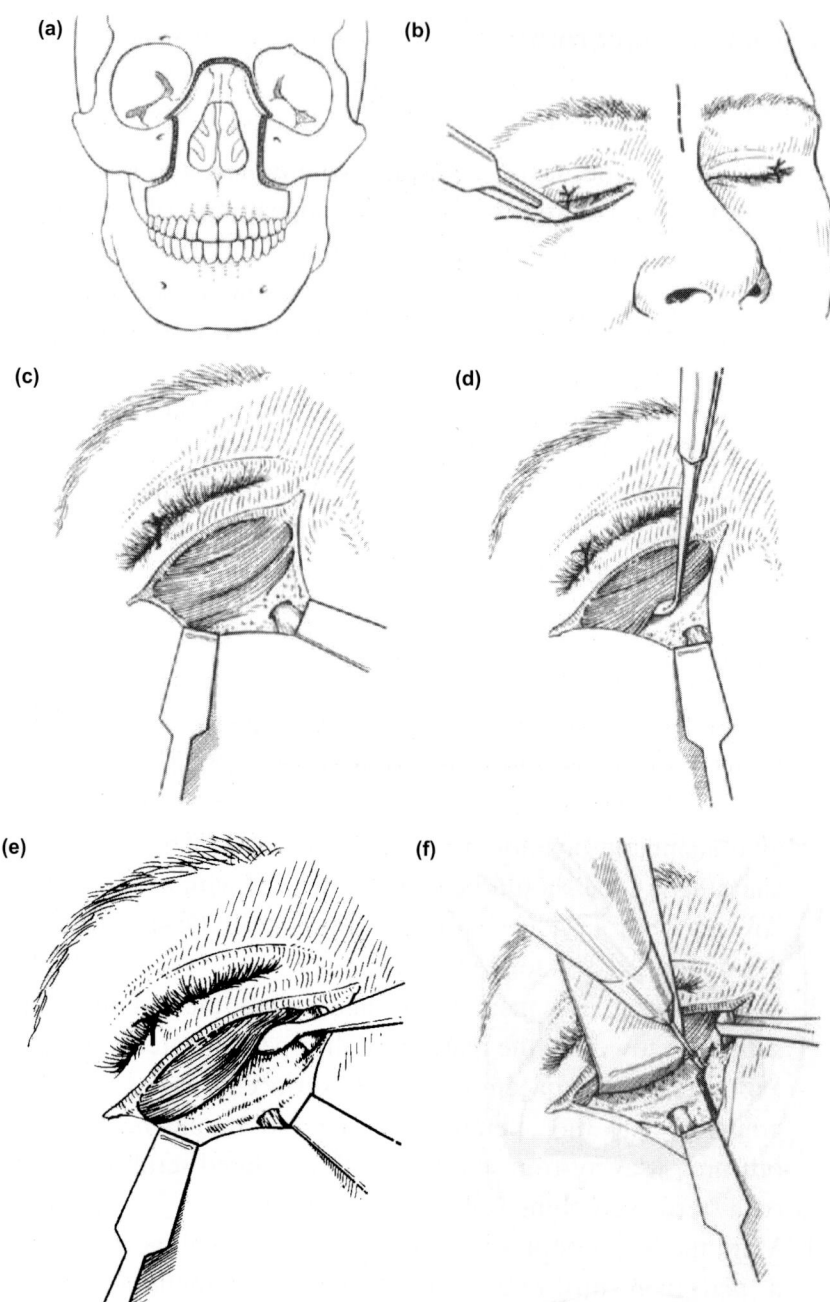

Figure 9.13   (a), (b), (c), (d), (e), (f)

are experienced with the procedure, The coronal incision is a lot of work for a limited exposure.

5. If the operation is part of a bimaxillary procedure with:

   a) an Obwegeser osteotomy: carry out this operation up to the splitting procedure, which is left until the maxilla has been repositioned;

   b) an intraoral subsigmoid osteotomy: carry out the soft tissue surgery exposing the rami but leave the osteotomy until after the maxilla has been repositioned.

6. The blepharoplasty incision should leave no detectable scar, although occasionally there is a minor degree of ectropion, which usually resolves. The incision is made 2–3 mm below and parallel to the eyelid margin until below the outer canthus. The skin is carefully elevated with a hook or fine forceps and then, with a sharp No. 15 blade, incise obliquely downwards through the orbicularis muscle, avoiding the orbital septum, i.e. outside and parallel to the fascial layer of the lower eyelid. Any breach in the septum is announced by a bubbling protrusion of fat which should be ignored. Later the defect can be repaired with a 4/0 resorbable suture. When the bony orbital margin is palpated, a round-ended copper strip or Lack's retractor is useful to retract the orbital contents whilst a firm clean incision through the periosteum is made.

7. Carefully raise the lower margin of the periosteum along the orbital margin and inferiorly down to the infraorbital foramen. This requires the detachment of the levator labii superioris alaeque nasi and the lower head of the orbicularis oculi, neither of which are recognisable (Figure 9.13c). Now extend the periosteal elevation upwards over the infraorbital margin with the spoon edge of a Mitchell's trimmer or a narrow, sharp, periosteal elevator such as a Freer or MacDonald, taking care not to breach the periosteum and release orbital fat. Elevate along the orbital floor posteriorly and then medially, supporting the orbital contents with an orbital floor retractor (Figure 9.13d).

8. Medially, the inferior orbital margin becomes narrow and sharp and is the so-called anterior lacrimal crest. Behind are the lacrimal sac and the nasolacrimal duct. Just lateral to the lacrimal sac one encounters a fine fibrovascular band which must be sacrificed in order to find the margin of the bony lacrimal fossa. The sac can be readily mobilised with a narrow dissector, first around the anterior, lateral and distal aspect, then medially around the back of the sac (Figure 9.13e). Finally extend the periosteal elevation up the frontal process of the maxilla towards the frontomaxillary suture.

   It is worth continuing the elevation at this stage, both upwards on to the down-facing convexity of the glabella and as far medially as possible on to the nasal bones. As the medial palpebral ligament is attached to the anterior lacrimal crest and the adjoining frontal process of the maxilla, this is also detached without disturbing the globe suspension.

9. The only remaining periosteal elevation is now inferiorly, passing medially and laterally to the infraorbital neurovascular bundle.

10. With a tapering tungsten carbide fissure bur cut through the inferior orbital margin, vertically downwards halfway between the nasolacrimal duct medially and the infraorbital bundle laterally. The orbital fascia and contents should be elevated and protected with a narrow, round-ended copper strip, Lac's retractor or orbital floor retractor. Extend the cut posteriorly along the orbital floor until it is distal to the lacrimal duct.

11. Now extend the cut medially behind the nasolacrimal duct, which is retracted with an elastic or nylon tape and protected with the narrow dissector (Figure 9.13f), and then continue the bur cut from the medial side of the duct (Figure 9.13g).

12. A vertical midline incision over the glabella is made down through the periosteum to bone. The tissues are firmly elevated widely, exposing the frontomaxillary suture and then passing

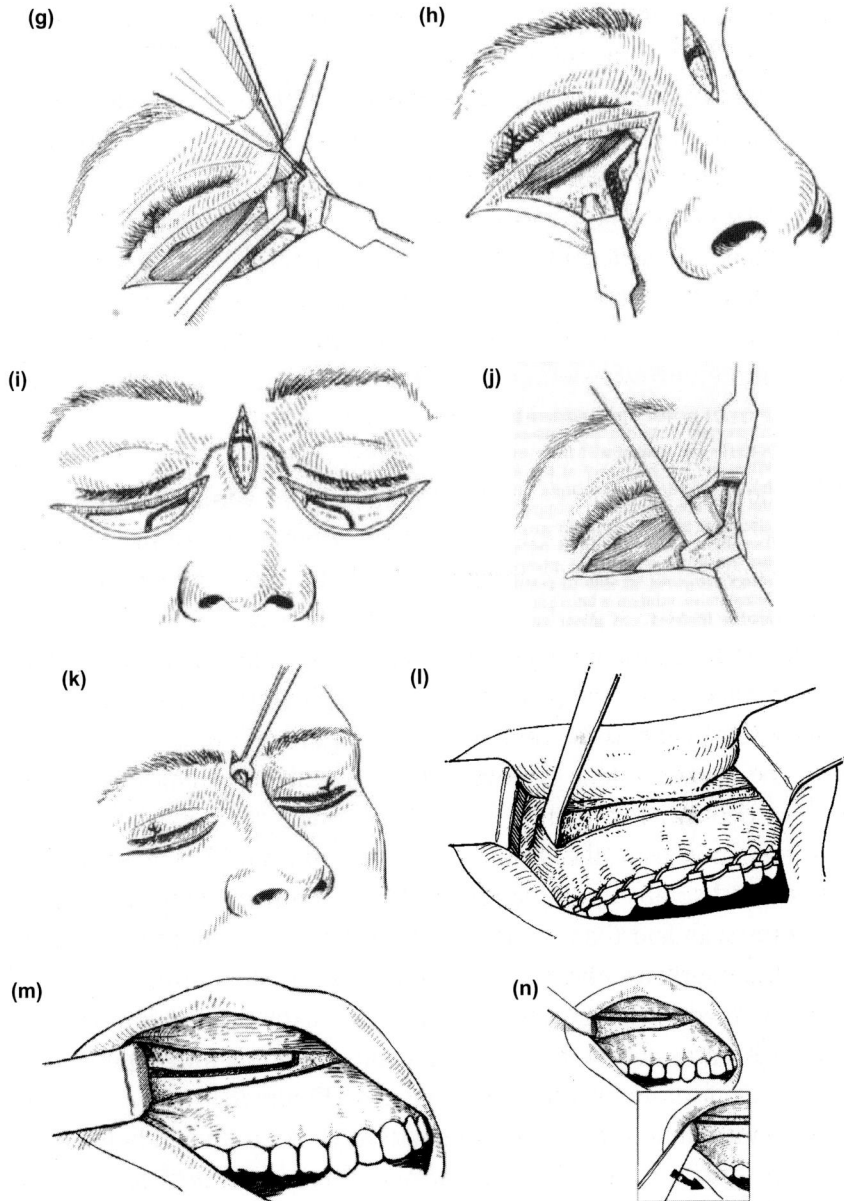

Figure 9.13   (g), (h), (i), (j), (k), (l), (m)

inferiorly and laterally in the direction of the suture line into the orbit behind the lacrimal fossa.

Using a Howarth periosteal elevator as a retractor and a tapering fissure bur, a horizontal cut is made below and parallel to the frontomaxillary suture. This suture is often the landmark of the floor of the anterior cranial fossa. The bur cut is extended posteroinferiorly into the lateral wall or the orbit behind the lacrimal sac (Figure 9.13h).

13. The two bur cuts may now be joined behind the lacrimal sac with a narrow osteotome inserted from the lateral side through the infraorbital incisions (Figure 9.13i).

14. This is repeated on the contralateral side.

15. The nasal septum is now divided through the vertical incision over the glabella. The Obwegeser nasal septum osteotome, with its convexity upwards, is inserted through the nasal bridge osteotomy cut. Once the septum can be felt firmly between the fork-like margins of the cutting edge, the osteotome is tapped diagonally downwards towards the posterior end of the hard palate, where it may be felt by the assistant's forefinger (Figure 9.13j).

16. The buccal sulcus is now infiltrated with local anaesthetic and vasoconstrictor solution and the incision made above the mucosal reflection from the distal aspect of the first molar around to the contralateral side (Figure 9.13k). This is reflected upwards with a dry swab and then periosteal elevator to reveal both the infraorbital neurovascular bundles and the lower ends of the osteotomy cuts medially (Figure 9.13l). The cut is extended downwards and backwards across the zygomatic buttress with a long tapering fissure bur or reciprocating sagittal saw (Figure 9.13m).

17. A flat bladed Lac's retractor will have been placed behind the posterior wall of the maxilla. As with the Le Fort I osteotomy, the cuts must be continued across to the posterior and medial wall of the antrum. Finally, the tuberosity is detached from the pterygoid plates with the curved pterygoid osteotome (Figure 9.13n).

(o)

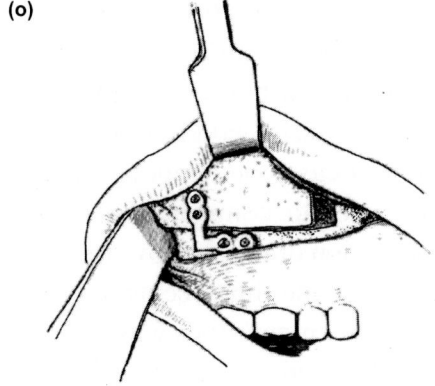

Figure 9.13   (o)

18. Mobilisation requires firm, bilateral, extraoral traction both downwards and forwards with the Rowe maxillary disimpaction forceps and then intraoral forward displacement with the Tessier maxillary retractors (Figure 9.13o). It is necessary to insert a broad osteotome in horizontally in the cut through the zygomatic buttress and carefully rotate it to mobilise the back of the maxilla. This part of the operation must be done with vigour if it is to succeed. With marked resistance the bone cut may need to be revised with a narrow osteotome. Gross haemorrhage can usually be controlled with hot gauze packs and tranexamic acid 1 g i.v.

19. Either during this procedure or at this stage, iliac crest bone is obtained to provide cancellous sheets to fill the osteotomy cuts. Always take too much rather than too little for a Le Fort II osteotomy.

20. The freely mobilised maxilla is repositioned and localised by relating it directly to the mandible, if it is not to be operated on, or with the intermediate wafer. Temporary intermaxillary tie wires are placed.

21. The cancellous bone is wedged between the osteotomy margins and secured with low profile plates. An inverted Y is useful at

the nasal bridge. With a grossly deficient bridge a pocket can be made downwards with small blunt scissors to the nasal tip to accommodate a cortical bone strut. Minature bone plates are readily inserted inferiorly and given excellent fixation.

22. With a bimaxillary case, the temporary intermaxillary fixation is removed in order to complete the mandibular osteotomy. Insert bilateral suction drains, remove the pack and suck out the pharynx and localise the final occlusion.

23. Carefully close the skin incisions with 3/0 subcutaneous polyglycollate and 5/0 subcuticular Prolene sutures.

The Kufner Modification of the LeFort III Osteotomy

Le Fort III procedures are outside the scope of this textbook as they are more appropriate for severe craniofacial deformities. However, a useful operation for malar-maxillary advancement is the Kufner modification of the Le Fort III osteotomy. This is particularly important when the nose is prominent. As can be seen from Figure 9.14, access and therefore the instrumentation are identical to the Le Fort II procedure.

However the malar maxillary advancement may now be corrected more effectively by distraction osteogenesis.

Indications

This operation can be used for patients with mild to moderate zygomatixomaxillary hypoplasia but with a normal nose. Gross malar and infraorbital augmentation is more easily achieved with a high Le Fort I osteotomy or distraction osteogenesis.

Technique

Follow the stages described for the Le Fort II osteotomy (steps 1–8) without mobilising the lacrimal sac.

1. Elevate the periosteum and facial tissues from the orbital margin downwards and medially on the anterior surface of the maxilla until the nasal pyriform fossa margin in reached.
2. Elevate the orbital periosteum distally and laterally to expose the anterior end of the inferior orbital fissure and the lateral orbital margin.
3. Extension of the blepharoplasty incision laterally will now give surprisingly good access to the malar bone itself, which must be exposed completely.
4. The bone cuts are made (Figure 9.14) with a tapering fissure bur. This is often easier from above the patient. Take care not to damage the infraorbital neurovascular bundle which can be seen through the thin orbital floor.
5. Take the lateral osteotomy cut horizontally through the base of the lateral orbital margin. Then make a vertical cut through the zygomatic bone two-thirds of the way back from the orbital margin. This will create an inverted L-shaped separation, giving

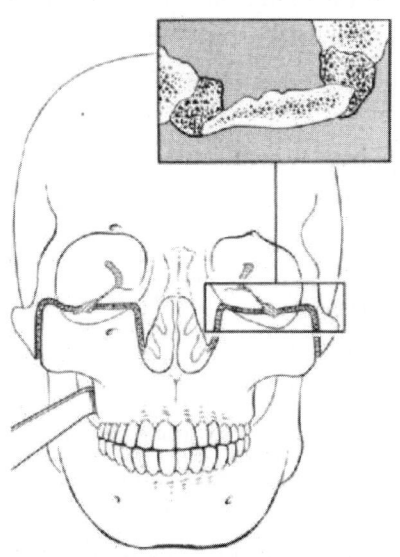

Figure 9.14

excellent access for placing a corticocancellous graft and for plating (Figure 9.14 inset).

6. Extend the medial cuts down into the pyriform margin. Repeat on the contralateral side.

7. The nasal septum and pterygoid plates are separated intraorally, as in the Le Fort I operation.

8. If distraction osteogenesis is not being used, mobilisation is carried out extraorally from above and behind the head ("slowly but strongly") with the Rowe's disimpaction forceps. Both a forward tilting and transverse rotation are required to achieve a completely mobile skeletal block. Intraoral traction with Tessier's maxillary retractors is also important.

9. Temporary intermaxillary fixation is applied, using an intermediate wafer in a bimaxillary case. The bone grafts are inserted at the osteotomy sites. The most important one is the malar cut, which is wedged open as shown in Figure 9.14 and fixed with bone plates.

10. All sharp bony margins are carefully masked with spare cancellous bone or smoothed with an acrylic bur.

11. At this stage the intermaxillary fixation is removed and, where necessary, the mandibular osteotomy completed, drains inserted and the intraoral wounds sutured.

12. The pharynx is sucked out and the pack removed.

13. The blepharoplasty wounds are closed after the insertion of miniature vacuum drains, with subcuticular 5/0 Prolene sutures.

Tongue Reduction

Indications

The enlarged tongue is an uncommon cause of anterior open bite and osteotomy failure. If it appears to be large and the incisor teeth are proclined and separated, surgical reduction is indicated and can be carried out prior to orthodontics or with segmental osteotomies.

Where there is any doubt, the patient should be informed that it may be necessary some time after the dental alignment or

osteotomy, and the case is carefully followed up at 3-monthly intervals to prevent any gross relapse. This will take the form of recurrent proclination and separation of the incisors. Once this is
obvious, reduction should be carried out and any dental relapse can
be corrected orthodontically. The tongue should always be reduced
in length and width, which can be achieved by a keyhole excision.

Technique (Figure 9.15)

1. Draw the tongue forwards with a towel clip or two heavy silk
    stay sutures and generously outline the tissue to be removed
    with a pen and Bonney's Blue.

    a) The full thickness wedge will determine the reduction in
        length and width at the tip (Figure 9.15a).
    b) A centrally placed ellipse overlapping the anterior wedge
        will reduce bulk and width, but will minimally increase the
        length. L = reduction in length. W = reduction in width
        (Figure 9.15b).

2. Infiltrate well with 0.5% bupivacaine and 1:200 000 adrenaline.
3. With a large blade (No. 20), first excise the anterior wedge,
    carefully arresting all bleeding points with mosquitoes and
    bipolar diathermy. Allis forceps or two heavy gauge traction

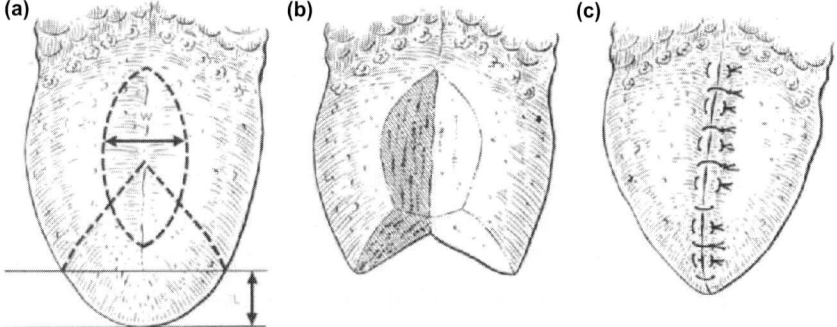

Figure 9.15 (a), (b), (c)

sutures can be used for immobilising the tongue while the central ellipse is excised with a triangular cross-section. Again careful haemostasis is important.

4. The tongue is sutured with 3/0 polyglycollate starting at the tip and working backwards with vertical mattress sutures from the depth to the mucosal suface. Simple sutures are then placed between each of the mattress sutures from behind working forward and continuing on to the ventral surface. (Figure 9.15c)

5. The combination of careful haemostasis and anti-oedema steroids (8 mg dexamethasone, 12-hourly, × 3) should prevent any gross swelling and obstruction.

6. Generous analgesia and nasogastric nutrition will be required for at least 3 days.

7. Postoperative speech therapy is useful to re-establish comfortable diction.

Bone Grafts

Indications

Bone may be required for an augmentation genioplasty and for the extensive maxillary osteotomies. It is used as cancellous bone chips or mush, cancellous bone slices or corticocancellous blocks. In order of value one can use:

1. Fresh autogenous bone, which is actively osteogenic and provides the best union.

2. Decalcified lyophilised bone (either autogenous or allogenous bank bone) as a satisfactory space filler which induces good union but is much improved when supplemented with autogenous cancellous mush.

3. Deep frozen or lyophilised whole autogenous bone, which may be rated only as satisfactory.

There is, of course, an increased risk of secondary infection and greater loss with the stored non-vital tissues.

Where fresh bone is employed, minimal storage outside the body is obviously desirable and the operation should therefore be planned to harvest the graft when it is needed. It should be kept in a blood-soaked swab. Immersion in saline and the application of antibiotic powders devitalise the fresh bone.

Iliac Crest

Technique (Figure 9.16)

Appropriate shaving and cleansing should be carried out on the ward.

1. In orthognathic surgery only portions of the iliac crest are required; therefore operate on the side which is most convenient. For right-handed surgeons, the left hip can be simultaneously approached by an assistant. A substantial sandbag should be placed under the buttock (ischium) to elevate the iliac crest.
2. Prepare the hip widely and carefully with a detergent-iodine solution. Square drape with 4 towels that are stitched into place with a heavy black silk (2/0) on a straight or 30 mm curved cutting needle, cover and seal the area with an adhesive drape, i.e. Opsite, Steridrape.

Note: Ensure the anterior superior iliac spine is at the inferomedial corner of the operative area and that the crest can be palpated along its whole length to the posterosuperior corner.

3. Clean and drape the head end for the osteotomy, and then cover the the patient with a large sheet, which can be rotated downwards to reveal the donor site when ready without reprepuration. The operator and assistant should change their gloves and gowns between mouth and hip.

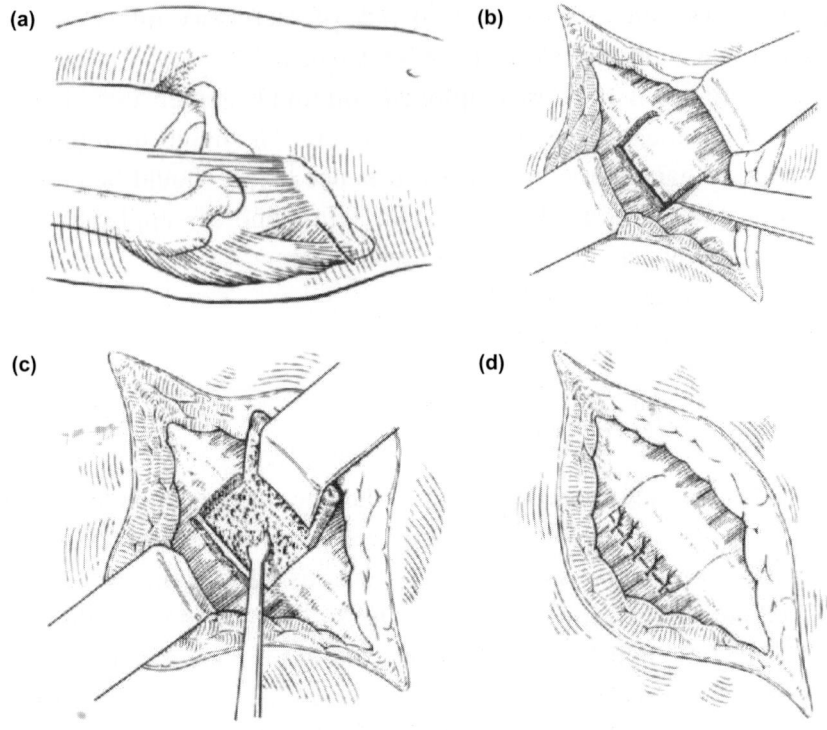

Figure 9.16   (a), (b), (c), (d)

4. For particulate cancellous bone/cancellous mush (the Flint technique).

    a) The assistant, standing on the contralateral side, pulls the skin medially so that the incision on to the iliac crest will ultimately fall below the bony surface (Figure 9.16a).

    b) A short incision of 6 cm is made down to the iliac crest with a No. 20 blade and the margins retracted. Diathermy will be required for bleeding points and the wound is enlarged.

    c) Once the periosteum-covered bone surface has been defined with a swab and knife, a 2.5 cm osteotome is used to outline a lid 5 cm wide on the superior and lateral aspects of the crest (Figure 9.16b).

d) This lid is elevated on its medial musculoperiosteal hinge and cancellous bone is removed using gouges and Volkmann spoon. The bone should be placed into a dry receiver and covered with a blood-soaked swab until used. Soaking fresh bone in saline kills the osteoblasts (Figure 9.16c).

e) The lid may be sutured into place with 1/0 polyglycollate, which is also used to oppose the muscle and for deep sub-cutaneous closure (Figure 9.16d). A continuous subcuticular 3/0 Prolene suture on a straight needle is used for the skin.

5. For blocks and sheets.

a) A 10 cm incision is made down to periosteum. Undermining the skin margins will give improved access. Dissection with a fresh blade will now define the periosteum-covered iliac crest.

b) A long lid (12 cm) may be outlined with an osteotome and lifted, pedicled on the inner periosteum and muscle in the same manner as described above, and block cut from the bone beneath. By outlining a rectangle on the outer surface of the ilium with the osteotome, a lateral cortical flap may also be rotated downwards, allowing sheets of cancellous bone to be cut from the centre. Some prefer to cut a medial cortical flap in order not to disturb the origin of the gluteal fascia and muscles (Figures 9.17a and 9.17b).

c) The cortical lids are replaced and sutured with 1/0 polyglycollate

   Note: It is easier to reflect the surface periosteum with a Farabeuf periosteal elevator and simply cut out cortico-cancellous blocks as required.

d) The muscle layer is closed with a 2/0 suture and a vacuum drain inserted. This ensures a marked reduction in haematoma formation and postoperative morbidity. The drain must be carefully sutured to the skin before wound clo-sure, ensuring 2 cm of non-perforated tube within the tissues.

(a)

(b)

(c)

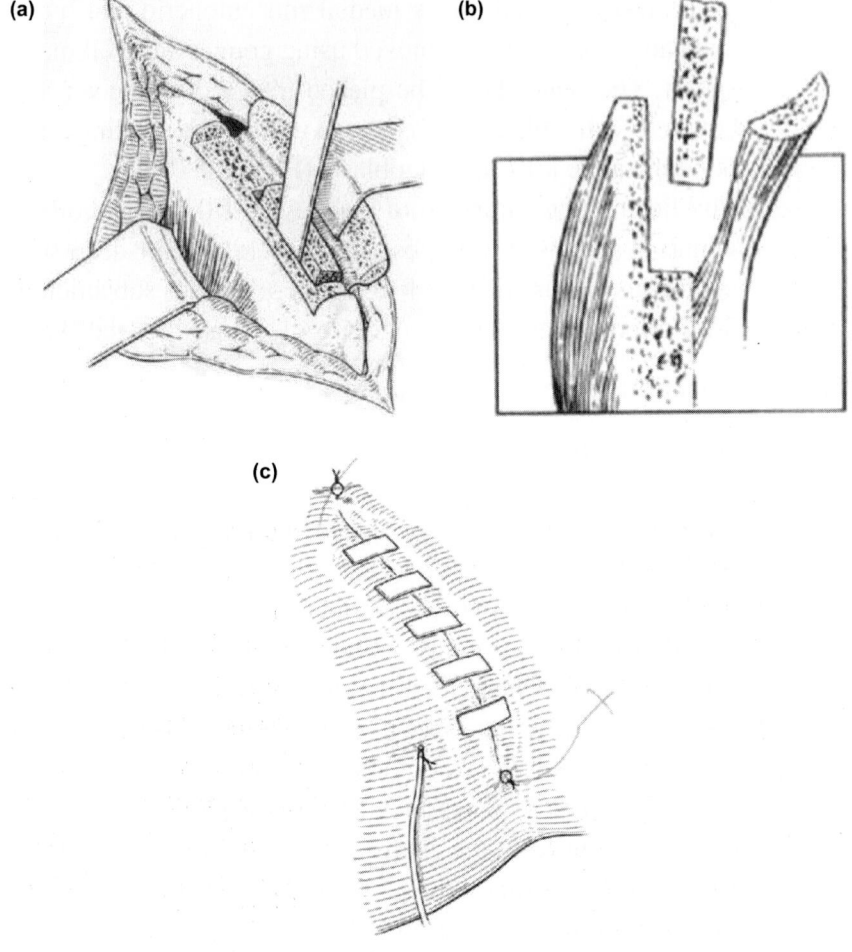

Figure 9.17   (a), (b), (c)

e)   Close the skin with a subcutaneous resorbable suture and
     then a continuous subcuticular 3/0 Prolene or polyglycol-
     late and Steri-strips (Figure 9.17c). If possible, cover the
     wound immediately with a sterile adhesive dressing
     (Demacel) and then complete the osteotomy.

     The drain is left in until it stops draining. The Prolene
     skin suture is removed after 10 days; the polyglycollate
     suture may be left to dissolve.

Rib (Figure 9.18a)

Rib is easier to remove than iliac crest, with considerably less morbidity for the patient, but provides less bone both qualitatively and quantitatively.

Rib may be split with an fine osteotome, separating the outer and inner cortices which are rendered pliable with Tessier rib forceps or a pair of straight extraction forceps. These strips can be laid over maxillary osteotomy cuts with the cortex facing "outwards" against the vascular soft tissues.

Technique

1. As with the hip, the chest wall must be carefully prepared with a detergent-iodine solution, dried, towelled and sealed with an adhesive drape.
2. Incisions must be planned to fall in the crease of the lower border of pectoralis major or beneath the breast. This may be done accurately using a marker pen, with the patient sitting upright, before the operation. A 6 cm incision with a No. 10 blade, once undermined, gives generous access to the 5th and 6th ribs. Coagulate bleeding vessels then incise the muscle layer, down to but not including the periosteum, with a cutting diathermy needle (Figure 9.18b).
3. The rib periosteum is incised with a fresh blade along its mid axis and then at right angles to this cut. Peel off the superficial periosteum, then carefully expose both rib margins (Figure 9.18c). The undersurface is then stripped with a curved rib rasperator (Figure 9.18d) as widely as possible and rib cutting shears are applied to cut the rib with the guillotine blade facing away from the graft to gain maximal length. It is then firmly grasped and carefully pealed off the underlying periosteum.
4. If the inner periosteum and pleura are torn, the lungs should be inflated by the anaesthetist as the defect is sutured with 3/0 Prolene or polyglycollate with a round-bodied needle.

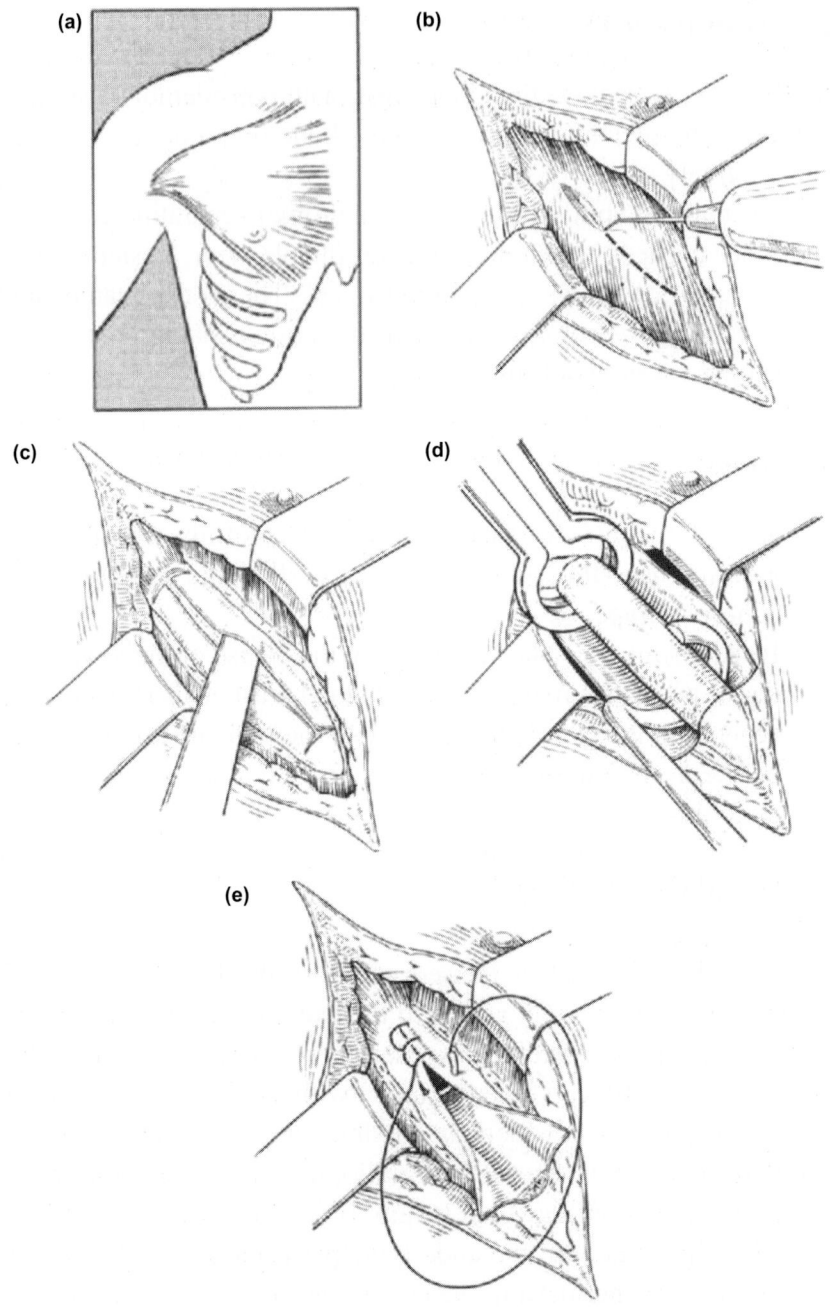

Figure 9.18   (a), (b), (c), (d), (e)

The periosteum is then closed with a continuous suture. The muscle layer and subcutaneous tissues are closed with the same needle, and the skin with a continuous subcuticular 3/0 Prolene or polyglycollate suture (Figure 9.18e). A drain is not necessary. Cover with an adhesive dressing (e.g. Opsite), and drape a towel over the area and continue with the osteotomy.

5. The costochondral graft; a minor modification is required for a costochondral graft. A 6 cm length of rib is exposed adjacent to the costal cartilage, but the medial right angle division of the periosteum is placed so as to leave a periosteal bridge between bony rib and cartilage. The lateral bone end is cut as above and the cartilage carefully incised with a No. 15 blade protecting the undersurface with a Howarth periosteal elevator. The cartilage is then trimmed to a round condylar like surface and the graft carefully stored until used.

6. A postoperative chest X-ray is essential the following day. Not uncommonly an effusion may result, especially where large quantities of rib have been taken. However, with antibiotic cover and physiotherapy no intervention will be required. The treatment of a pneumothorax is dealt with in Chapter 14.

Distraction Osteogenesis

Introduction

Distraction osteogenesis is the alternative to some conventional orthognathic procedures but is already too complex to cover in a short section of this book. The Hyrax screw appliance which is still used for expanding a narrow hard palate was probably the first distraction osteogenesis procedure and was used as a tooth borne appliance both with and without an osteotomy in the 1920s. At the time the expansion was considered to be a separation of the midline palatal suture than a stimulation of new bone formation. The problem with this tooth borne appliance is that compression of the abutment teeth, against the buccal perimeter of their periodontal membranes activates the release of bone resorbing factors, so that the teeth not only tip outwardly but also lose their overlying buccal plate. This has been overcome by bone borne expansion appliances for both the maxilla and mandible, and now many well designed distraction protocols have become established in the field of craniofacial surgery, to be used in maxillary, mandibular and dentoalveolar deficiencies.

Distraction osteogenesis is designed to lengthen and create new bone by stretching the callus of an osteotomy site. Following an appropriately designed osteotomy, carefully controlled tensile forces are gradually applied to the callus increasing the regenerative immature bone laid down between the cut ends. Over time, the bone remodels into mature bone and the surrounding soft tissues adapt to their new content and length. This remarkable process is made possible by the extensibility of the skin, fascia and muscle in response to gradual elongating traction. Muscle fibres have been shown to add on sarcomeres in response to carefully controlled extension.

The Cell Biology

Preosteoblasts, osteoblasts and fibroblasts are sensitive to mechanical deformation such as the tensile stress of osteodistraction and respond by the release of a complex soup of cellular factors. These include osteogenic cytokines transforming growth factor (TGF β1), bone morphogenic proteins (BMPs) including BMP 2 and 4 and angiogenic factors such as basic fibroblast growth factor (BFGF). In addition osteoclastogenesis is also upregulated by the release of tumour necrosis factor-alpha (TNFα), RANKL (receptor activator for nuclear factor kappa B ligand) and interleukin 1β (IL1β) which recruit and activate osteoclasts. Both of the remodelling processes are upregulated but the balance between bone formation and resorption is probably determined by the rate of separation and ischaemia in the callus. This overall increased activity may explain why teeth moved into the consolidating callus (osteoid) undergo marked root resorption indicating increased osteoclast/cementoclast activity at this stage. The maturation process of the osteoid to bone takes place during the retention phase.

The Clinical Technique

This is divided into the following phases.

1. Osteotomy.
2. Period of latency. In the craniofacial region this is usually about 4–5 days to allow callus formation and primary wound healing.
3. Distraction phase. This is carried out at a constant rate (1–2 mm per day) until the desired length or volume of bone has been created. Despite this slow rate of distraction the procedure can be painful at each turn for up to 20 minutes duration and adequate analgesia is recommended on a daily basis before the procedure.
4. Retention phase. Retention of the distracted bone is necessary to allow for calcification and remodelling of the osteoid. In the craniofacial region this will usually be a minimum of 6–8 weeks but may be longer.

The Procedure

Early reports on craniofacial distraction mention corticotomies rather than osteotomies. While a corticotomy in young children with soft bone may suffice to allow mobilisation of the bone fragments, it is essential to carry out a complete osteotomy in adolescents and adults. Most distraction in adults in the craniofacial region is carried out at the rate of 1 mm per day. Rates of less than 0.5 mm a day may result in ankylosis and rates of more than 3 mm a day may result in non-union. Children may tolerate faster rates of distraction than 1 mm a day with the production of good quality distraction bone, however the more gradual the distraction rate the more predictable is the generation of vascular distraction bone. Therefore a distraction rate of a 0.5 mm twice a day or a 0.25 mm four times a day is more satisfactory than a single movement of 1 mm a day.

The Vector of Distraction

The vector or direction of distraction will determine where the length and volume of bone is obtained. The resolution of the optimum vector may be estimated using plain radiographs or more accurately 3D modelling computer programmes which simulate virtual surgery and distraction of the case preoperatively. Simulated distraction can also be carried out for the more complicated cases prior to surgery with stereolithic models. The many distractors available can be intraoral or extraoral and experienced supervision is essential.

Types of Distractor

The first cases were carried out using external distractions only. External distractors in the oral and facial area besides being visible and bulky, have the disadvantage of producing visible scars where the fixation pins enter the skin as they move during the distraction phase (Figures 9.19a and 9.19b). Internal distractors were subsequently developed and there are now many types of both external and internal available to suit most deformities. Multidirectional distractors allow for one or more osteotomies to be carried out simultaneously and the bone distracted in more than one direction.

In general, internal distractors are more readily accepted by patients. There are now a number of slimline internal distractors with a variety of designs and sizes to accommodate most clinical situations (Figures 9.20a and 9.20b).

Some indications for distraction include:

• craniofacial abnormalities, e.g. Crouzons;
• hemifacial microsomia;

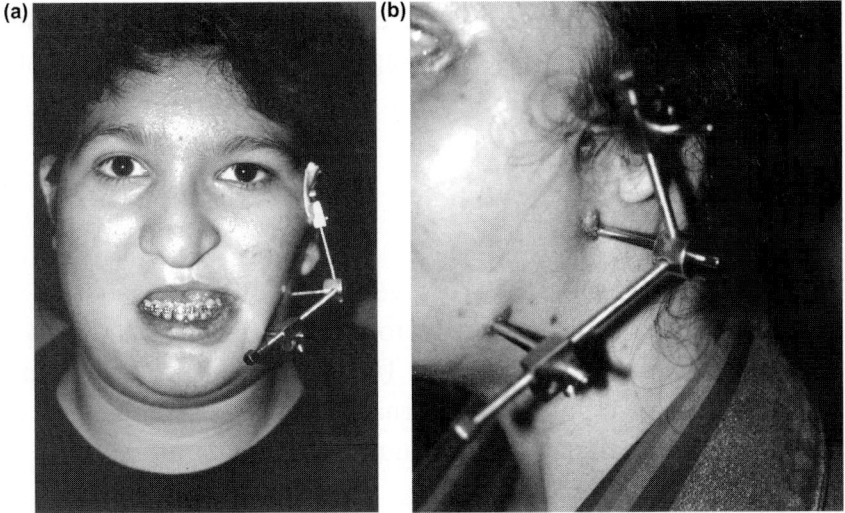

Figure 9.19   (a), (b)

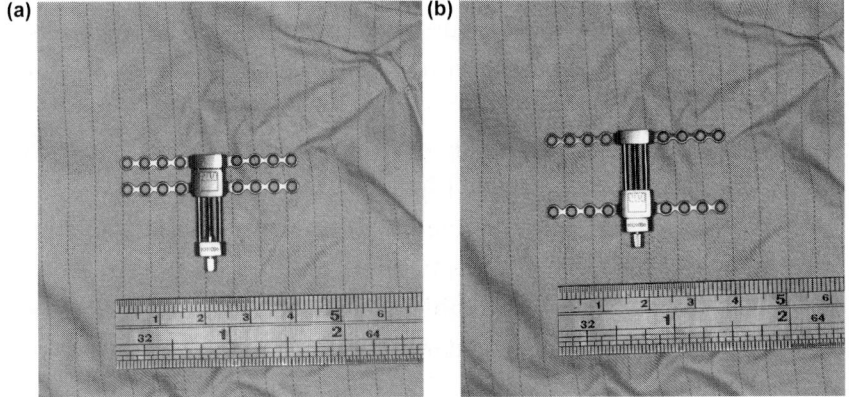

Figure 9.20   (a), (b)

- maxillary hypoplasias due to previous cleft palate surgery;
- palatal and mandibular expansion;
- dentoalveolar hypoplasia for implant insertion;
- tumour/trauma reconstruction; and
- TMJ ankylosis.

Some of the applications of the technique are illustrated by the following cases and also in Chapter 11 on cleft lip and palate deformity.

The Hypoplastic Mandible

The common management of a severely hypoplastic mandible is an inverted L advancement osteotomy with a ramus bone graft and an augmentation genioplasty. The L or horizontal osteotomy of the ascending ramus with internal distraction osteogenesis is a simpler and assured way of achieving the same correction.

Case 1. This patient presented with a mandibular hypoplasia and rudimentary condyles. The cause of the lack of condylar development was unknown but could have been early childhood trauma. The patient was seen at 15 years where the degree of hypoplasia was becoming more apparent with increasing facial growth (Figures 9.21a and 9.21b)

Radiographs demonstrate a mandible which is both short in ramus height and body length (Figures 9.21c and 9.21d).

The maxilla was also deficient, especially in posterior height presumably secondary to the mandibular hypoplasia, but it was decided to treat only the mandible at this stage. Bilateral horizontal osteotomies of the mandibular ascending rami were carried out above the level of the lingulae. The choice of this site would allow subsequent conventional sagittal osteotomies to be carried out should the need arise when the patient was mature. Distractors with universal joint mechanisms were used (KLS Martin) (Figures 9.21e and 9.21f).

An oblique vector was chosen to provide both a downward and forward direction of distraction. This increased the vertical ramus height bilaterally and at the same time achieved forward projection

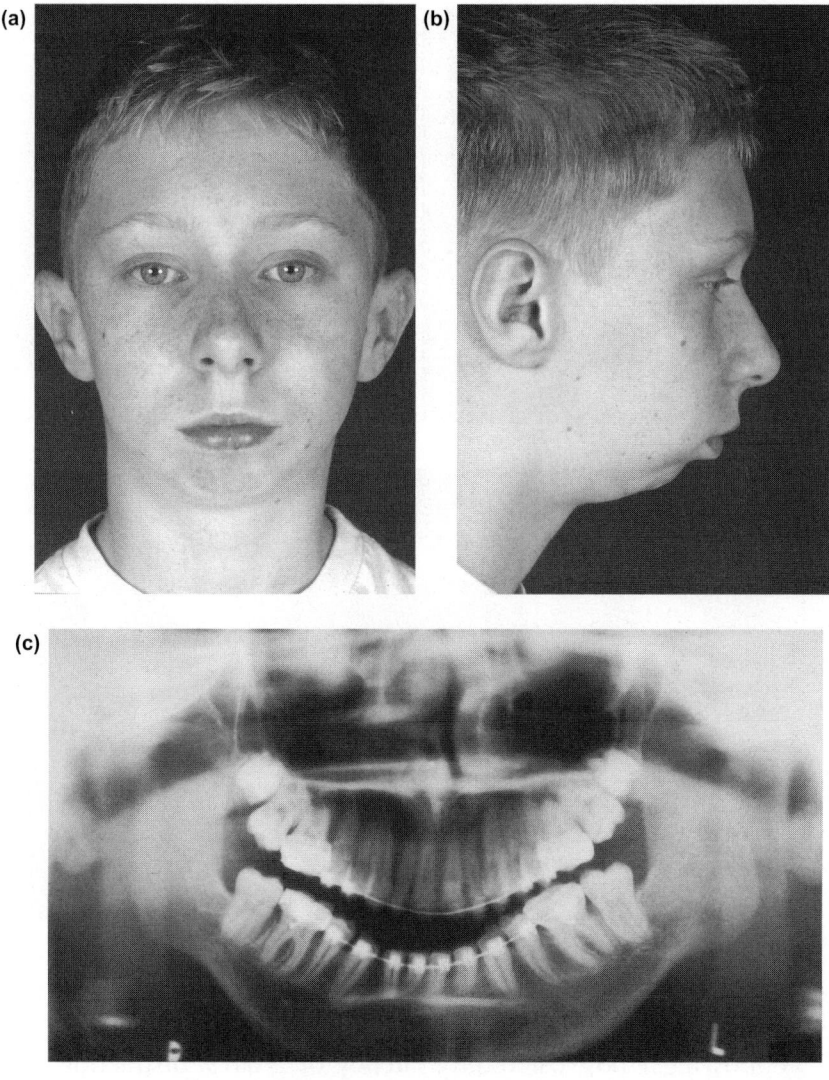

Figure 9.21 (a), (b), (c)

of the mandible. The immediate postoperarative OPG shows the distractor closed. The apparent osteotomy line below the distractor is an oropharyngeal shadow artefact, the true oseotomy line is above the distractor and less evident (Figure 9.21g).

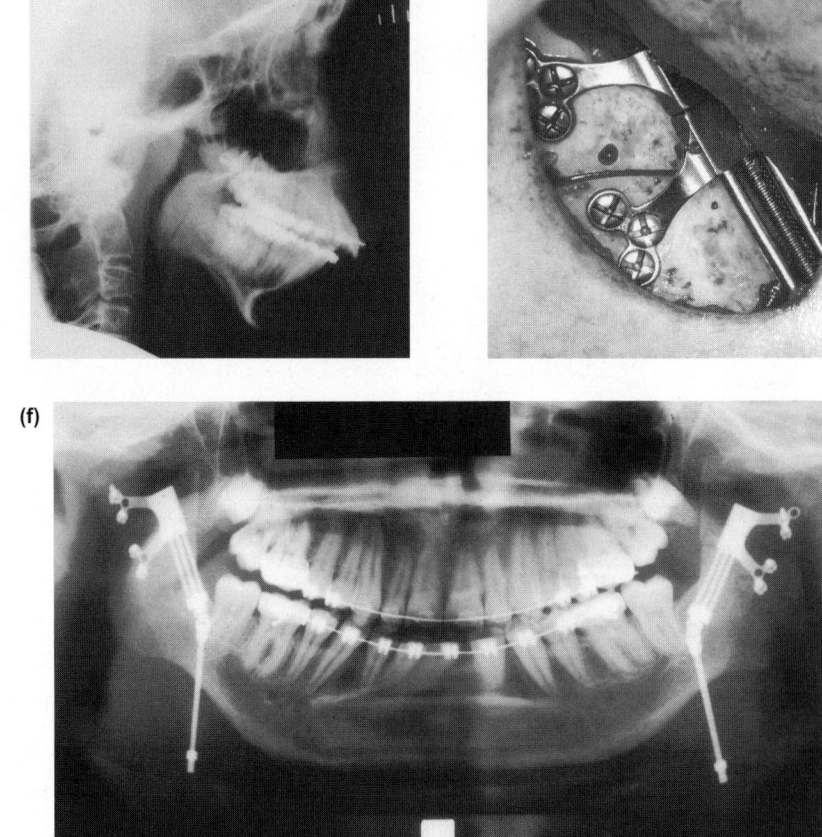

Figure 9.21   (d), (e), (f)

Following a post-osteotomy latency of 5 days, distraction was commenced at the rate of 1 mm per day (0.5 mm, 12-hourly). Distraction was continued for 15 days. At the end of 15 days the distractors were maintained *in situ* for a period of 8 weeks before surgical removal. Figures 9.21h and 9.21i show the postoperative X-ray appearance with the distractors fully extended and the clinically improved lower facial height and mandibular profile (Figures 9.21j and 9.21k).

(g)

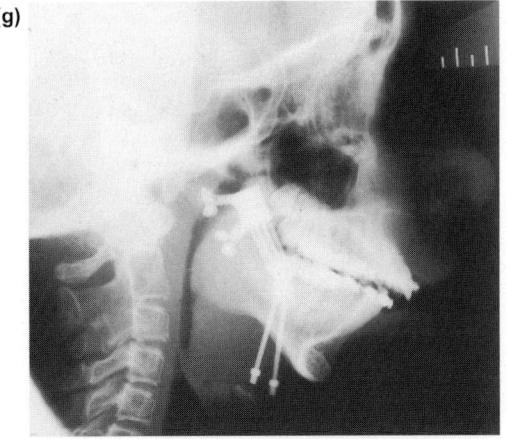

(h)

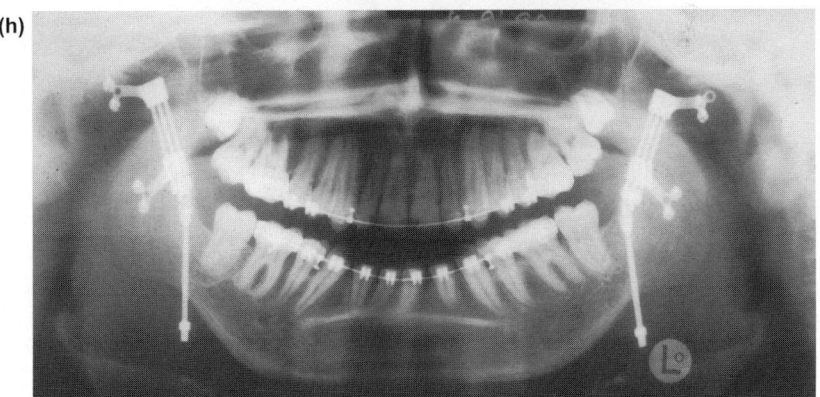

(i)

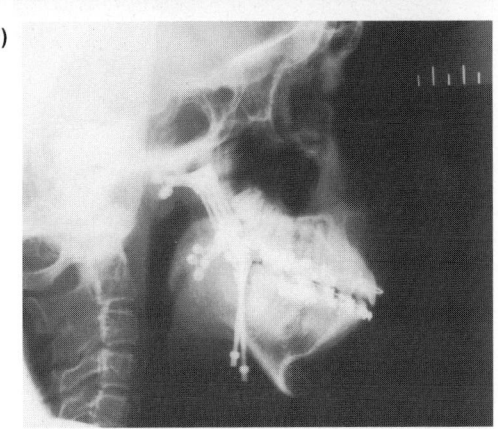

Figure 9.21 **(g), (h), (i)**

(j)

(k)

(l)

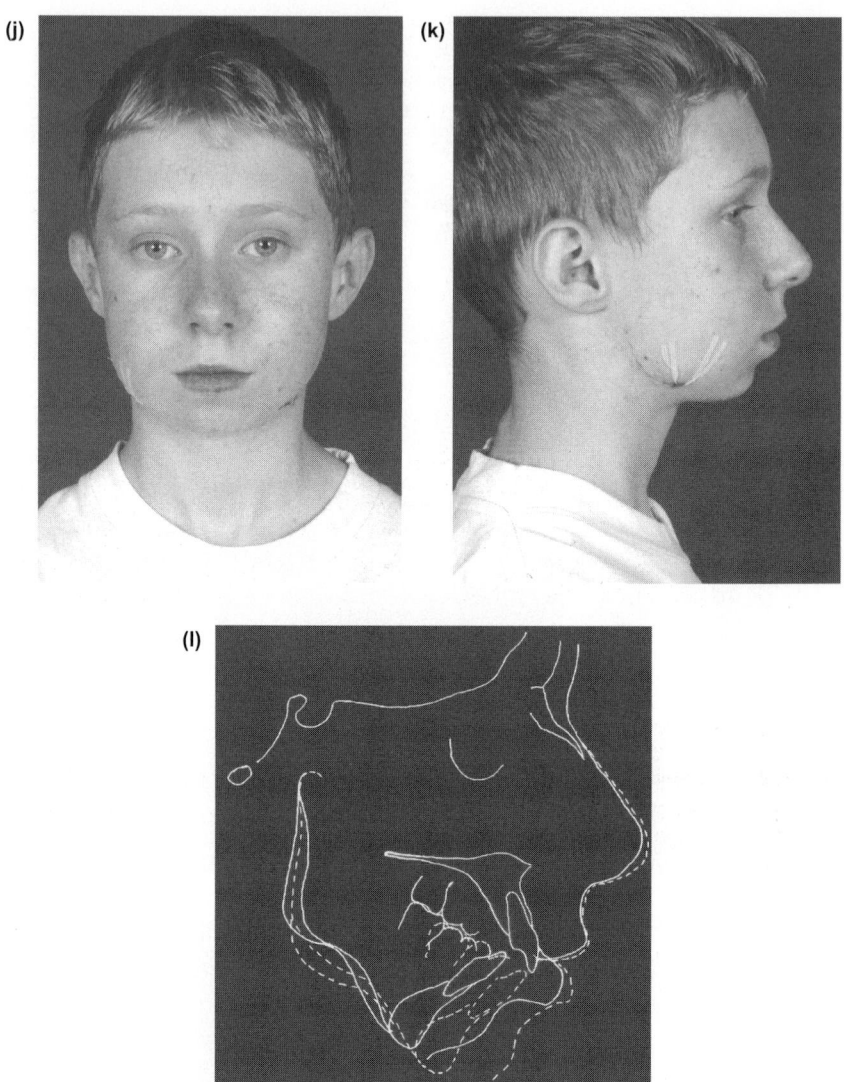

Figure 9.21   (j), (k), (l)

The cephalometric tracing (Figure 9.21l) shows that the vertical ramus height had increased 8 mm and the forward projection of the mandible increased by approximately 11 mm. The final pictures (Figures 9.21m and 9.21n) show the patient after an

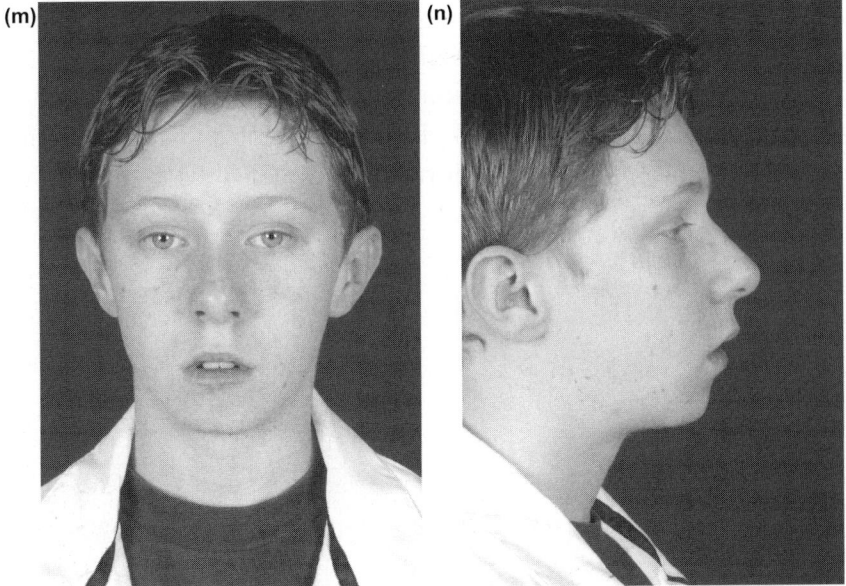

Figure 9.21   (m), (n)

additional advancement genioplasty. It is worth noting that all short mandibles require a supplementary genioplasty after a lengthening procedure.

Temporomandibular Joint Ankylosis (See Also Chapter 11)

The established treatment is to divide the condylar fusion at the base of skull, create an arthroplasty with a costochondral graft growth centre and a temporalis myofascial interpositional membrane, and perform bilateral coronoidotomies or coronoidectomies as temporalis myotomies to release the restraining muscular contractures. Distraction osteogenesis has the potential to make up the growth deficiency and provide the lost ramus height and mandibular length in a more predictable way.

Case 2. This patient presented with ankylosis of the right temporomandibular joint present since childhood and presumed to be due to middle ear infection. She had an opening of only 4–5 mm interincisally. The ankylosed right side showed the characteristic straight contour with reduced dimensions compared to

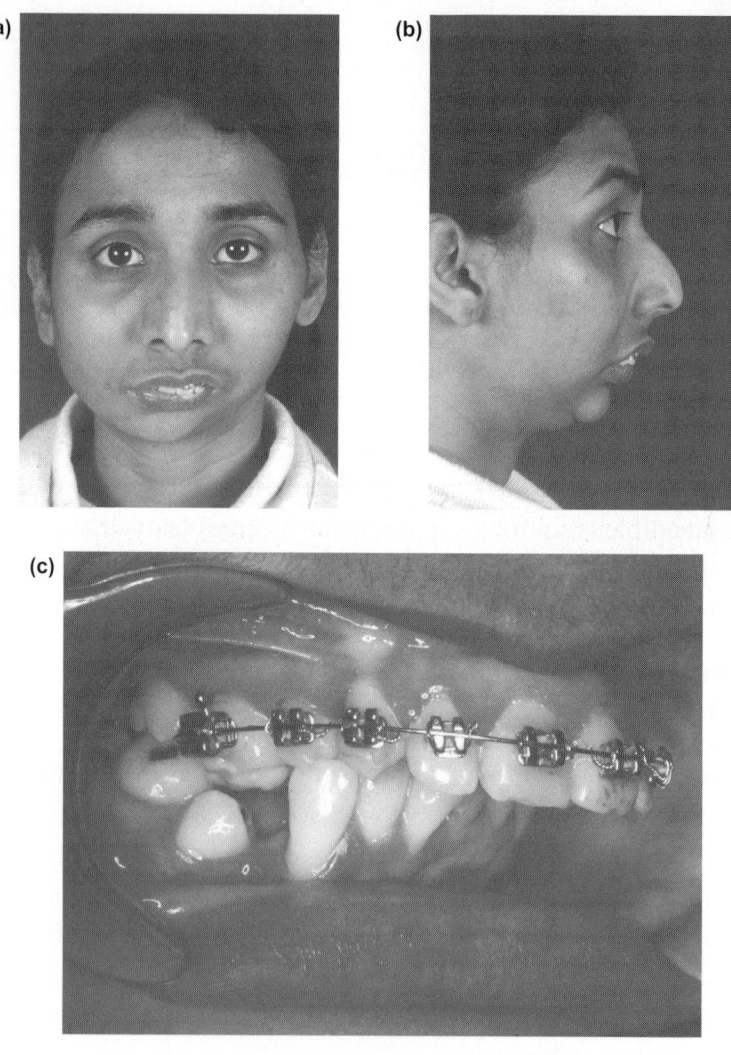

(a)

(b)

(c)

Figure 9.22   (a), (b), (c)

(d)

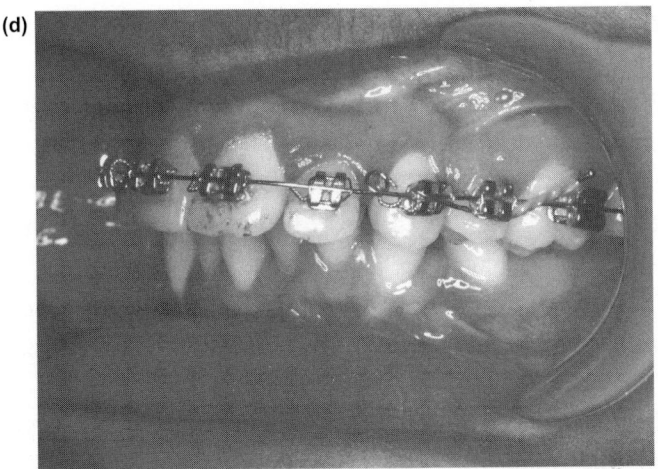

(e)

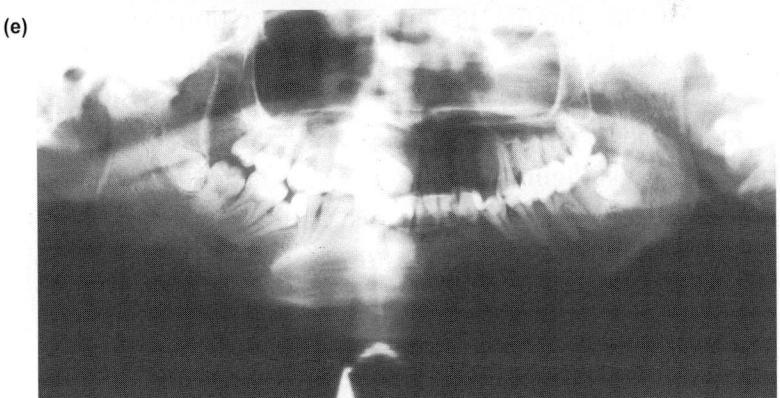

(f)

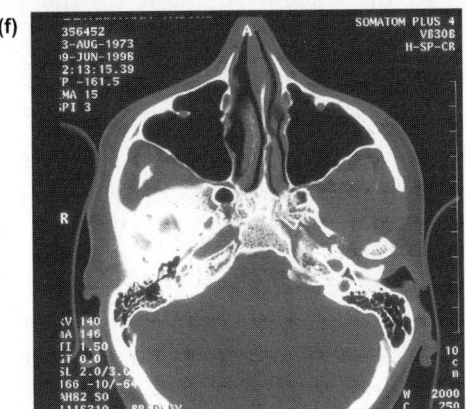

Figure 9.22   (d), (e), (f)

the contralateral side with its distorted deviation towards the ankylosis (Figures 9.22a and 9.22b).

There was a complete crossbite of the buccal teeth on the unaffected side, and with the limited opening it was not possible to access the lower teeth on the left side to place an orthodontic appliance (Figures 9.22c and 9.22d). The inverted mushroomlike ankylosed condyle may be seen on the OPG (Figure 9.22e). The degree of hypoplasia of the mandible is best appreciated on the axial views of the 3 dimensional CT scan. (Figures 9.22f to 9.22h).

A simple osteotomy was first performed on the right side at the angle of the mandible preserving the inferior dental bundle. Because of the limited opening, access required an extraoral approach and the impacted third molar was removed at the same time. The vector chosen was parallel to the lower border and a 15 mm distractor (Liebinger & Co.) was activated after a latent period of 5 days. Figures 9.22i and j show the patient's radiographs at the beginning and end of the distraction phase. Figures 9.22k and 9.22l show the distractor *in situ*, with an increased symmetrical appearance and chin projection. Figures 9.22m and 9.22n demonstrates the improved occlusal relationship. As the opening was now 20 mm it was possible to place an orthodontic appliance on the lower teeth as the buccal segment on the left side was no longer in crossbite.

A second phase of distraction using bilateral internal distractors was carried out 3 months later to correct the marked Class II relationship. It was now possible to place the second phase distractors from an intraoral route. The distractor on the right hand side was placed with a vector parallel to the lower border of the mandible, and the left hand distractor was placed with an oblique vector to increase mandibular height and take the posterior teeth out of premature contact. Distraction was continued for 15 days bilaterally at a rate of 1 mm per day following the

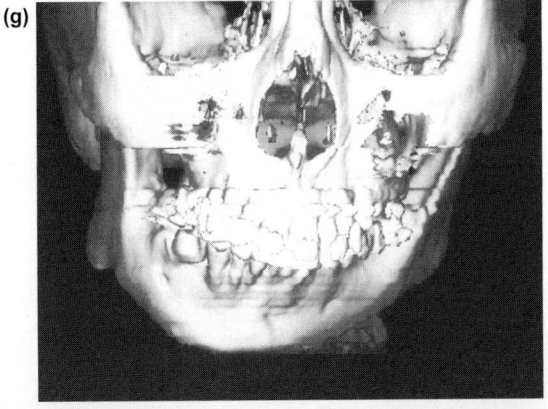

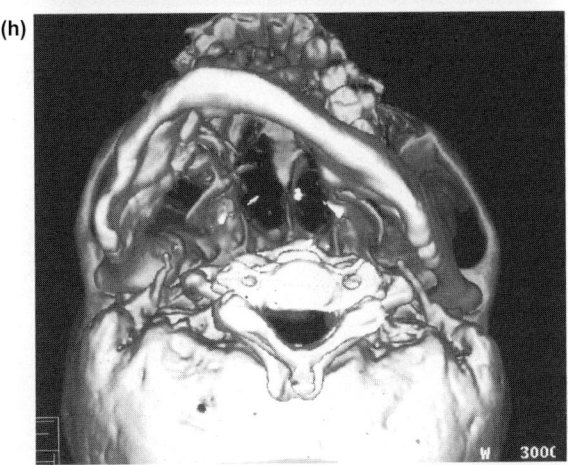

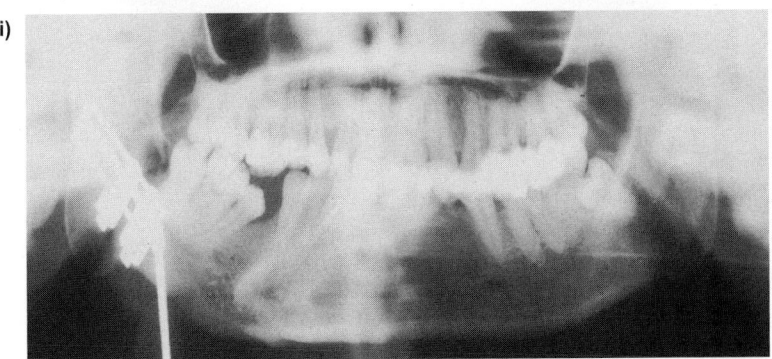

Figure 9.22   (g), (h), (i)

(j)

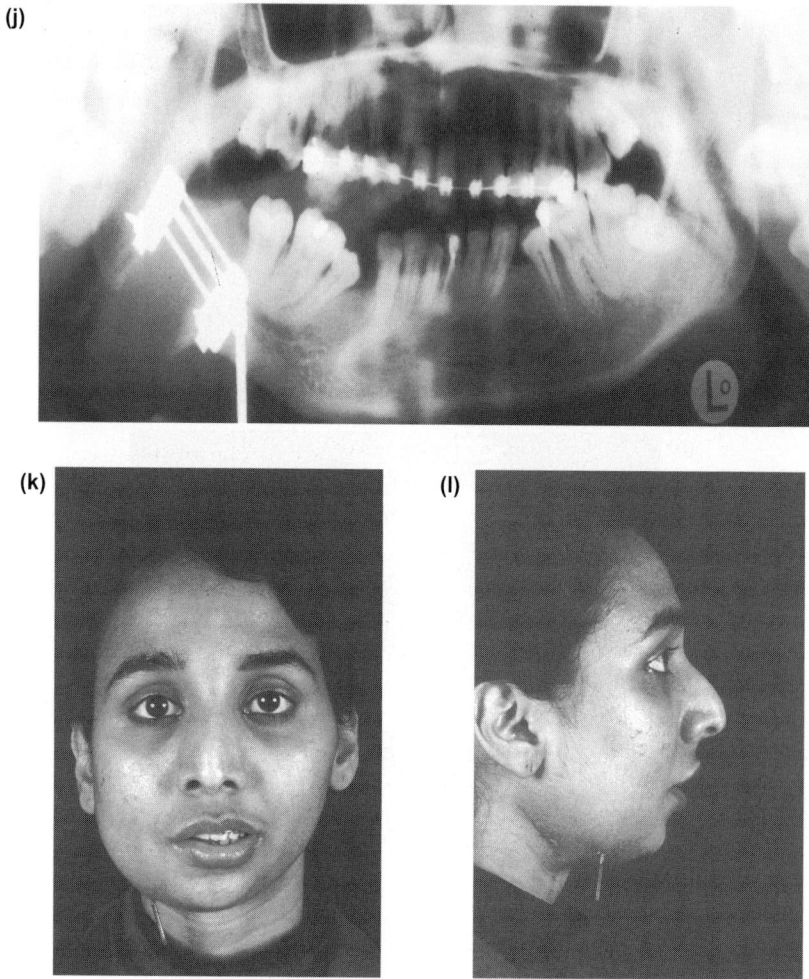

Figure 9.22   (j), (k), (l)

latent period. Figures 9.22o and 9.22p show the OPGs before and after distraction.

At the end of this period, the patient had an overcorrected edge to edge incisor occlusion to accommodate relapse, and an interincisal opening of 22 mm (Figures 9.22q and 9.22r). The final post orthodontic views are Figures 9.22s to 9.22u.

(m)

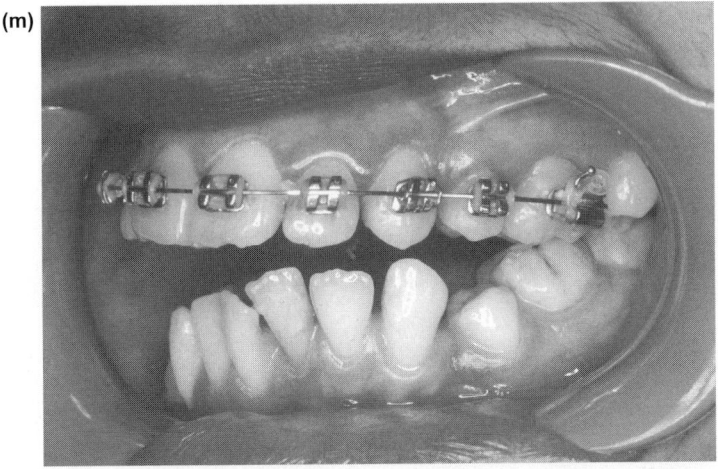

(n)

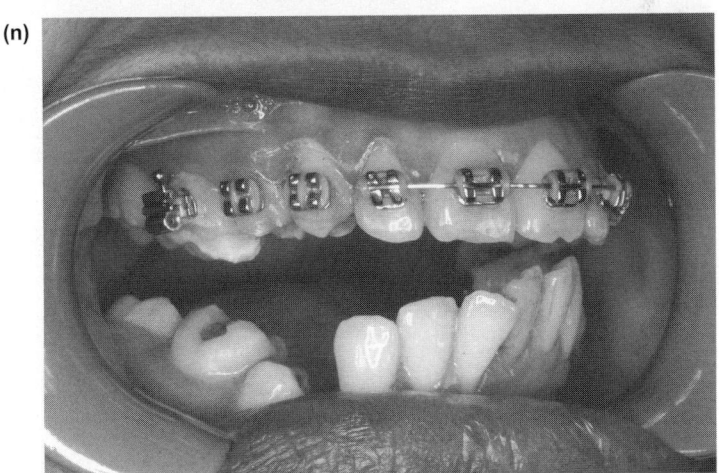

Figure 9.22   (m), (n)

Comment

An obvious question in this case is how has the jaw opening improved? The final opening of 22 mm is greater than can be expected from the innate elasticity of a fused craniomandibular complex. Placement of the second distractor confirmed complete healing of the first osteotomy site, hence a degree of pseudarthrosis may have formed

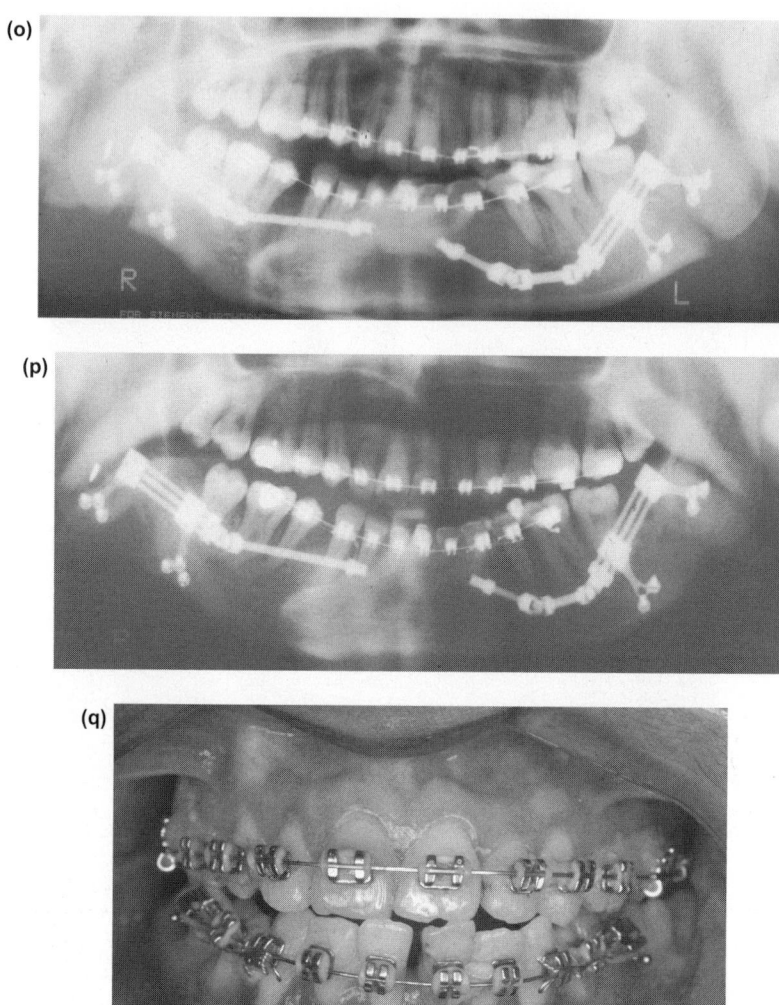

Figure 9.22   (o), (p), (q)

in the second osteotomy sites. Ideally, division of the joint ankylosis but conserving the residual condyle to create an arthroplasty, and coronoidectomies/otomies should be done at the same time as a vertical subsigmoid distraction osteotomy, with the placement of internal

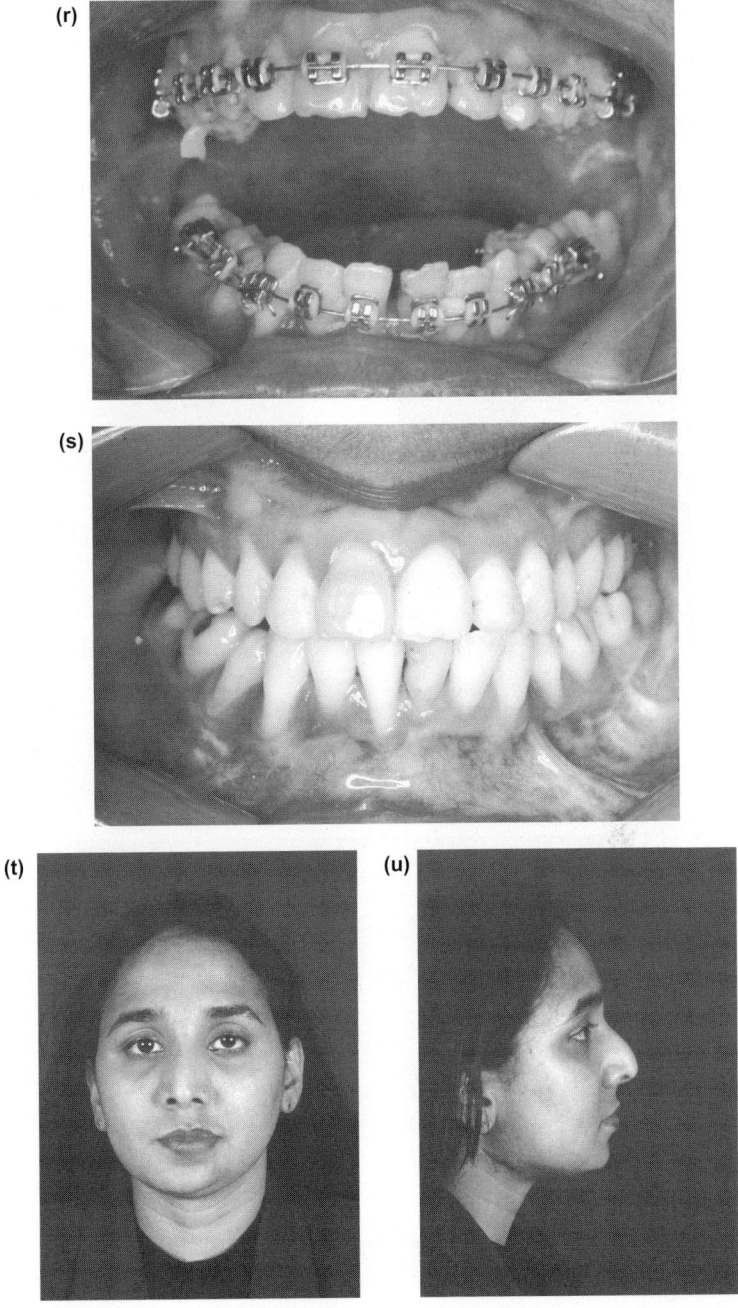

Figure 9.22   (r), (s), (t), (u)

distractors. However this case shows the significant correction possible with only a combination of distraction and orthodontics.

Maxillary Hypoplasia Due to Cleft Surgery

Early surgery for the repair of the cleft palate can damage the mid face growth potential giving rise to marked hypoplasia which with scarring of the integument renders conventional surgical

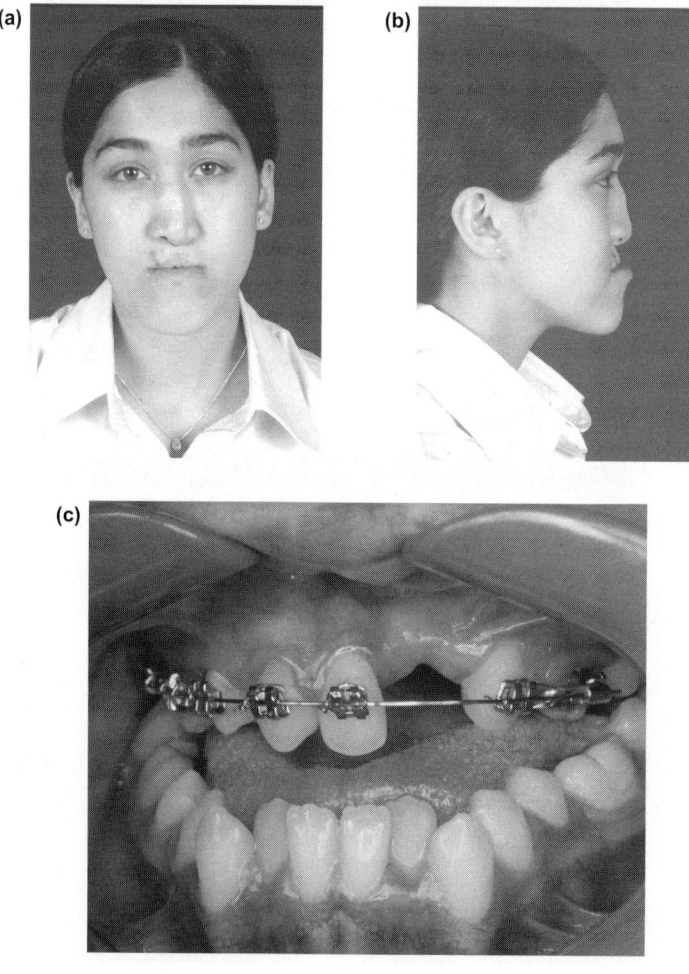

Figure 9.23   (a), (b), (c)

(d)

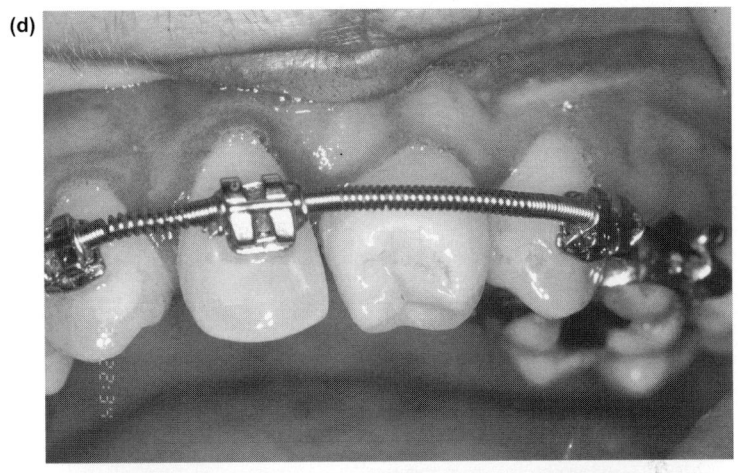

(e)

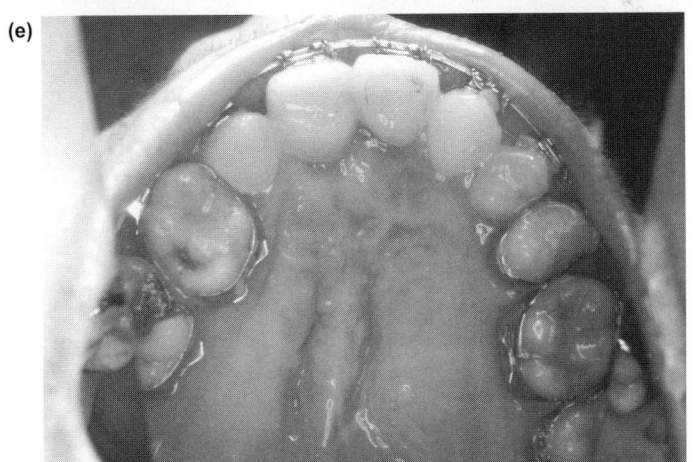

Figure 9.23   (d), (e)

advancement difficult and subject to relapse. Distraction osteogenesis requires a limited osteotomy and the gradual controlled traction can overcome the restraint of the scar tissue.

Case 3. This patient had a severe maxillary hypoplasia secondary to a cleft lip and palate deformity, with nasal hypoplasia due to absence of much of the septum (Figures 9.23a and 9.23b). There was

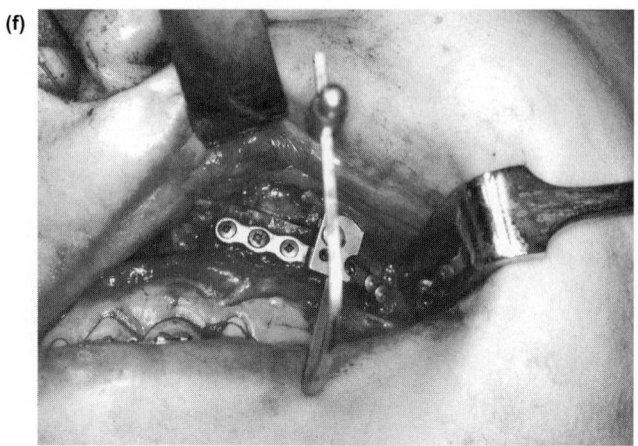

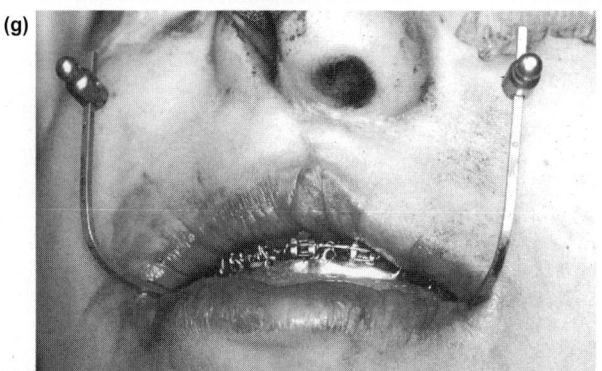

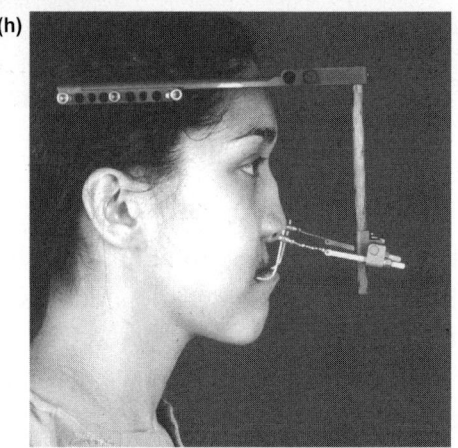

Figure 9.23   (f), (g), (h)

(i)

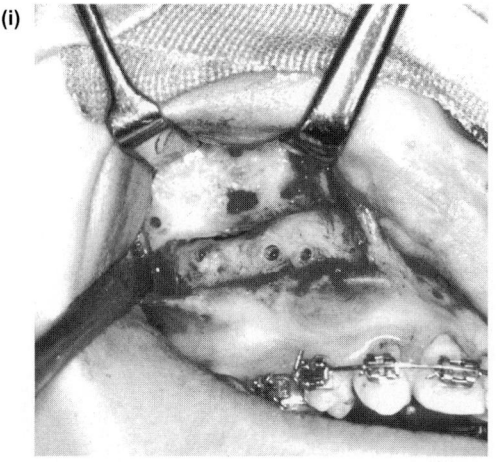

(j)

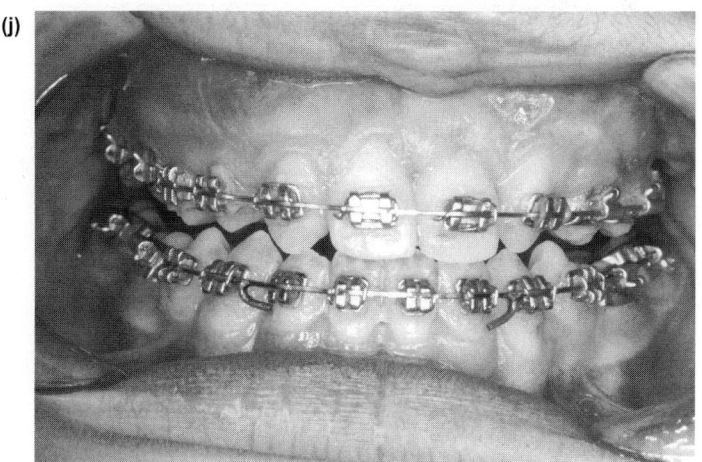

Figure 9.23   (i), (j)

also mild mandibular elongation. Dental radiographs confirmed the absence of both the upper central and lateral incisor on the cleft side. As orthodontic extractions were necessary in the lower arch one of the lower second premolars was transplanted into the upper left central incisor alveolar region. Figures 9.23c to 9.23e show the presurgical orthodontics, and the transplanted premolar contoured to simulate a central incisor.

(k)

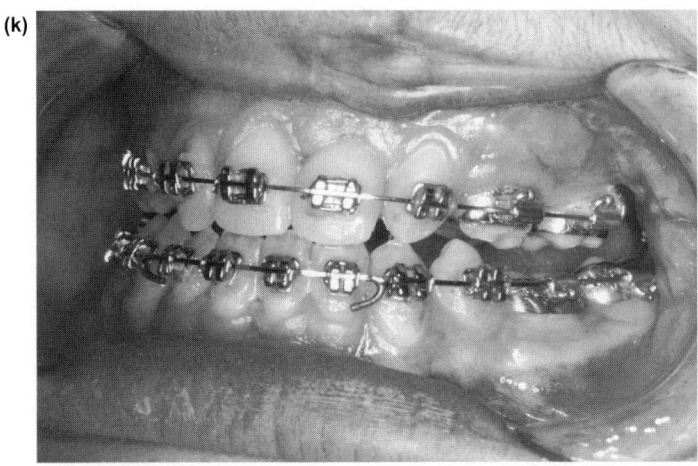

(l)

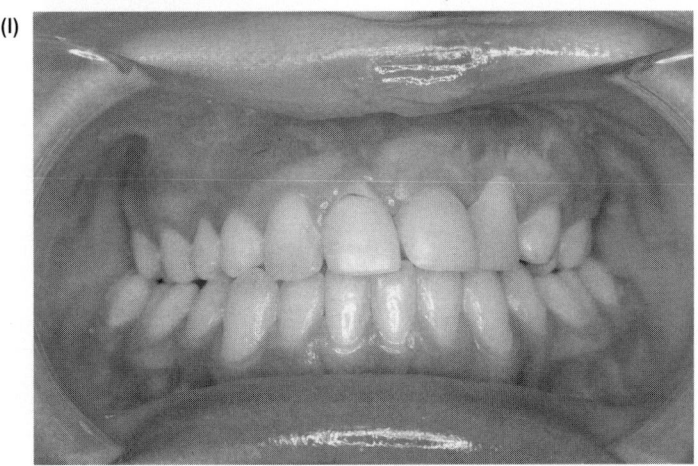

Figure 9.23   (k), (l)

A Le Fort I osteotomy was carried out with mobilisation, and an external halo distraction system was placed (Figures 9.23f and 9.23g) (Martin MLS/Red System). Following a latent period of 5 days, maxillary distraction was commenced at the rate of 1 mm a day and was continued for approximately 19 days. The halo (Figure 9.23h) was removed after a consolidation period of 6 weeks. At the time of removal very good bone regeneration at the

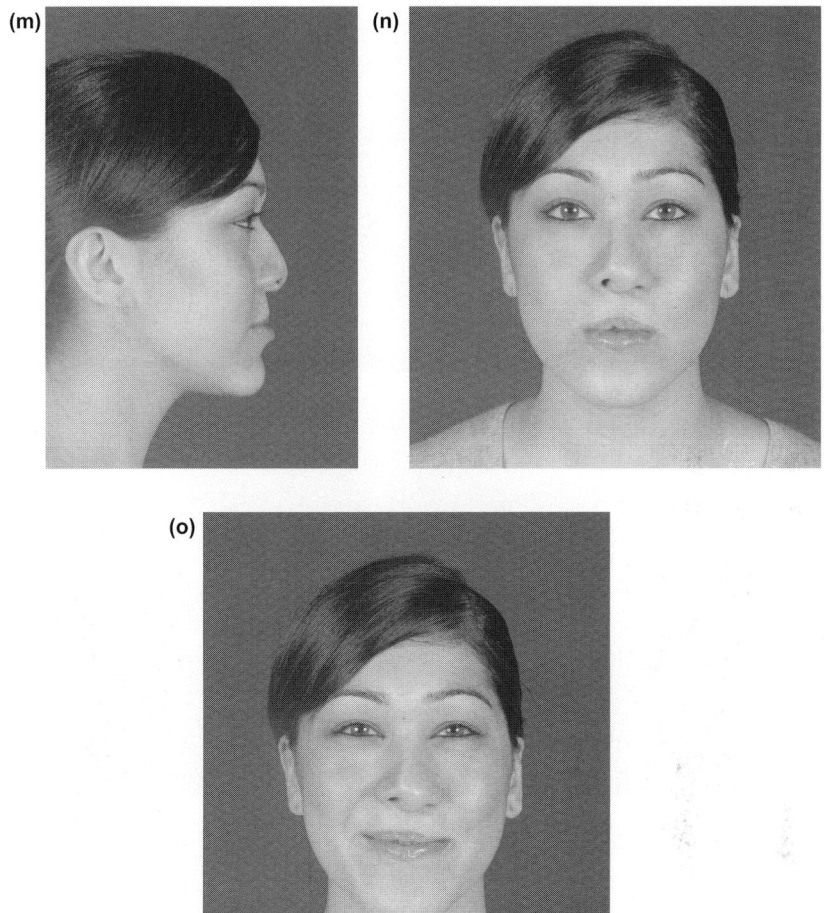

Figure 9.23   (m), (n), (o)

osteotomy site was noted (Figure 9.23i). Clinical photographs demonstrate the occlusion, full face and profile at the end of distraction (Figures 9.23j to 9.23o).

The patient subsequently had a rhinoplasty and a 5 mm mandibular pushback approximately 9 months after the end of maxillary distraction.

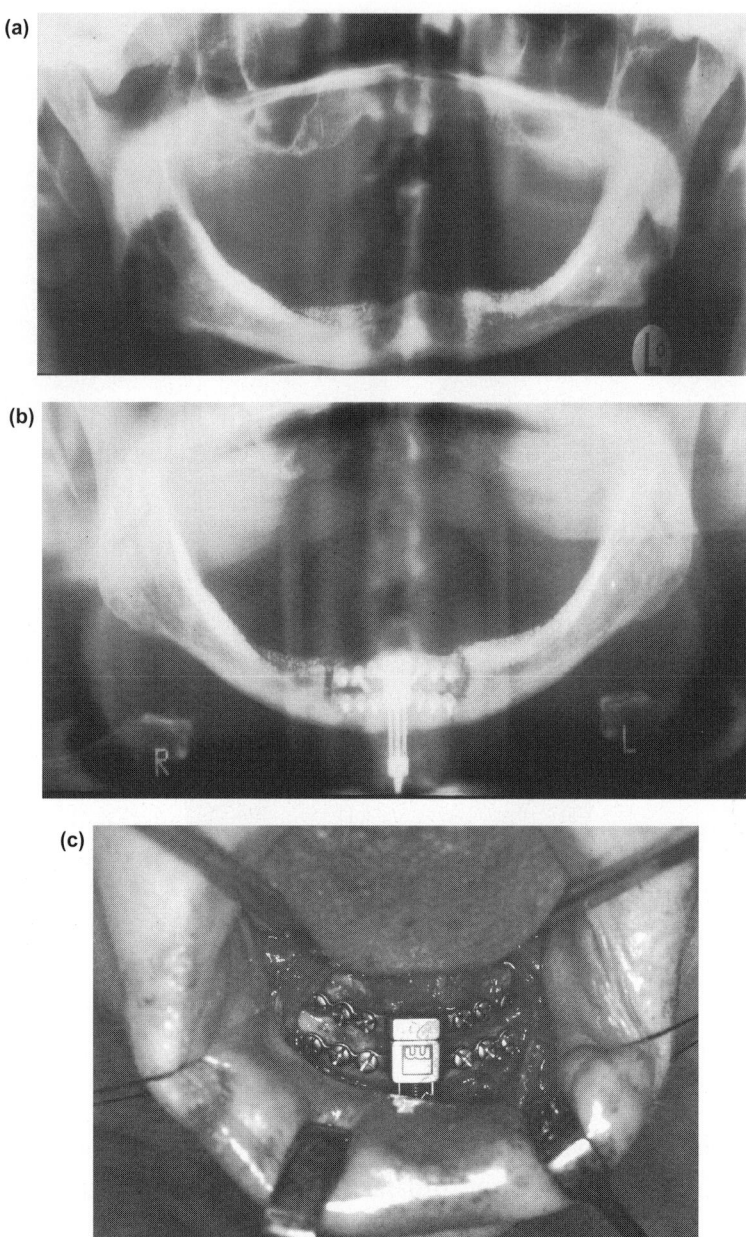

Figure 9.24   (a), (b), (c)

(d)

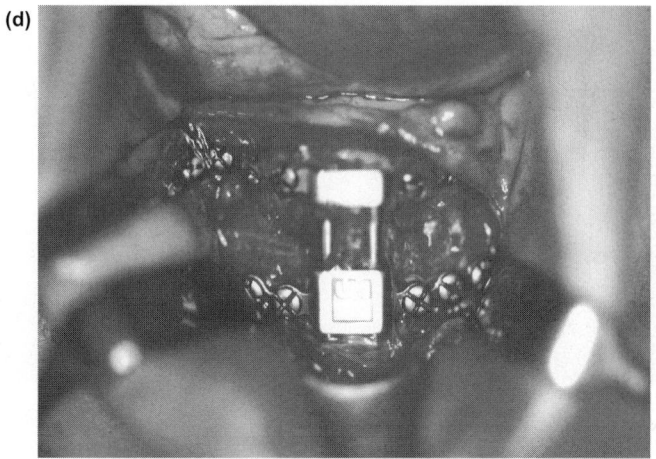

(e)

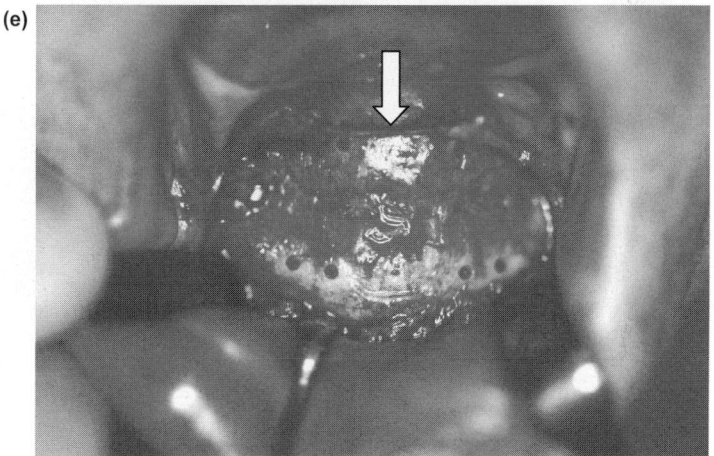

Figure 9.24 (d), (e)

Dento-Alveolar Distraction

Augmentation of the alveolus by onlay grafting is often difficult. It will provide increased width but not height, and in very atrophic cases it is subject to failure due to mucosal dehiscence leading to the loss of the graft material. Figure 9.24a shows the orthopantomograph

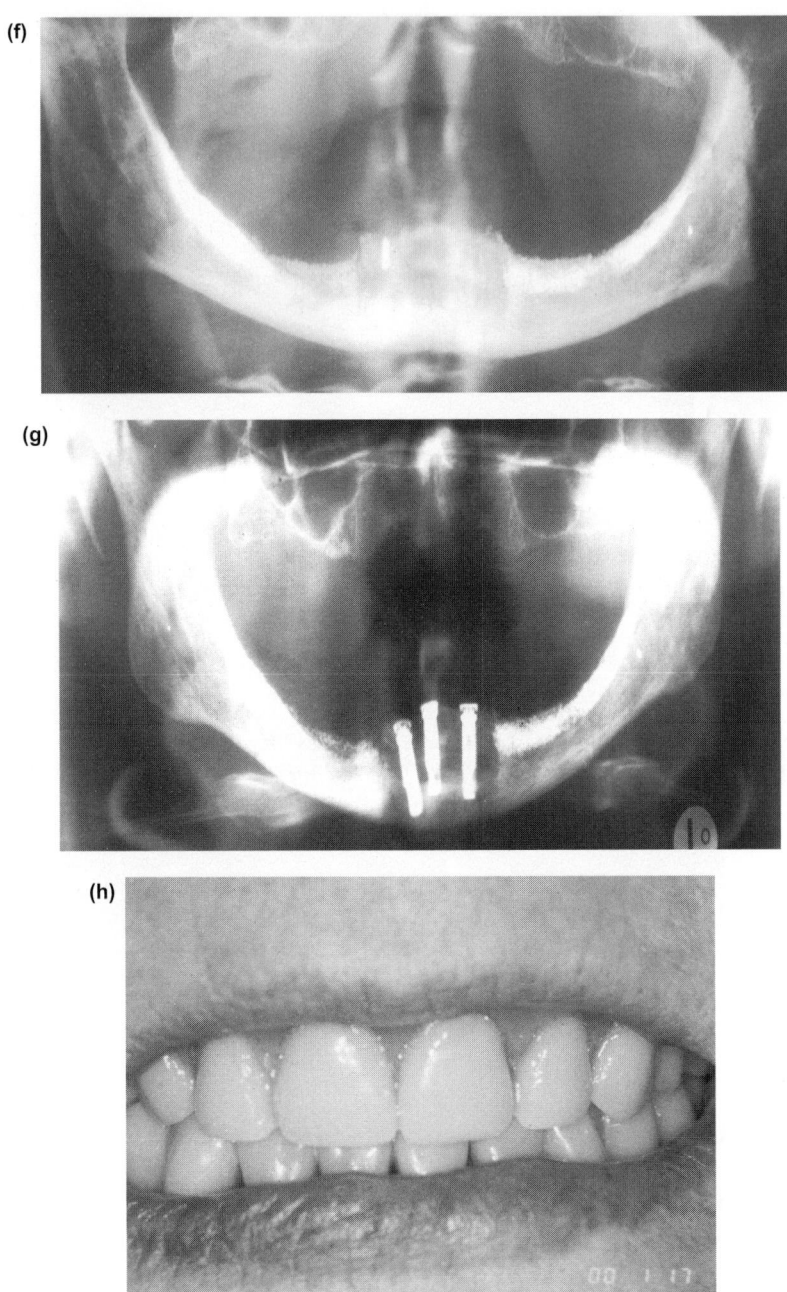

Figure 9.24 (f), (g), (h)

of an atrophic sharp ridge in the mandibular incisor region which made the wearing of a denture intolerably painful and unstable. Figures 9.24b and 9.24c show the alveolar osteotomy and the distractor in position. Figures 9.24d and 9.24e show the height of the distraction and the increased postdistraction bulk of bone both in height and width, completely eliminating the tender knife edge ridge. Figures 9.24f and 9.24g show radiographs of the distracted area and the insertion of three implants to support and stabilise the lower denture (Figure 9.24h).

Summary

Distraction osteogenesis can achieve multidimensional bone formation in situations where grafting is unsuitable or has failed. With rapidly improving mechanics the procedure is becoming more patient friendly and cost effective.

10

The Surgical Correction of Common Deformities

- **_Single Jaw Deformities_**
  Mandibular prognathism
  Mandibular asymmetry
  Mandibular retrognathism
  The chin
  Mandibular incisor proclination
  Maxillary hypoplasia
  Nasomaxillary hypoplasia
  Malar-maxillary hypoplasia
  Maxillary prognathism

- **_Bimaxillary Deformities_**
  Gross mandibular prognathism
  The deep overbite
  Bimaxillary proclination
  The long face
  The open bite (apertognathia)
  The large tongue
  The short face
  Maxillary asymmetry

- Unfortunately, the diagnosis of a facial deformity does not always suggest an operative solution. There may be a choice of procedures or the complexity requires several simultaneous osteotomies. This chapter considers both single jaw and bimaxillary deformities. As will be seen, there is usually an overlap and what appears to be a major single jaw problem invariably requires a bimaxillary solution.

• It is also impossible to classify all cases under one treatment group. For instance, a patient with a long face may have an open bite. Both treatment sections in this chapter should therefore be consulted.

• Although it is possible to describe horizontal and vertical deformities separately, they are surgically interdependent, in that a vertical osteotomy will produce a horizontal change and *vice versa*.

Timing

The choice of age for any orthognathic procedure can be difficult. The optimum age is when facial growth has finished. This is approximately 16 years for girls and 18 years for boys. Later maturation of the face can undo the benefit of a well-intentioned osteotomy. This is particularly true if the prognathic mandible is treated too early. The only exception is the rare unilateral condylar hyperplasia which may require ablation of the articular growth cartilage during adolescence to prevent a major degree of secondary deformity. As all young patients with jaw deformities require orthodontic treatment, this provides a period of scrutiny to monitor continued growth with study models and lateral skull radiographs, at yearly intervals. Wrist radiographs when considering abnormal facial growth and sequential technetium-99m bone scans are unhelpful.

Presurgical orthodontic treatment not only simplifies the operative procedure but also improves the occlusal and profile outcome.

However a decision must be made if surgery is to be the ultimate treatment of choice. The orthodontic decompensation for surgery for a jaw disproportion will be different from the pure orthodontic compensatory management to conceal the deformity, and will start later to reduce the period in appliance retention. Therefore, please read Chapter 4 (Orthodontic Preparation).

The neglected details of planning and data transfer and fixation are to be found in Chapters 7 and 8 and those for each operation are described in Chapter 9.

Single Jaw Deformities

Mandibular Prognathism

This is characterised by elongation of the mandible producing a negative overjet, with compensatory retroclination of the lower incisors, and proclination of the upper incisors. Both the dentition and jaws show a marked Class III relationship. Some patients also have an increased lower facial height which is automatically reduced when the mandible is displaced backwards, up an inclined occlusal plane (Figure 10.1).

Beware of seeing all negative overjets as cases of mandibular prognathism. With a mild mandibular protrusion in a man, the preferred aesthetic solution is often a forward movement of the maxilla, leaving a "strong chin". This profile correction may be predicted by padding out the upper lip with cotton wool or wax. The same cephalometric values in a female usually require a mandibular setback for aesthetic harmony. The occlusal correction is identical in both cases.

Most prognathous mandibles are associated with a degree of maxillary retrognathism with the need for a bimaxillary correction. This becomes clear after presurgical orthodontics with incisor decompensation (see below, Bimaxillary Deformities).

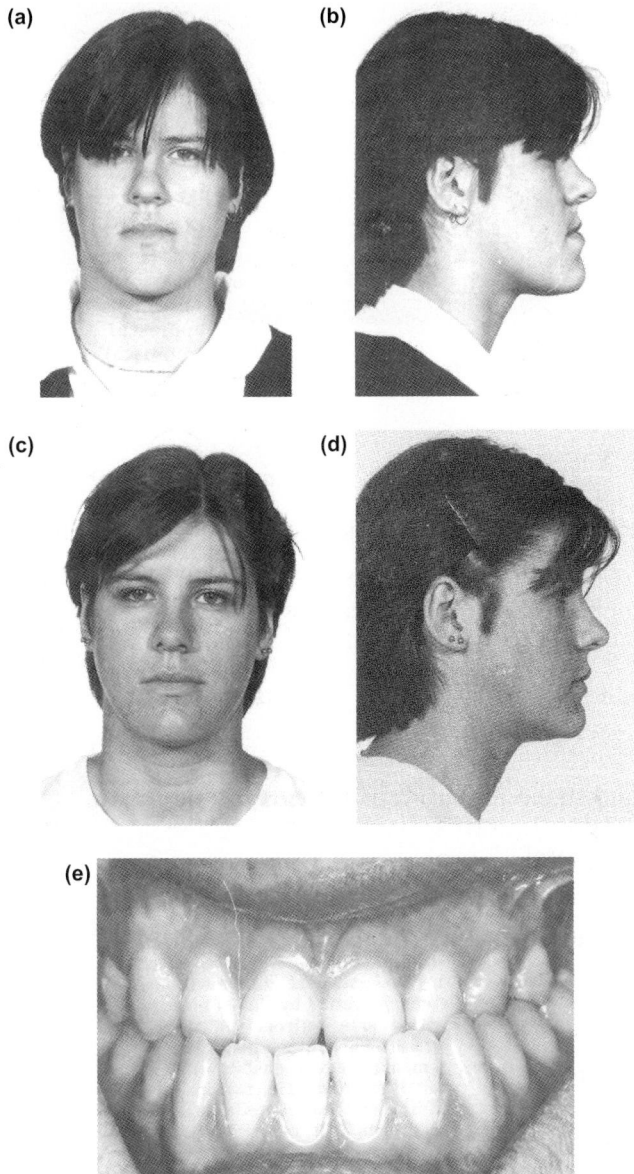

Figure 10.1 Mandibular prognathism requiring moderate orthodontic decompensation of the incisors followed by a sagittal split pushback. **(a)**, **(b)** and **(e)** Preoperative. **(c)**, **(d)** and **(f)** Postoperative.

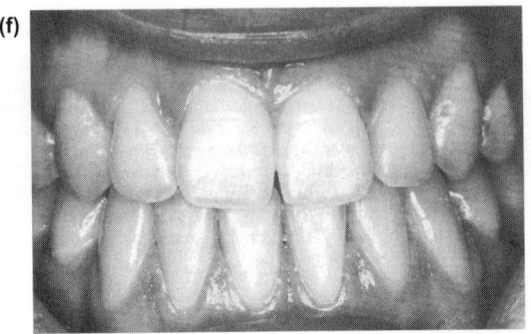

Figure 10.1   (*Continued*)

Treatment

Presurgical orthodontics will be required to correct arch size discrepancy, overcrowding and to decompensate the incisors. Posterior displacement of the mandible can be achieved by a:

1. sagittal split osteotomy,
    and less commonly,

2. oblique subcondylar (subsigmoid) osteotomy

    a) extraoral,
    b) intraoral (buccal approach), and
    c) intraoral (medial approach).

Mandibular Asymmetry (Unilateral Hyperplasia and Hypoplasia of the Mandible)

Introduction

There are two distinct types of asymmetrical overgrowth, but hybrid forms are occasionally found with both abnormalities merged on one side or even one of each deformity on opposite sides. Each deformity is frequently attributed to condylar hyperplasia. However, in both types the increased dimension arises beyond the accepted localised area of condylar growth.

Unilateral hypoplasias will be treated in the same manner as mandibular retrognathism, except when part of a hemifacial microsomia deformity, which will require additional attention to the difficult problem of soft tissue deficiency.

Beware of diagnosing asymmetry where a malocclusion is really causing a unilateral displacement of the mandible on closure.

Hemimandibular Elongation

This asymmetry presents with an increased ascending ramus width and length of the body on the affected side, with deviation of the dental and jaw midline to the contralateral side and a crossbite (Figure 10.2). The condylar head may be minimally enlarged compared with the normal side but the neck is elongated. The occlusal plane is undisturbed. Surgical correction should be delayed until the end of adolescent growth particualrly as some cases "creep on" to the end of the second decade.

Treatment

Presurgical Orthodontics

Insufficient maxillary intercanine width to accommodate the lower arch is not uncommon. Surgery should therefore be preceded by maxillary expansion. Where there is a gross discrepancy between the arches the maxillary arch may be expanded with a quadhelix appliance, which increases the width from behind forwards over a period of three to five months. However in such cases, tipping of the molars may relapse postoperatively and produce an anterior open bite. For this reason with large discrepancies surgical expansion of the maxilla may be the treatment of choice or distraction osteogenesis with a bone borne expansion appliance.

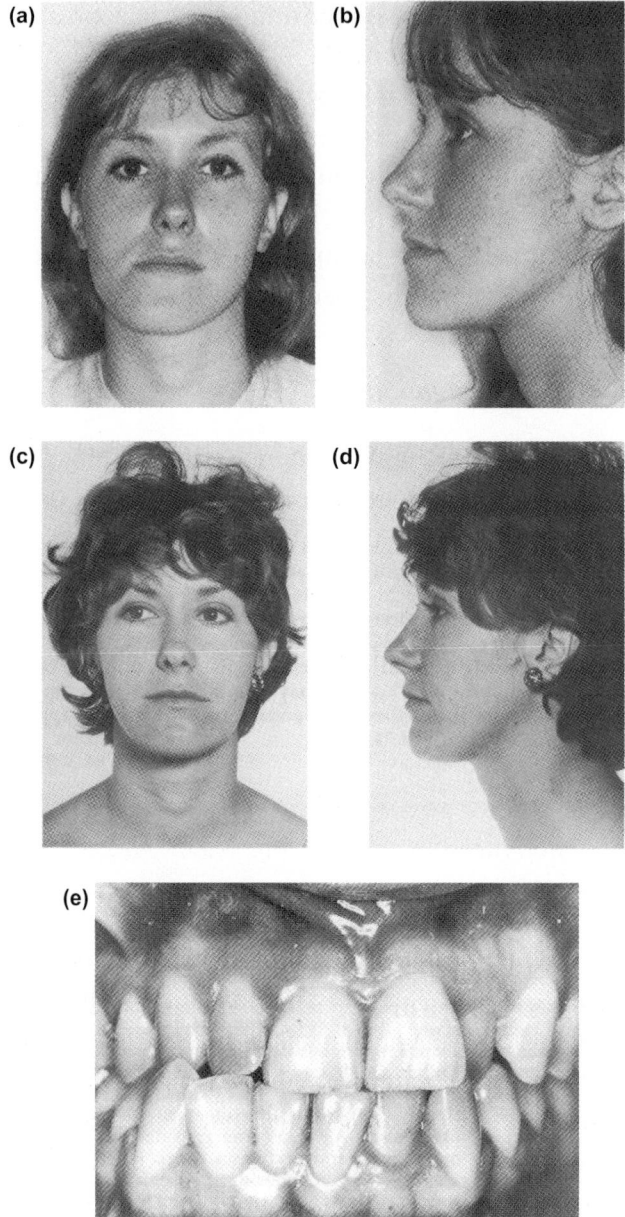

Figure 10.2   Left hemi-mandibular elongation with prognathism and deviation of the midline to the right, corrected by a bilateral sagittal split osteotomy. **(a)**, **(b)** and **(e)** Preoperative. **(c)**, **(d)** and **(f)** Postoperative.

(f)

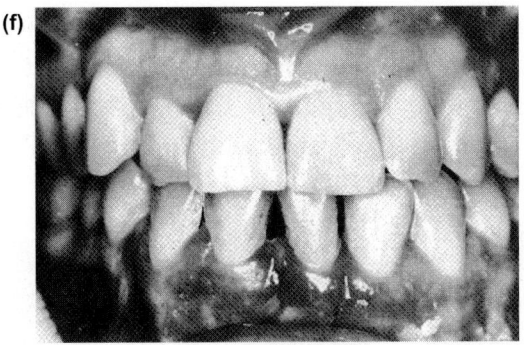

Figure 10.2 (*Continued*)

Surgery

Asymmetry, with or without prognathism, can be corrected by a bilateral ramus osteotomy, such as the sagittal split, which shortens the affected side and allows rotation at the contralateral angle.

Although correction of the bony deformity produces a marked improvement in appearance by eliminating both the unilateral deviation and prognathism, there is often a persistent asymmetry of the face in movement.

Recurrent growth creates a difficult decision and will require a careful high condylar shave preserving the meniscus.

Hemimandibular Hyperplasia

This type of mandibular asymmetry often starts dramatically with the pubertal growth spurt, although it is detectable earlier. Other cases appear to develop insidiously during adolescence. Another enigma is the principal site of overgrowth. Although often considered to be a condylar hyperplasia, there is, in addition to the considerably enlarged condylar head and ascending ramus, a convex downward growth of the lower border of the mandibular body which extends as far forward as the midline. Initially this creates an ipsilateral lateral open bite followed by secondary maxillary alveolar growth. When all mandibular growth is complete, there is an overall hemimandibular hyperplasia and an occlusal cant down to the affected side but no deviation of the midline (Figure 10.3). The inferior dental neurovascular bundle is carried downwards with this growth. This seems to be

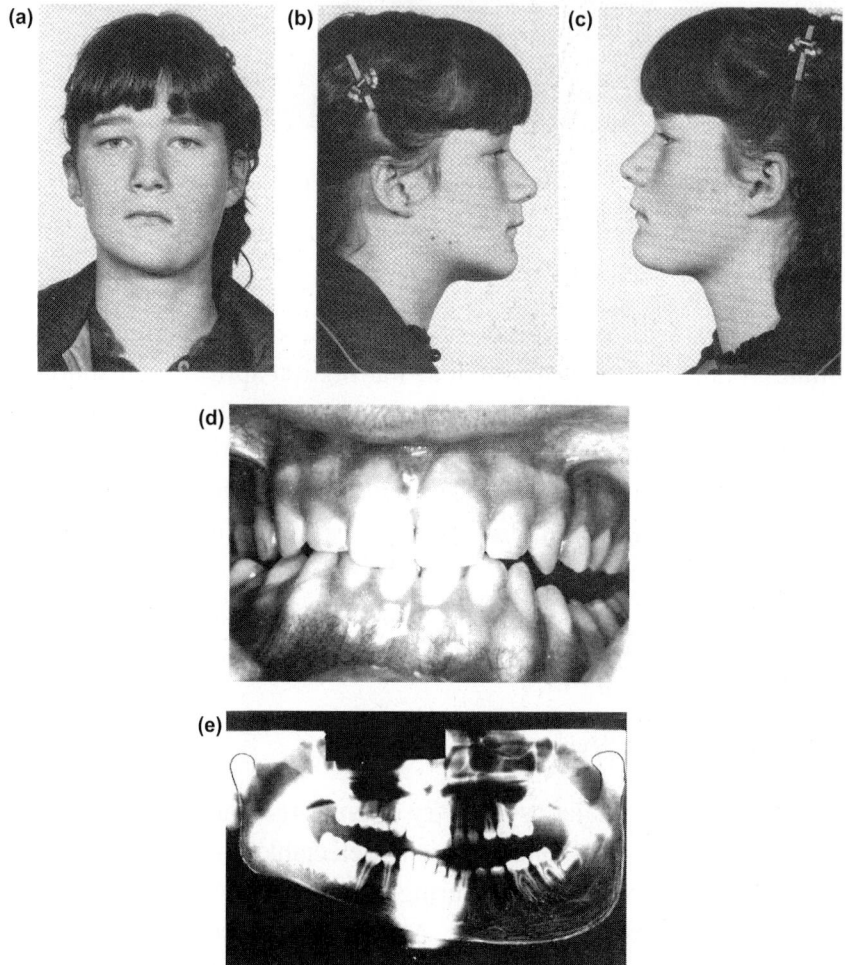

Figure 10.3 (a) to (e) This left hemi-mandibular hyperplasia dramatically occurred over 6 months at the onset of puberty. There is no horizontal displacement of the lower midline despite the increase in vertical dimensions producing a lateral open bite.

associated with hyperplasia of the associated mylohyoid muscle in the same way as masseteric hyperplasia produces an enlarged square gonial angle. Excess growth appears to cease in most cases at the end of puberty. It is interesting to see the ipsilateral antral floor is also lower due to remodelling following the alveolar downgrowth.

Treatment

Early

When seen early, the aim of surgery is to reduce ramus height before the secondary alveolar growth creates a permanent asymmetry with an oblique cant of the occlusal plane. It is tempting to remove part or all of the condyle to ablate the growth centre, i.e. a partial condylectomy. However, not only does the excess growth take place throughout the hemimandible beyond the influence of the condylar growth area, but it has usually finished by the time the deformity is diagnosed. Therefore, at this stage, surgical damage to the joint mechanism would seem unwarranted. A simple approach is a subsigmoid osteotomy, either intraorally or extraorally, to bring the teeth into occlusion. Later the increased depth of the body of the mandible can be corrected with trimming of the lower border and this can be done extraorally through a skin crease incision (see below) or if access permits, intraorally. However the displaced neurovascular bundle must be protected.

Late

Where compensatory alveolar growth has taken place, bringing the separated buccal segment teeth into occlusion, the most economical correction is simply reducing the lower border convexity. This improves the facial appearance and corrects the obliquity of the mouth, but not the occlusal plane (Figure 10.4). However, if desired, the downward tilt of the occlusal plane can be corrected with a bimaxillary procedure elevating the maxilla with a Le Fort I osteotomy (see Maxillary Asymmetry) and the mandible must then be adjusted to this horizontal occlusal plane, either by a sagittal split or subcondylar osteotomy. Finally, the convex lower border will still need to be trimmed. This is sometimes possible intraorally but is more easily achieved in conjunction with an external subcondylar osteotomy through the same skin incision.

Rarely, when all growth seems to have ceased and the deformity has been corrected, the condylar cartilage may suddenly spring to life again. This justifies a condylar cartilage trimming procedure with careful preservation of the meniscus.

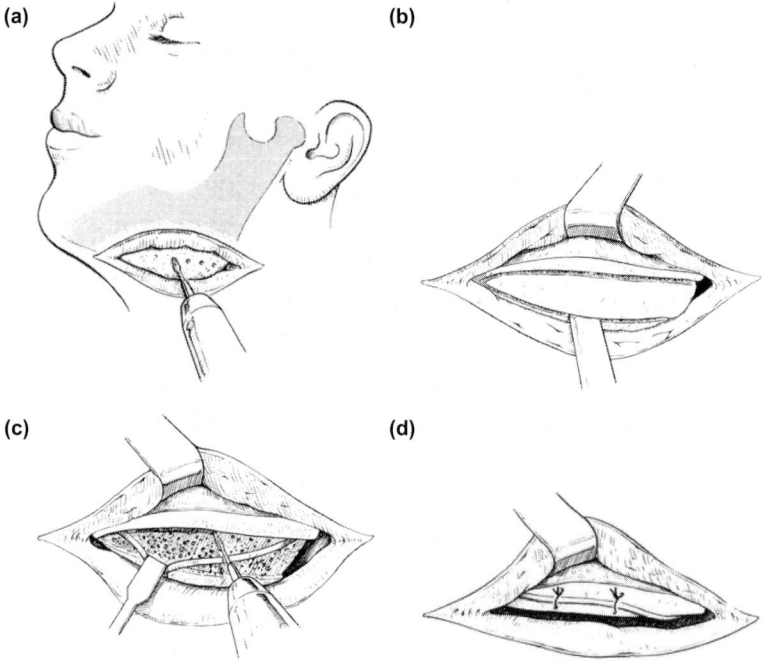

Figure 10.4 Lower border cortical split to expose and preserve the neurovascular bundle prior to trimming the excess depth of mandible. **(a)** The outer cortical plate is removed. **(b)** If the neurovascular bundle is found within the hyperplastic lower border, it is dissected from its canal and retracted prior to resection of the inner cortical plate **(c)** and **(d)**. An adult left-sided hemimandibular hyperplasia where the lateral open bite has closed spontaneously

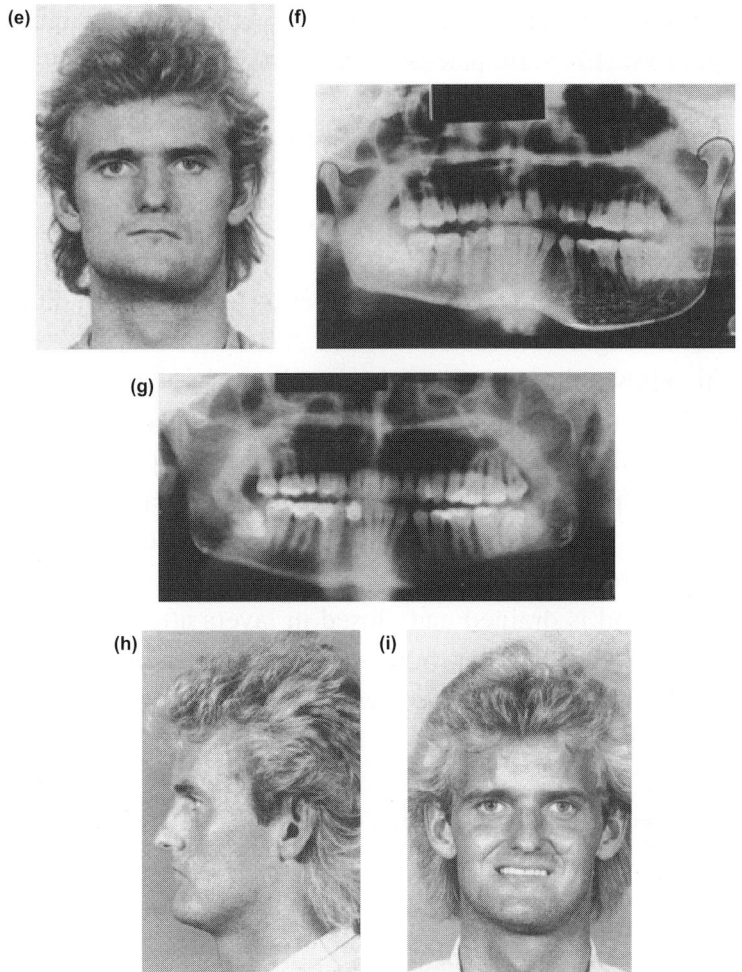

Figure 10.4 (*Continued*) leaving an ipsilateral downward slope of the occlusal plane. The external deformity has been corrected by trimming the lower border of the mandible through an external approach. (**e**) and (**f**) Preoperative. (**g**) to (**i**) Postoperative.

Trimming the convex mandibular lower border (Figure 10.4).

1. An aesthetic incision is made in a low skin increase, or where a crease might be anticipated. The mandible is exposed subperiosteally.

2. The lower border excess is outlined with bur holes, using the normal side for comparison (Figure 10.4a).
3. These holes are then joined together, cutting only through the outer cortex so as not to damage the inferior dental neurovascular bundle, which is invariably near the lower border.
4. A similar cortical bur cut is then made along the lower and posterior border and the excess outer cortex can then be split off with an osteotome, which is inserted in the lower cut, and rotated (Figure 10.4b).
5. This allows the neurovascular bundle to be exposed by carefully trimming off its overlying shell of compact bone.
6. The bundle is retracted and the excess lingual plate is trimmed off and the margins smoothed (Figures 10.4c and 10.4d). The neurovascular bundle is then left loosely sutured above the new lower border.
7. The wound is drained and closed in layers after loosely suturing the neurovascular bundle into the deep aspects of the wound. The skin is sutured with a continuous subcuticular 3/0 Prolene suture.

Figures 10.4e–10.4i shows such a case.

Condylar Hypoplasia

Occasionally it can be difficult to decide whether the asymmetry is the result of unilateral overgrowth or contralateral deficiency. Most unilateral hypoplasias appear to follow neonatal or childhood condylar damage with preservation of the meniscus. In addition to deviation of the chin to the affected side, the condyle is usually short, flattened or deformed. An exaggerated antegonial notch is present on the affected side. As the deficiency in ramus height gives rise to a secondary restriction in maxillary growth, the asymmetry is also reflected in the transverse occlusal plane. This is tilted downwards towards the normal side. Loss of the meniscus through a fracture displacement or destruction by infection or juvenile arthritis may lead to joint ankylosis and an even greater asymmetry due to the lack of functional stimulation to the growing mandible. Such cases require reconstruction of the joint with a costochondral graft (see Chapter 13).

Treatment

Moderate degrees of hypoplasia may be treated like an asymmetrical hyperplasia, with a bilateral sagittal split osteotomy. This will lengthen the affected side and provide a rotation adjustment on the normal side. However, the maxillary occlusal plane has to be levelled first. In adolescence this can be achieved orthodontically after the mandibular surgery by creating a lateral open bite intraoperatively with a unilateral thickened occlusal wafer or splint. The lateral space to be created may be estimated by examining the models mounted with a face-bow on an anatomical articulator. In most cases, a little excess is desirable. Following the sagittal split osteotomy the buccal teeth are brought into occlusion orthodontically (Figure 10.5).

With a large unilateral deficiency, or where there has been previous ramus surgery, the downward and forward mandibular reconstruction can only be achieved with an inverted L osteotomy and interpositional bone graft or distraction osteogenesis (see Chapter 9). Again, the maxillary occlusal plane will also require correction. If the patient is an adult, a Le Fort I osteotomy will be necessary to level the transverse occlusal tilt, and precedes the mandibular correction as part of a bimaxillary operation (see also Maxillary Asymmetry).

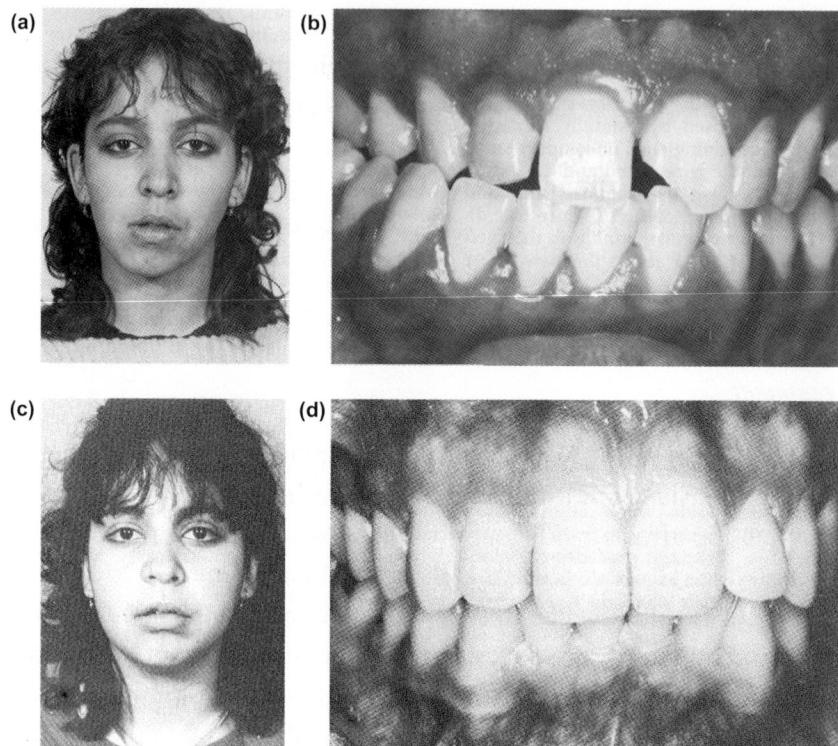

Figure 10.5   Post-traumatic right condylar hypoplasia treated with an inverted L bone graft to increase ramus height and correct the midline deviation. Postoperative orthodontics is used to achieve a horizontal occlusal plane. **(a)** and **(b)** Preoperative. **(c)** and **(d)** Postoperative.

Mandibular Retrognathism or Hypoplasia

The retrognathic mandible is either too small, i.e. a short Go-Pg, or set too far back with an increased saddle angle (NSAr) or a combination of both.

These cases may be classified as mild to marked skeletal Class II division 1 malocclusions. However, as with unilateral hypoplasias, there are both congenital and acquired forms of this deformity. The more severe, "bird face" deformity can be inherited, or acquired *in utero* as in the congenital Robin syndrome. One of the common features of this inherited form is a beak-shaped nose, which may also require reduction. In all cases the lower lip and tongue produce a secondary deformity of the maxilla, with dentoalveolar proclination and a narrow arch.

The severe acquired form follows bilateral loss of the condylar growth centres and is usually due to childhood trauma, in which case the condyles are small with no neck, and stigma of a submental scar may be found (Figure 10.6). Occasionally, the patient may have suffered juvenile rheumatoid arthritis (Still's disease).

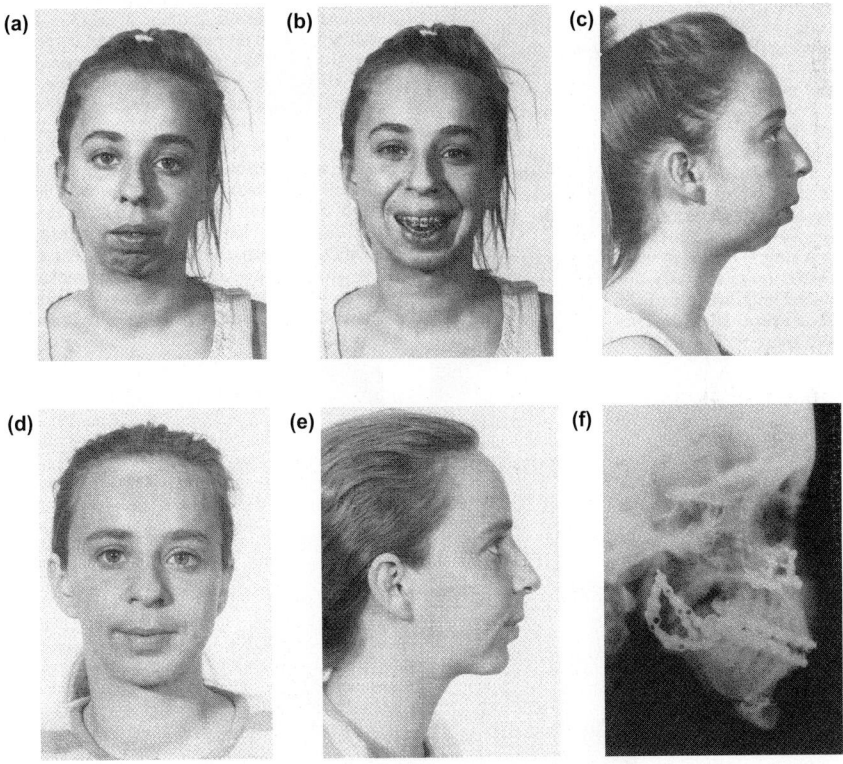

Figure 10.6 Marked retrognathia and an anterior open bite due to bilateral condylar damage in childhood **(a)**, **(b)** and **(c)**. Correction by a combination of a Le Fort I posterior impaction to close the open bite, and a bilateral inverted L advancement with interpositional bone grafts. The augmentation genioplasty was carried out simultaneously **(d)**, **(e)** and **(f)**.

Ankylosis only occurs when the meniscus is also displaced or destroyed, allowing the condyle to proliferate against the surface of the condylar fossa. In such cases the lack of function leads to a greater loss of mandibular development. The management of temporomandibular joint ankylosis will be discussed in Chapter 13.

Clinically there is an increased overjet which is usually exaggerated by the lower lip being trapped behind the upper incisors, increasing their proclination and spacing (Figure 10.7). Externally this is seen as an everted lower lip exaggerating the labiomental groove.

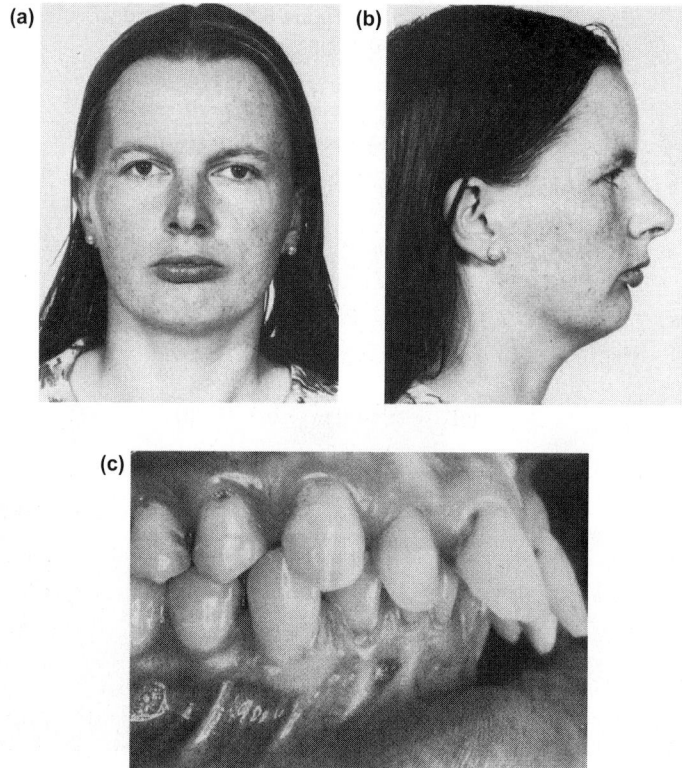

(a)   (b)   (c)

Figure 10.7 Surgical correction of mandibular retrognathism by a sagittal split advancement, after orthodontic incisor retroclination and levelling of the occlusal plane. Note to dramatic improvement of the lower lip contour as well as the skeletal profile. **(a)** to **(c)** Preoperative and preorthodontic therapy. **(d)** to **(f)** Postorthodontic therapy and surgery.

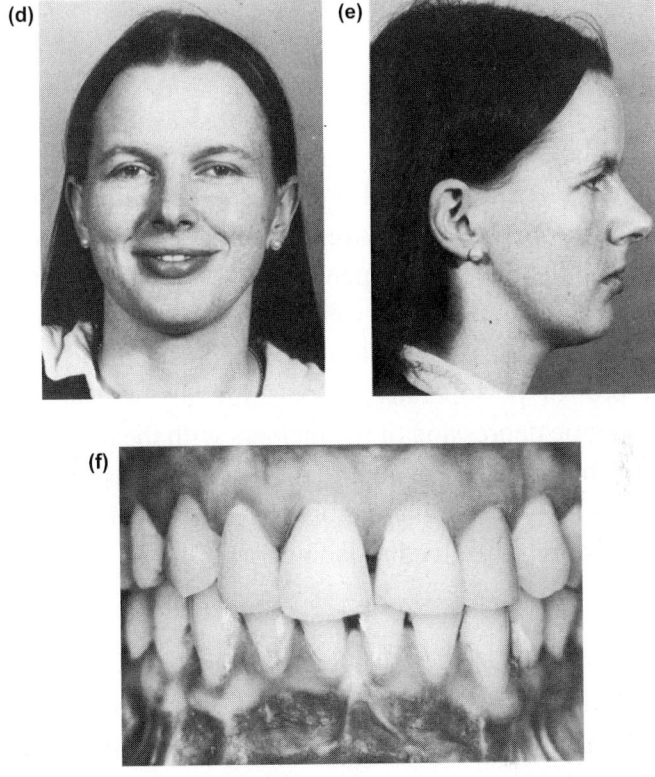

Figure 10.7 (*Continued*)

With unopposed occlusal drift (overeruption) of the lower incisors, the overbite is also increased.

The reduced lower facial height is a secondary aesthetic defect which may be self-correcting with the forward repositioning of the mandible.

A simple means of visualising the surgical correction is to study the face and profile before and after protruding the mandible. Before protrusion the chin will be set back and there will be a relatively low anterior facial height. With forward movement, not only does the profile improve but there is also an aesthetic gain from the increased lower facial height as the mandible moves downwards and forwards on the occlusal plane.

Treatment

The Occlusion

1. As will be seen clinically and on the study models, the over erupted lower incisors will prevent the mandible being moved forward into a satisfactory relationship without a lateral open bite. In adults this lateral open bite will not be self-corrected by postoperative compensatory eruption of the molars and premolars. Some means of levelling the occlusal plane orthodontically pre- or postoperatively, or surgically will be necessary. Orthodontic depression of the incisors with the associated eruption of the posterior segments may not be possible to achieve preoperatively in adults without the lower incisors being proclined through the alveolar labial cortex.

    The choices are:

    a) Decompensation of the incisors and a forward osteotomy of the mandible to an overcorrected edge to edge incisor relationship, giving a three-point contact occlusion, i.e. incisors and distal molars, followed by orthodontic closure of the lateral open bites. However, this is only possible if there is sufficient interdental space in the buccal segments to allow the premolars and molars to erupt from the perimeter of a curve into the shorter horizontal straight line.
    b) Separate orthodontic levelling of the canine and incisors, and the buccal segments. This will be followed by a lower anterior mandibulotomy setdown carried out at the same time as the mandibular lengthening procedure. This has the advantage of providing an additional supplement to the lower facial height. Figure 10.8 shows the increase in lower facial height and improved lip and chin profile after forward repositioning of the mandible with a lower incisor setdown achieved by an anterior mandibulotomy.

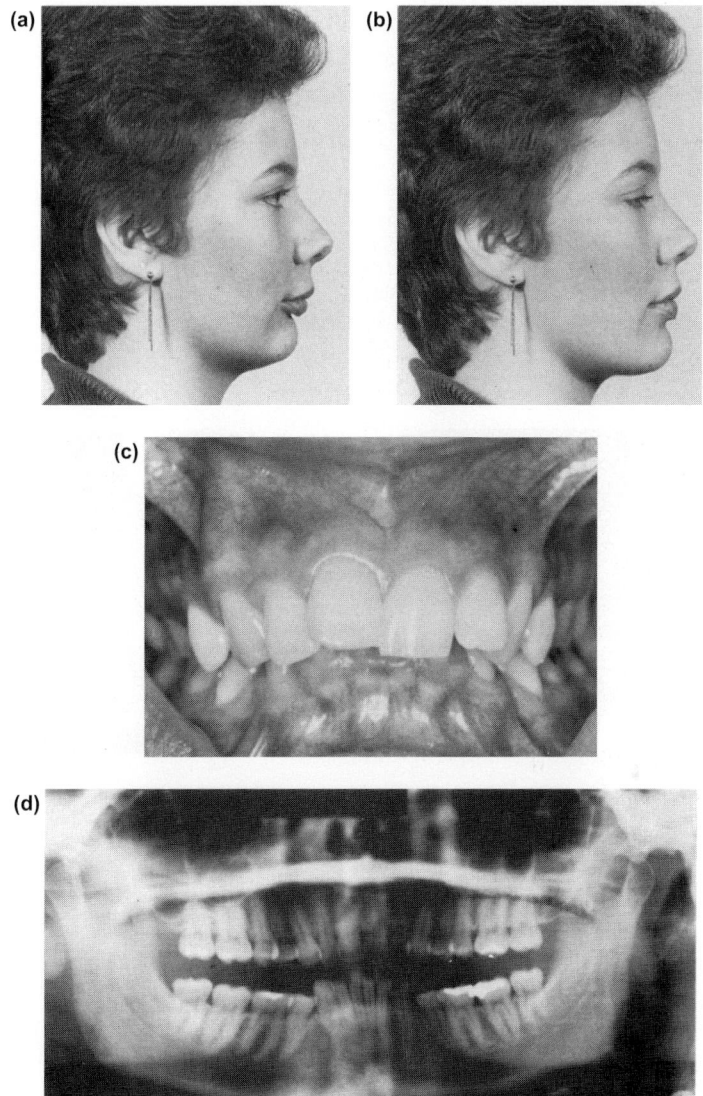

Figure 10.8 An anterior mandibulotomy combined with a forward osteotomy not only flattens the occlusal plane but also increases the chin depth. (**a**) Shows the preoperative profile in occlusion and (**b**) with the mandible postured forwards stimulating the surgical advancement. (**c**) to (**e**) The preoperative occlusion and radiographs before orthodontics and (**f**) after levelling the incisor and buccal segments independently. (**g**) to (**k**) Postoperative results. (**k**) The immediate postoperative orthopantomogram which shows the mandibulotomy cuts and set down.

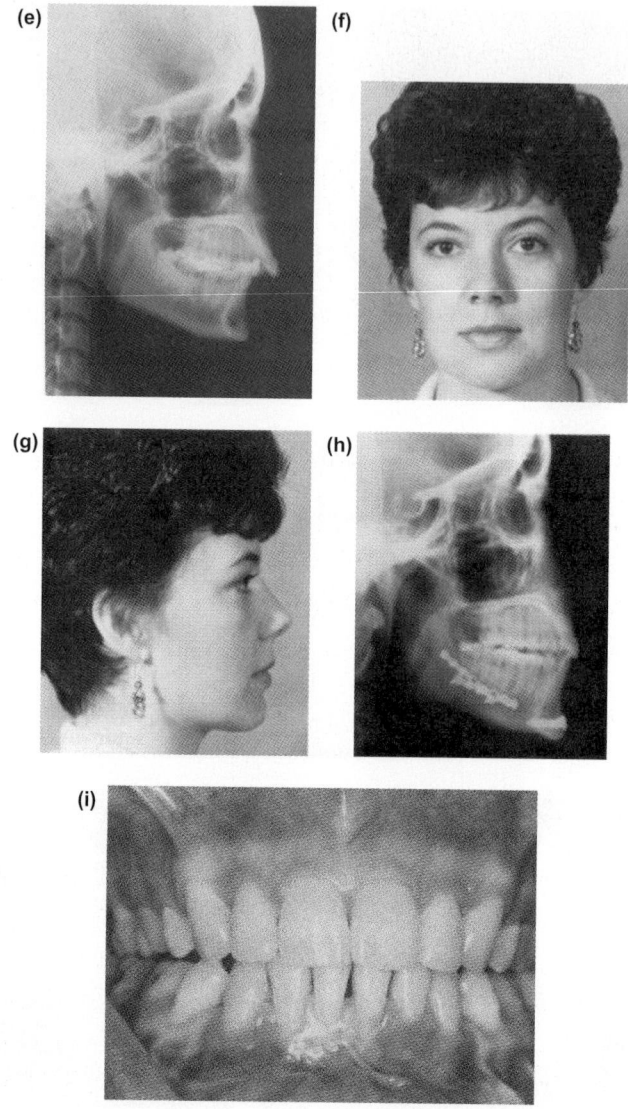

Figure 10.8   (*Continued*)

2. In all cases, preoperative orthodontic decompensation, coordination of the arches and closure of any spaces, is essential preparation for surgery (Figure 10.7). This may reveal an unsatisfactory upper lip incisor relationship requiring a Le Fort I impaction.

(j)

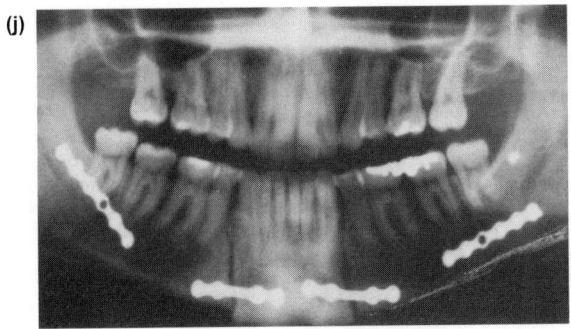

Figure 10.8 (*Continued*)

Lengthening the Mandible and the Chin

Most marked Class II division 1 cases require not only a forward repositioning of the mandible to an overcorrected edge to edge incisor relationship by a sagittal split but also a sliding augmentation genioplasty. Always resist the temptation to wait and see if a genioplasty is also required — it is! (Figure 10.9).

The Chin

As described earlier there are aesthetic and ethnic variations in the profile. In most cases the chin point, i.e. the soft tissue pogonion (Pg), should lie within 6 mm of a vertical drawn downwards from subnasale at right angles to the Frankfort horizontal plane (Figure 10.10). Retrogenia is a receding chin and must be differentiated from the more common retrognathia, where the mandible is set too far back and is too short. The increased overjet of retrognathia is not usually found in pure retrogenia.

The chin depth (anterior inferior dentoalveolar height) from the incisor edge to the bony menton is 40 ± 2 mm for women and 44 ± 2 mm for men. This usually equals the distance of the lower lip margin to the soft tissue menton. Chin depth is often overlooked and may also require augmentation or reduction.

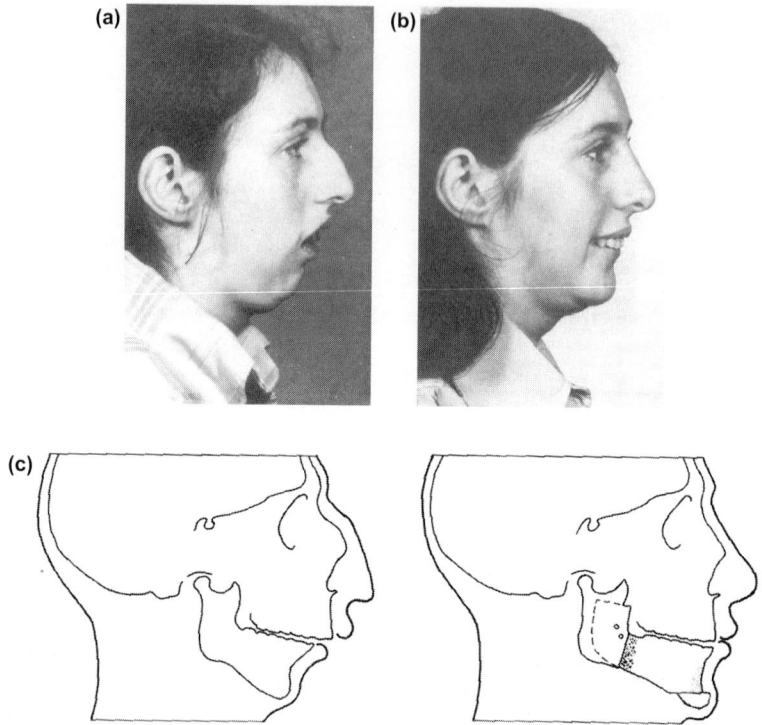

Figure 10.9   Severe "bird face" retrognathism corrected with a forward sagittal split osteotomy and genioplasty followed by a rhinoplasty. **(a)** Preoperative **(b)** postoperative, and **(c)** diagrammatic representation of change.

Unfortunately these estimations will be complicated by changes brought about by other osteotomies. For instance:

- after a Le Fort I elevation the chin will advance with the forward autorotation of the mandible, simultaneously reducing the apparent chin depth;
- forward movements of the mandible will have a predictable effect on the chin point (Po), but will simultaneously increase the lower facial height as the mandible moves down the occlusal plane;
- with backward correction of a prognathous mandible the distalisation of the chin is usually desirable, but occasionally it may require a paradoxical augmentation forward slide;

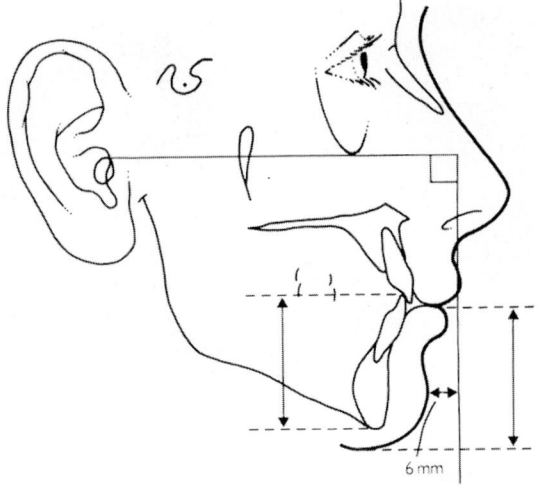

Figure 10.10 The vertical and horizontal parameters of the chin in relation to the vertical from the Frankfort mandibular plane (see text).

- bimaxillary osteotomies will also influence the chin profile if the occlusal plane is altered. By increasing the occlusal plane angle, the chin will rotate backwards and downwards. With a decreased occlusal plane, the chin will rotate forwards and become more prominent.

In all these cases a planning tracing on which the mandibular outline may be moved in the anticipated direction will enable the outcome to be predicted. Only in this way can any supplementary surgical addition or subtraction of the chin be confirmed.

Figure 10.11 shows the result of augmentation with a sliding genioplasty. Reduction and augmentation of chin depth will be discussed with the Long Face, and the Short Face.

Lower Lip Sag: A Warning

With some cases of augmentation genioplasty, especially when carried out with a Le Fort I elevation (upward impaction), the lower

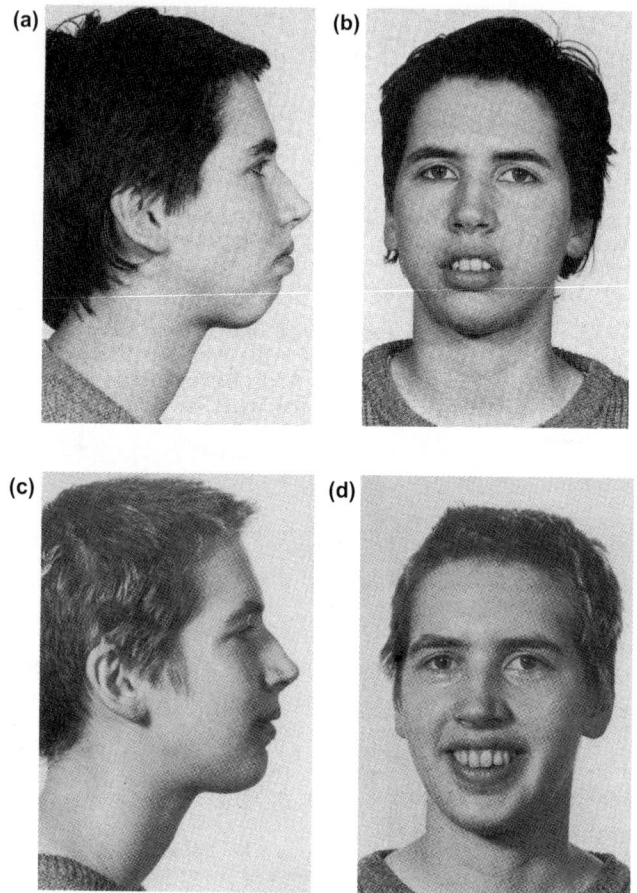

Figure 10.11 Retrogenia treated with a sliding genioplasty. **(a)** and **(b)** Preoperative. **(c)** and **(d)** Postoperative.

incisor occlusal plane rises above the lower lip line. Poor adaptation of the soft tissue and mentalis function leaves an unsightly display of lower incisor and gingival margin (Figure 10.12). This may be avoided by

1.   Extensive undermining of the soft tissues of the neck to accommodate the advanced chin,

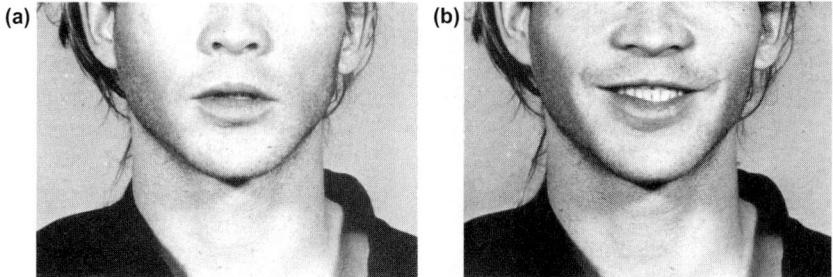

Figure 10.12   Lower lip sag following augmentation genioplasty. **(a)** at rest. **(b)** smiling.

2.   Careful suturing of the divided origin of the mentalis to the depths of the periosteal aspect of the degloved chin.
3.   External elevation by an adhesive pressure dressing for a week, followed by active "upward" lip exercises by the patient to restore upward muscle tone.

Mandibular Incisor Proclination

Proclination of the lower incisors with a normal jaw-base relationship is an uncommon deformity. The incisors are usually spaced, suggesting the tongue as the cause of the problem.

Treatment (see Figure 10.13)

- Where orthodontic retraction is not practicable, the first premolars can be extracted and the canine-incisor segment brought backwards with a Kole subapical (labial segmental) osteotomy.
- If the tongue looks large, reduce it with the osteotomy. If there is any doubt, warn the patient that should incisor proclination relapse occur, tongue reduction may be necessary (see also Bimaxillary Proclination).

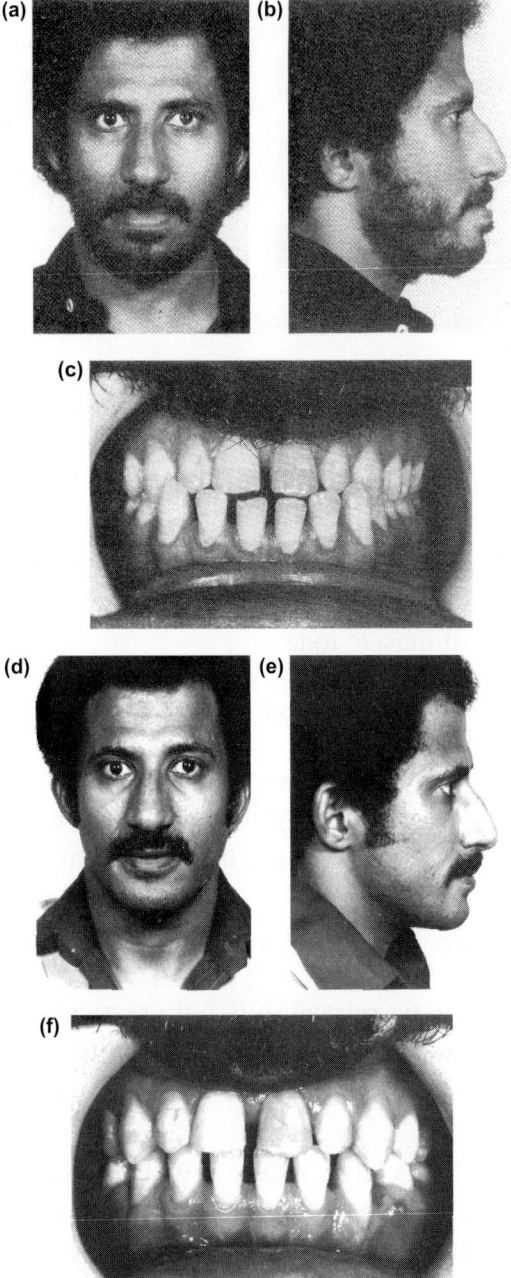

Figure 10.13   Segmental setback of lower incisors and canines. (**a**) to (**c**) Preoperative. (**d**) to (**f**) Postoperative.

The Maxilla

Maxillary Hypoplasia

- Although one would expect to recognise a maxillary deficiency, many cases are diagnosed and operated on as a mandibular prognathism. The result is a flat face, which is more noticeable in a man than a woman. This is particularly likely to occur if the SNA is artificially high, i.e. more than 82°, due to a high sella or a short cranial base, i.e. a short SN.
- Cleft cases require special consideration. One important factor is the misconception that the cleft hypoplastic maxilla is associated with an enlarged mandible. Cleft patients often have a small mandible, which rarely may be elongated with the maxilla advancement for an ideal correction of the profile.

Treatment

The treatment of choice is a Le Fort I osteotomy with a forward movement of 3, 6, or 9 mm. depending on the degree of deficiency. (Figure 10.14). In addition to correcting the occlusion, the maxillary forward movement will elevate the nasal tip but does not usually decrease the nasolabial angle. A narrow intercanine width will have to be increased orthodontically (Figure 10.14) or surgically at operation after the down-fracture (Figure 10.15).

Where there is marked hypoplasia of the inferior orbital margins a Le Fort II osteotomy is necessary or a high Le Fort I with a bone onlay (see below). However, with a good nose the Kufner modification of the Le Fort III osteotomy produces an advancement of the malar bones and infraorbital margins (see Malar-maxillary Hypoplasia).

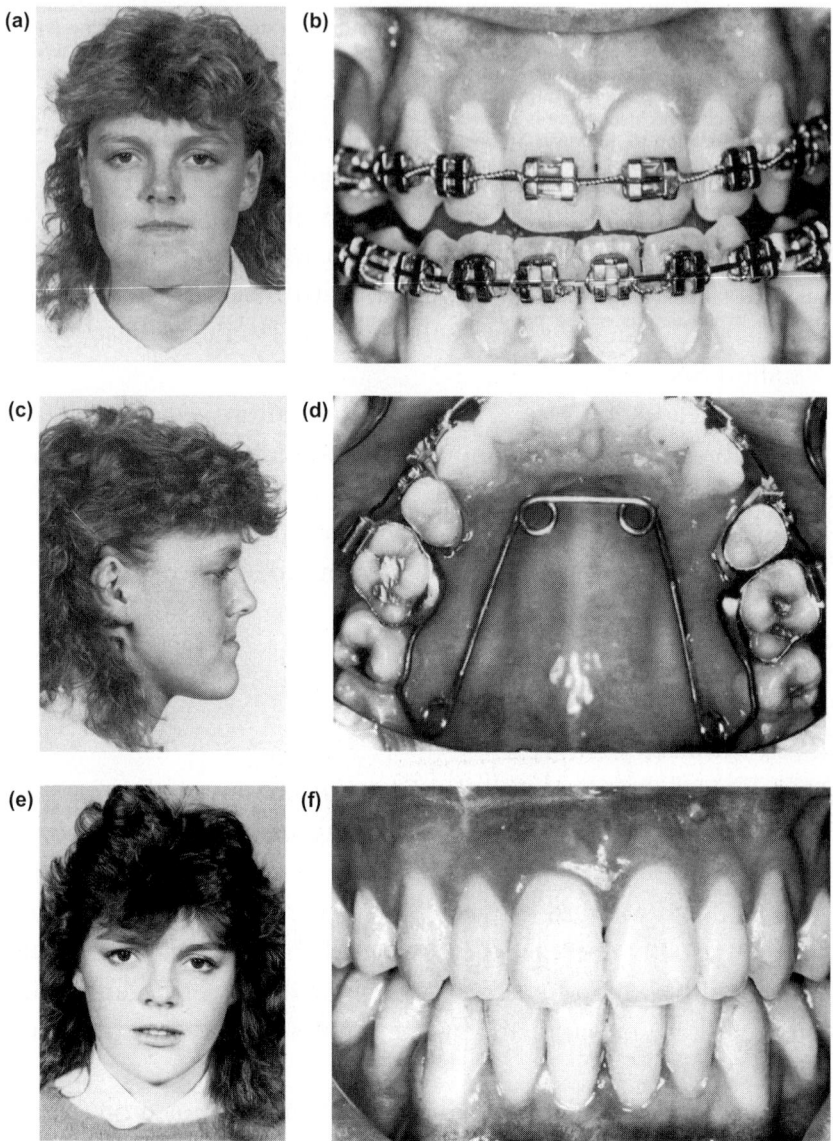

Figure 10.14   Maxillary retrusion corrected by a Le Fort I advancement. This was facilitated by preoperative upper arch expansion with a quadhelix appliance. (**a**) to (**d**) Preoperative. (**e**) to (**g**) Postoperative.

(g)

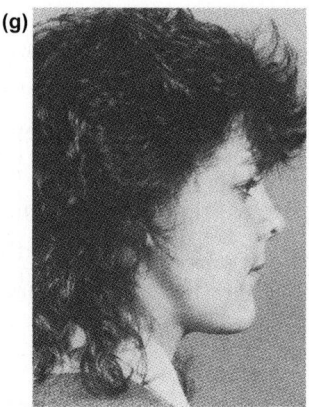

Figure 10.14 (*Continued*)

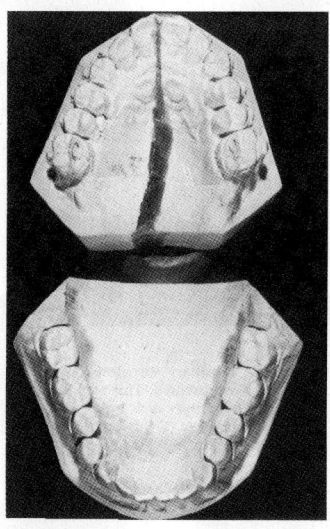

Figure 10.15 Planning model for surgical expansion of maxillary arch.

Major movements, i.e. more than 9 mm, require carefully sited plates with bone grafting of the osteotomy gaps. However, where significant movements appear necessary, especially in non-cleft cases, a bimaxillary procedure is needed. This will divide the distance between the two jaws (see Bimaxillary Deformities).

Nasomaxillary Hypoplasia

With nasomaxillary hypoplasia, especially with a deficiency of the infraorbital margins, a Le Fort II osteotomy is required. There may be a noticeable band of white sclera below the limbus of the iris, and in profile there is some degree of pseudoproptosis, i.e. the globe protrudes more than 2–3 mm beyond the infraorbital margin. Figure 10.16 shows the result of a combined Le Fort II advancement and mandibular pushback.

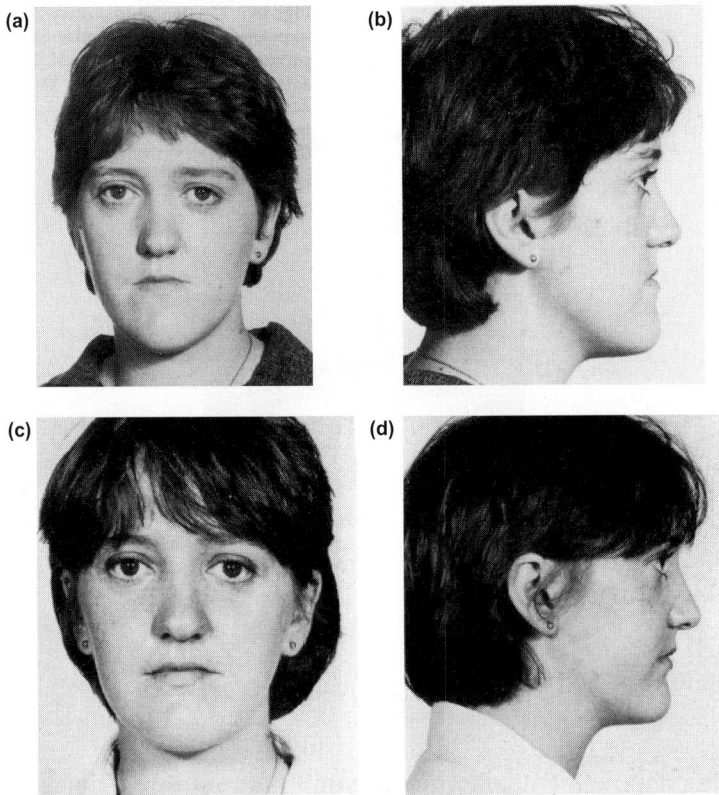

Figure 10.16   Nasomaxillary hypoplasia and mandibular prognathism corrected with a Le Fort II advancement and mandibular setback. **(a)**, **(b)** and **(e)** Preoperative. **(c)**, **(d)** and **(f)** Postoperative.

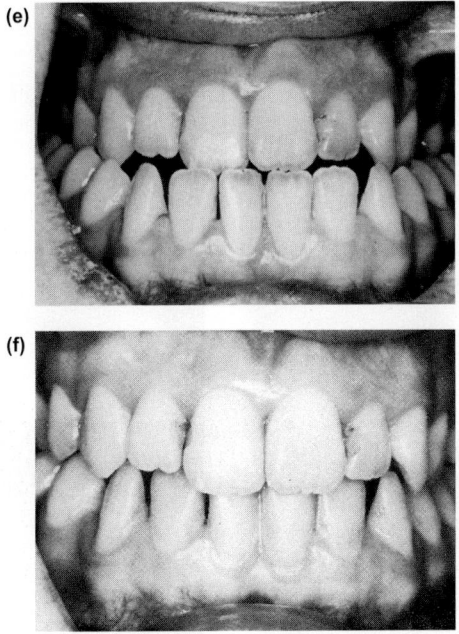

Figure 10.16   (*Continued*)

Malar-Maxillary Hypoplasia

The presentation is very similar to the previous case, requiring a Le Fort II correction, except that the nose is either good or prominent. Here, the treatment of choice is:

i)   A malar-maxillary advancement, leaving the nose undisturbed. This procedure is the Kufner modification of the Le Fort III osteotomy (Figure 10.17).

ii)   The alternative solution is a Le Fort I advancement with simultaneous alloplastic malar onlays.

iii)   The Kufner osteotomy followed by distraction osteogenesis.

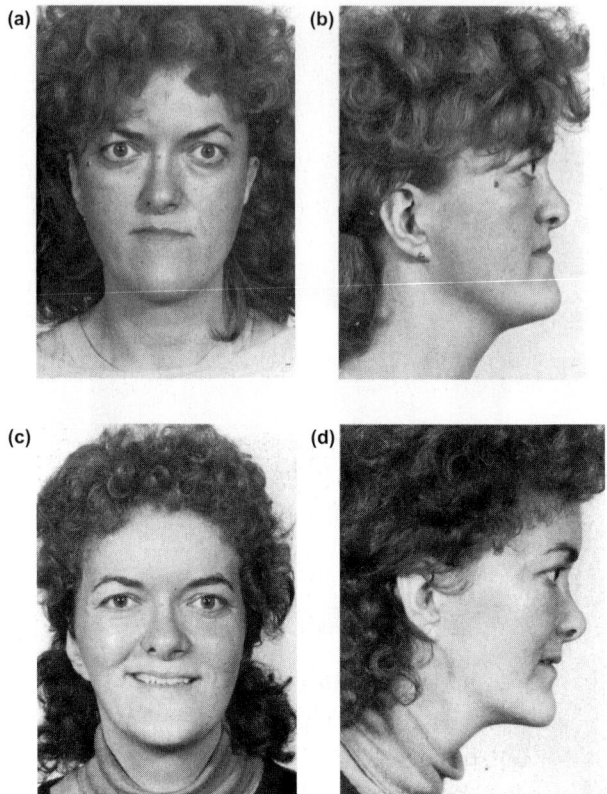

Figure 10.17 Malar-maxillary hypoplasia and mandibular prognathism corrected by a Kufner modification of the Le Fort III osteotomy and a mandibular setback. **(a)** and **(b)** Preoperative. **(c)** and **(d)** Postoperative.

Maxillary Protrusion

Patients with this deformity are usually severe Class II division 1 cases that have had failed orthodontics or refuse orthodontic treatment. As they also present with deep overbite problems, they are discussed in detail in the next section. Occasionally the uncomplicated maxillary prognathism may be treated with an anterior segmental osteotomy (Wassmund/Wunderer). This is usually an adult patient who is unwilling to undergo orthodontic treatment (Figure 10.18). The canine-incisor segment is set back after extraction of the first

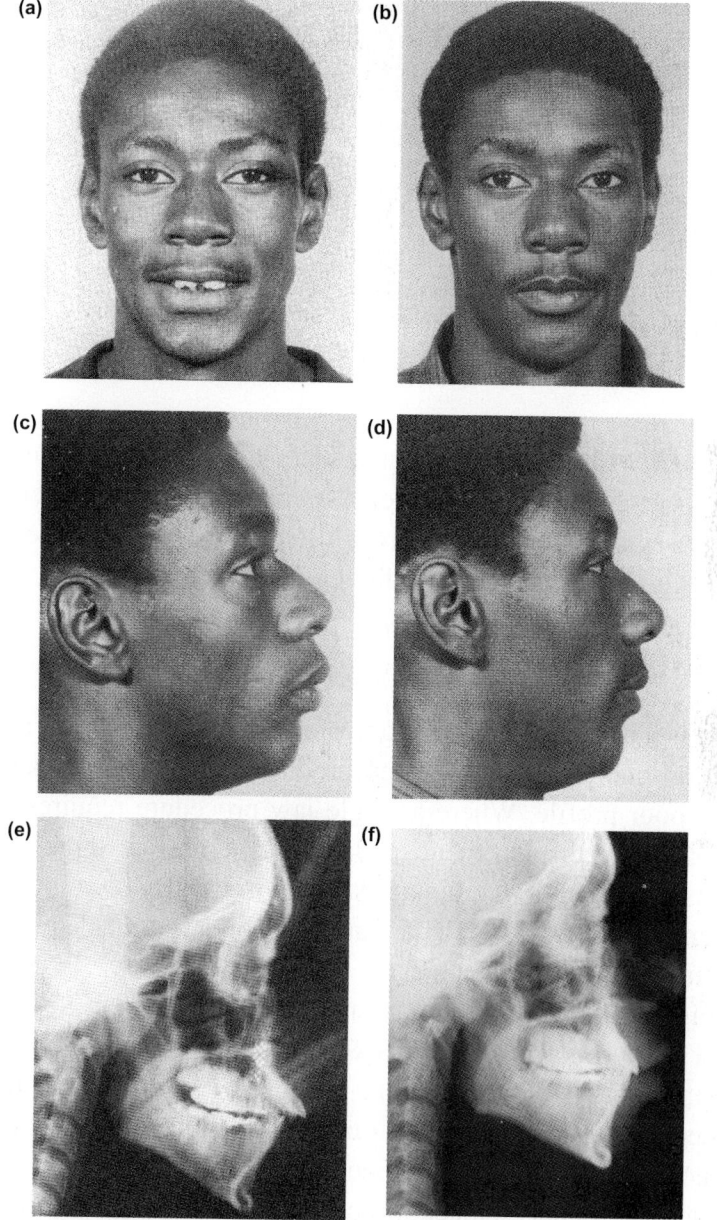

Figure 10.18   Maxillary prognathism with increased overjet and proclined incisors corrected with an anterior segmental setback. **(a)**, **(c)** and **(e)** Preoperative. **(b)**, **(d)**, **(f)** and **(g)** Postoperative.

(g)

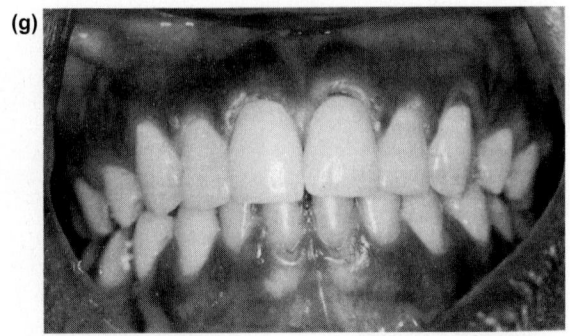

Figure 10.18   (*Continued*)

premolars. A midline split is necessary to maintain a natural dentoalveolar arch. Where premolar extractions have shortened the buccal segments the best approach to achieve optimum aesthetics and occlusion is to correct with a Le Fort I setback.

Bimaxillary Deformities

There is a natural temptation to treat most deformities with an operation on one jaw, but this often produces an acceptable occlusion and a poor profile. Where a single jaw procedure requires a large dentoalveolar displacement of 6 mm or more, one should always reconsider the case as a bimaxillary deformity. By dividing the displacement into two complementary components, a stable result with a better profile will be achieved.

Figure 10.19 shows how a small maxilla, with an SNA of 72° and a large negative overjet (SNB = 90°), has been "successfully" treated with a large mandibular pushback. Unfortunately, this has created a flat mid-face with an obtuse nasolabial angle. The surgery of choice should have been a combination of a forward Le Fort I and a mandibular setback procedure (see below). Furthermore, before this is done, orthodontic decompensation of the incisors with arch coordination, provides a considerably better postoperative dental occlusion and profile. Incisor decompensation always reveals the

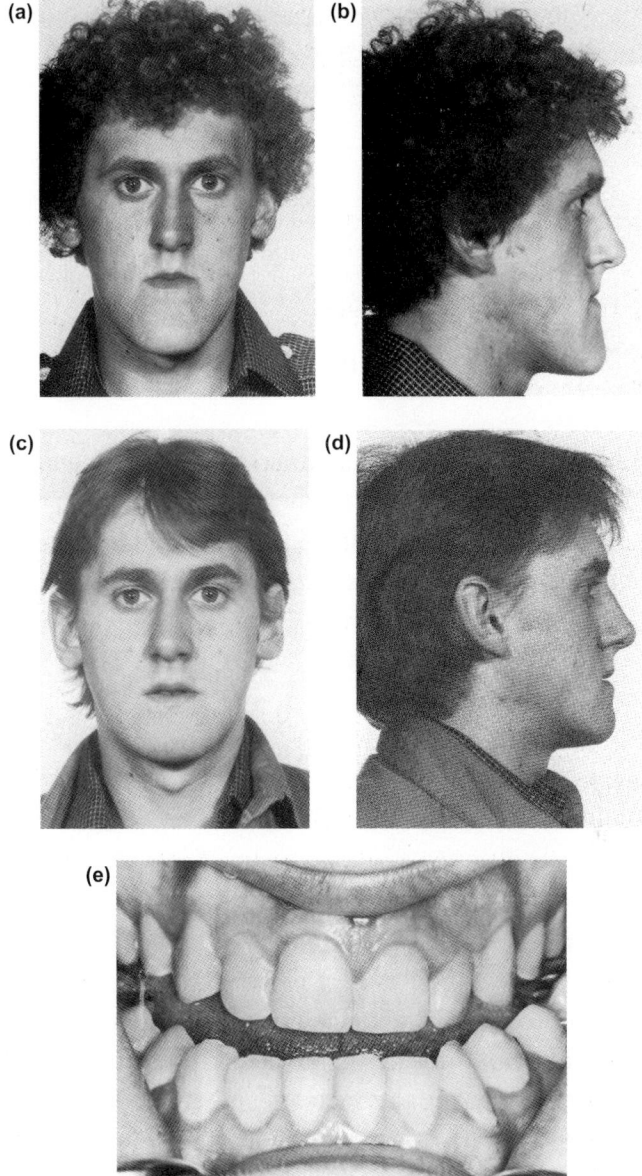

Figure 10.19 Marked mandibular prognathism treated with a pushback osteotomy but no orthodontic decompensation produced a satisfactory occlusion, but an unsatisfactory flat profile. **(a)**, **(b)** and **(e)** Preoperative. **(c)**, **(d)** and **(f)** Postoperative.

(f)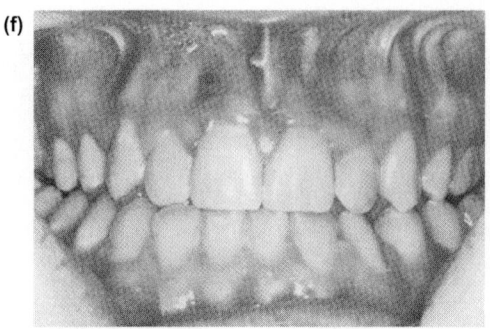

Figure 10.19   (*Continued*)

true discrepancy between the upper and lower arches and facilitates greater surgical movement and the best profile.

With all bimaxillary osteotomies, care should be taken to maintain or achieve a normal occlusal plane which is 8 ± 4° to the Frankfort plane. This will ensure:

- a good chin profile
- optimum function, and
- occlusal stability.

Gross Mandibular Prognathism

As stated all cases of gross mandibular prognathism have an element of maxillary hypoplasia (Figure 10.19) which should be defined in order to plan an advancement in addition to the mandibular setback. This can only be achieved by presurgical orthodontic treatment decompensating the incisors and arch coordination.

The surgery is done as one combined procedure in the following way.

1. The sagittal split osteotomy cuts are carried out as far as, but not including, the ramus split.
2. The maxillary osteotomy, which is usually a Le Fort I, is completed and positioned with an intermediate occlusal

wafer designed to relate the forward movement of the repositioned maxilla to the unchanged mandible. Bone plates provide stable fixation both during and after the mandibular surgery.

3. The mandibular osteotomy is completed and repositioned distally to the planned overcorrected postosteotomy occlusion with the maxilla.

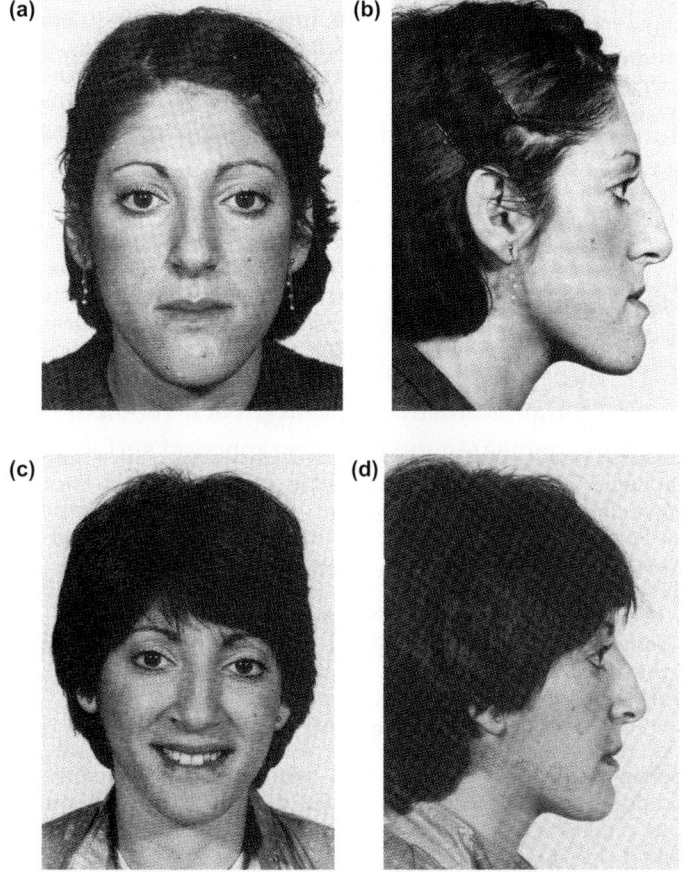

Figure 10.20 Combination of maxillary hypoplasia and mandibular prognathism treated with a Le Fort I advancement and an intraoral subcondylar pushback. Note how the prominence of the nose dimishes with the corrected facial drape. **(a)** and **(b)** Preoperative. **(c)** and **(d)** Postoperative.

Operating time can be reduced by using one of the intraoral subsigmoid osteotomies. The operative sequence, including a subsigmoid osteotomy, is as follows (see Figure 10.20):

i)   A medial (or lateral) intraoral subsigmoid osteotomy is performed, cutting only the posterior border of the mandible.
ii) The maxillary osteotomy is carried out and repositioned with the intermediate wafer designed to relate the postosteotomy maxillary position with the unchanged mandible.
iii) The intraoral subsigmoid osteotomy is completed and the final occlusal relationship determined and fixed with elastics.

Unfortunately this loses all the advantages of internal fixation with the elimination of intermaxillary fixation and immediate rehabilitation.

The Deep Overbite

Patients with a deep overbite are neglected because they do not usually complain of an aesthetic deformity. Their problem consists of incisor attrition damaging the opposing mucosal surface, leading to bone and tooth loss. The lower incisor over eruption also leads to premature loss with the onset of periodontal disease. Conventional solutions are an overlay or bite guard, or extractions with the provision of a denture. Orthodontics and orthognathic surgery can readily eliminate these problems without a prosthesis and with preservation of the dentition.

The patients fall into the two Angle Class II groups, each with subgroups.

Class II Division 1

Here the damage is on the palatal aspect of the upper incisors, leading to increased proclination and separation with progressive bone loss.

Treatment

1. With a poor profile, consisting of a retrognathic mandible, reduced lower facial height and the lower lip trapped behind the upper incisors (Figure 10.21), treatment comprises orthodontic decompensation of the incisors followed by a combination of a lower anterior dentoalveolar setdown with an anterior mandibulotomy, and a sagittal split osteotomy to bring the whole mandible forward to an overcorrected edge to edge incisor relationship.

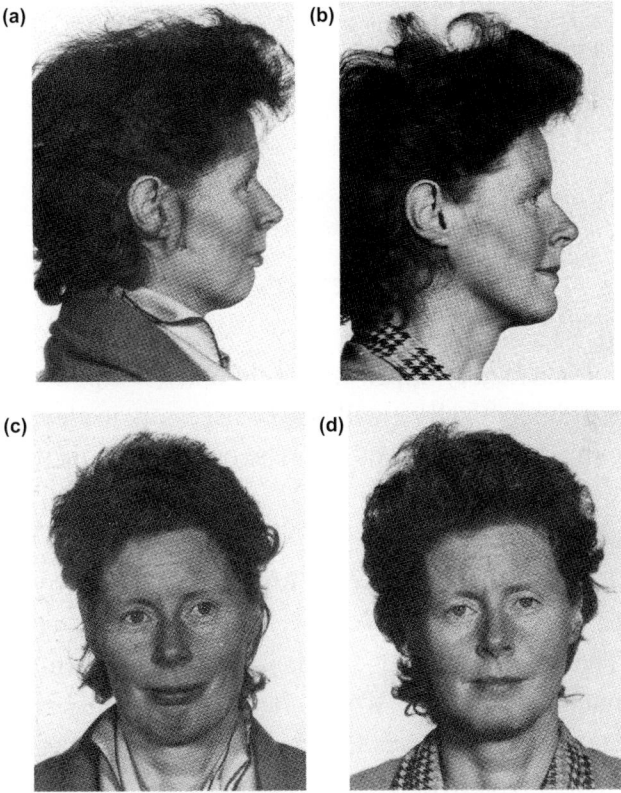

Figure 10.21 A forward sagittal split osteotomy combined with an anterior segmental setdown to correct a marked Class II, division 1 skeletal disproportion. The spaced proclined maxillary incisors were aligned preoperatively. (**a**), (**c**) and (**e**) Preoperative. (**b**), (**d**) and (**f**) Postoperative.

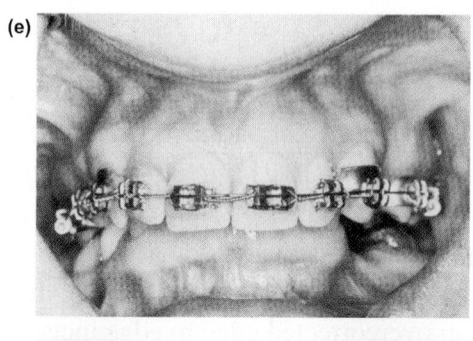

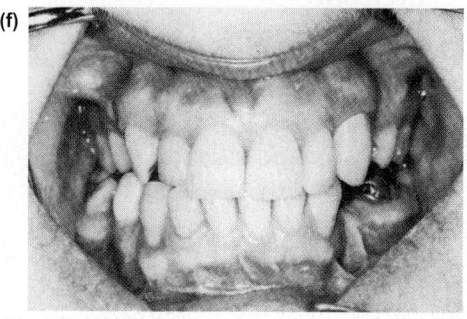

Figure 10.21   (*Continued*)

If a satisfactory upper incisor lip relationships cannot be corrected orthodontically it will also be necessary to elevate the maxilla with a Le Fort I osteotomy. The operative sequence will be:

a) The sagittal split cuts, but without splitting.
b) The maxillary Le Fort I impaction osteotomy with rigid fixation.
c) The lower anterior segmental setdown with an anterior mandibulotomy. A Kole subapical osteotomy is more challenging and reduces the chin depth which may not be aesthetically desirable.
d) Completion of the sagittal split and anterior movement to an overcorrected edge to edge incisor relationship. Relapse is a natural tendency and is avoided by the forward overcorrection.

The Class II Division 2

Here the incisor trauma affects both the buccal and palatal gingivae leading to loss of the lower incisor bony support and secondary periodontal disease. Cases may be divided into two groups:

1. Uncommon patients with a satisfactory profile and upper incisor inclination. Relief of the traumatic occlusion may be

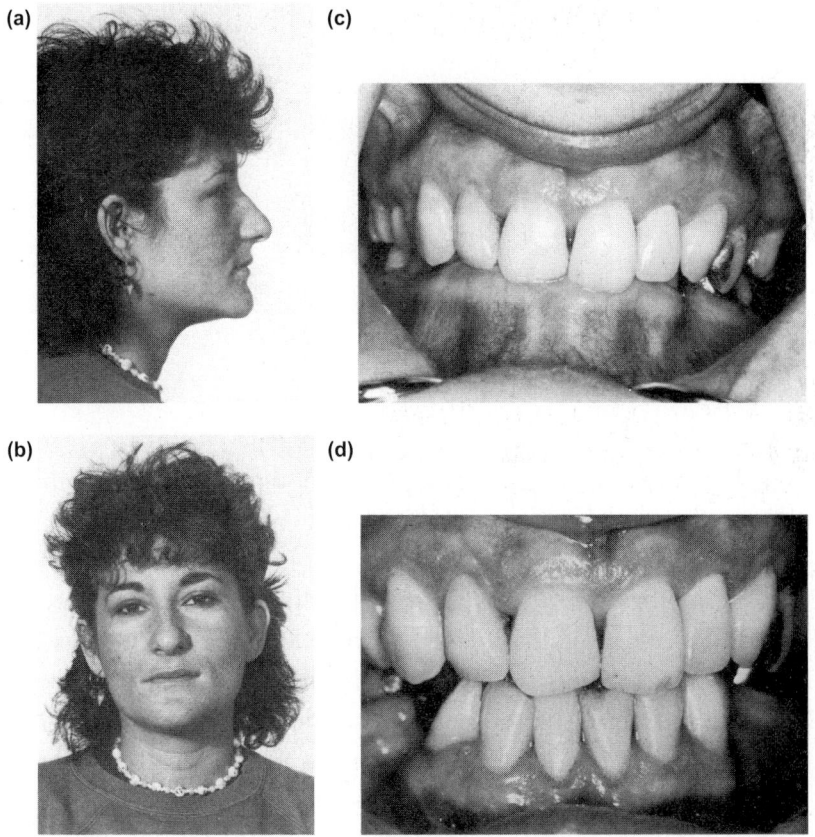

(a)

(c)

(b)

(d)

Figure 10.22 Elimination of a deep class II division 2 overbite by a lower segmental setdown. **(a)** to **(c)** Preoperative. **(d)** Immediate postoperative. **(e)** Note the lower incisor eruption and imbrication two years after operation. **(f)** The final restoration with fixed bridgework.

(e)

(f)

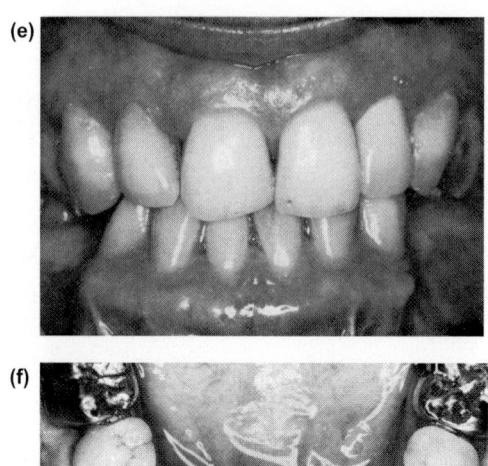

Figure 10.22 (*Continued*)

achieved by a lower segmental setdown alone. For stability, an edge-to-edge relationship must be established (Figure 10.22).

2. The majority of cases have retroclined upper incisors and orthodontic proclination must precede the surgery. This converts the case into a Class II division 1 problem over a period of 18 months. It is then treated surgically, as described above for the poor profile Class II division 1 deep overbite, i.e. (a) the upper lip-incisor relationship correction, (b) a lower anterior setdown, and (c) a forward slide mandibular osteotomy (Figure 10.23).

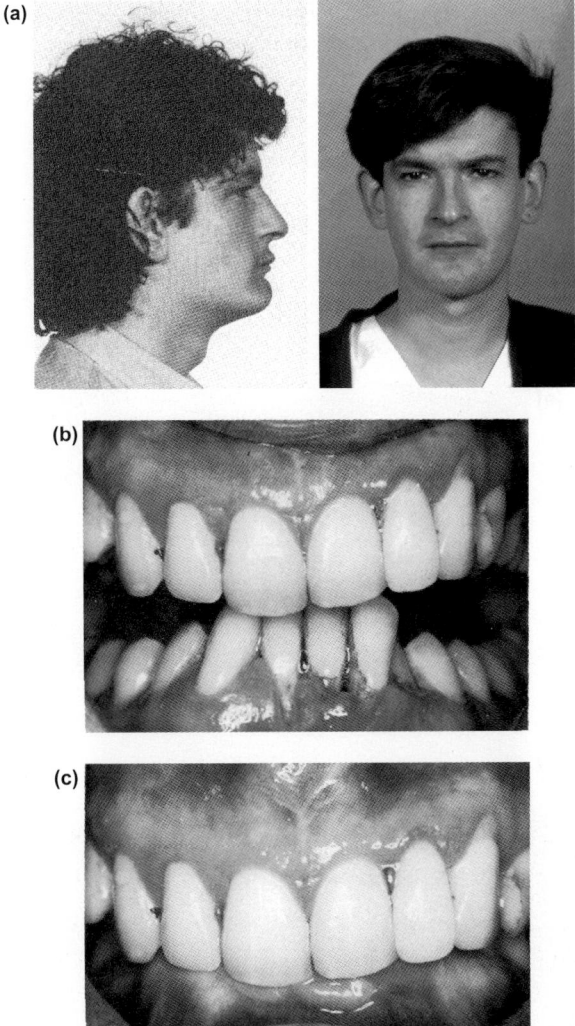

Figure 10.23 Class II, division 2 deep overbite with marked periodontal breakdown due to gingival trauma and poor oral hygiene. **(a)** to **(c)** Preoperative. Models show orthodontic "conversion" to Class II, division 1, **(d)** and **(e)**, which was then treated surgically with a lower segmental setdown and a mandibular advancement. **(f)** to **(h)** Postoperative. Note the increase in the postoperative lower facial height seen on the profile, and the marked change in the interincisal occlusion.

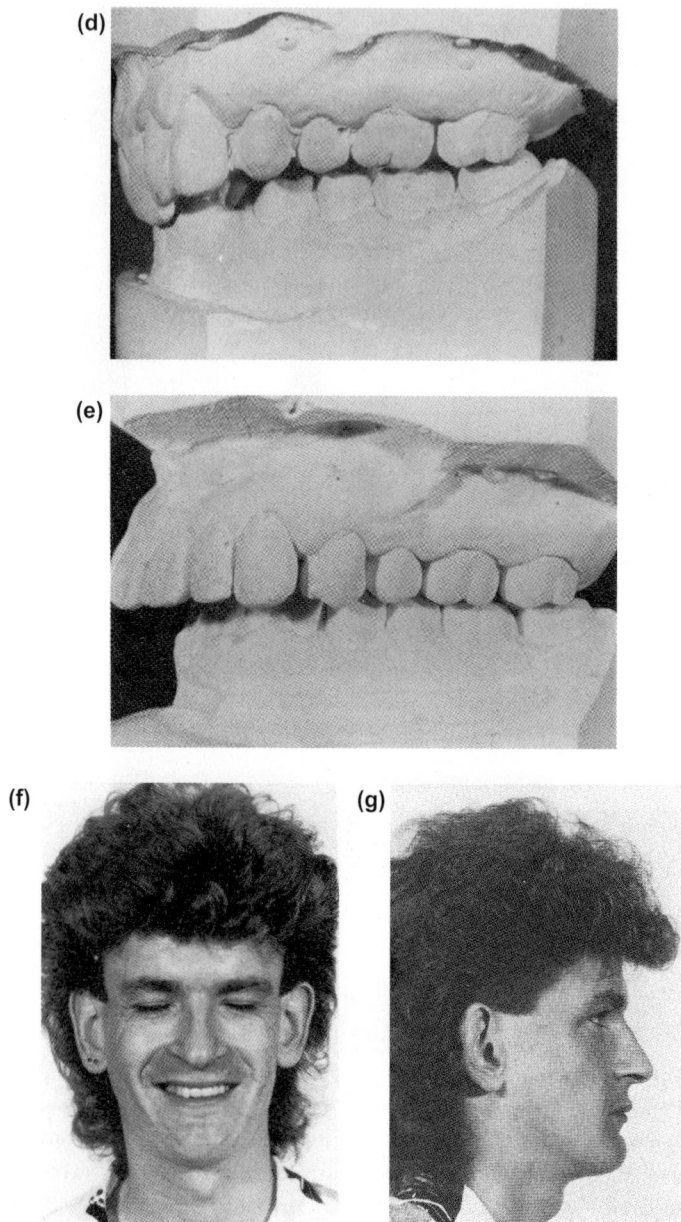

Figure 10.23   (*Continued*)

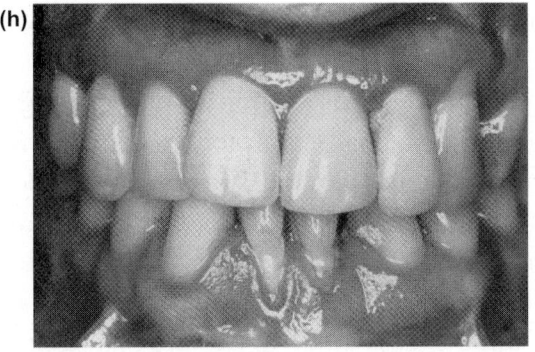

(h)

Figure 10.23 (*Continued*)

The Long Face Syndrome ("Vertical Maxillary and Chin Excess")

Although the mean facial heights for males and females are quoted as 130 mm and 120 mm respectively, the standard deviation of 8 mm, i.e. a range of 32 mm, indicates a very wide normal variation. However, in terms of vertical facial aesthetics, the most important diagnostic factors are:

1. labial competence at rest,
2. the upper lip-incisor relationship, and
3. the upper/lower facial proportions.

The soft tissue profile can be roughly divided into thirds (see Figure 1.3) from hairline to nasion, nasion to subnasale, i.e. the junction of philtrum and columella, and then to the lower border of the chin. The lower facial height can also be subdivided into a third and two thirds by the line of labial contact, the one third being the upper lip, which is 20 ± 2 mm in females and 22 ± 2 mm in males. However for surgical planning, the best guide is the underlying skeletal ratio of 45:55 between the upper facial

height (N to ANS) and the lower facial height (ANS to Me) (see
Figure 1.4).

Patients with long faces exhibit a variety of growth disturbances which are principally, but not exclusively, in the vertical
plane (Figure 10.24). It is obviously important to identify the true
vertical maxillary excess (VME) case. Clinically this will present
as labial incompetence with a poor incisor-lip relationship, i.e. an
excess of incisor showing at rest. This will be exaggerated on
smiling, revealing excess gingiva. Be sure that such a discrepancy
is not due to a short upper lip. If this is misinterpreted as VME and
treated exclusively with a superior maxillary impaction, the end
result will be a short mid face. Therefore any maxillary impaction
must be proportional to lip length. The longer the lip length, the
greater the upward impaction and *vice versa*. Standard cephalometry will help to clarify the skeletal proportions, and a template
such as the Jacobson or Bolton Standard will also show whether
there are discrepancies in the levels of the maxillary (palatal) and
occlusal planes.

This will reveal an increased alveolar depth with (a) a normal
maxillary plane, whereas the rest have (b) a low, or (c) postero-
inferior tilted maxillary planes with or without alveolar overgrowth.

Many VME cases also have a degree of vertical chin excess
(VCE). In men, the anterior inferior dentoalveolar height measured
from lower incisor tip to bony menton is 44 ± 4 mm and in women
40 ± 4 mm. Note that this is remarkably similar to the lower lip margin to soft tissue menton depth.

An important 25% of patients with a long face have a normal
maxilla but vertical chin excess, or an anterior open bite (or
both).

The four basic varieties of a long face are shown in
Figure 10.24 where the shaded areas indicate skeletal excess.

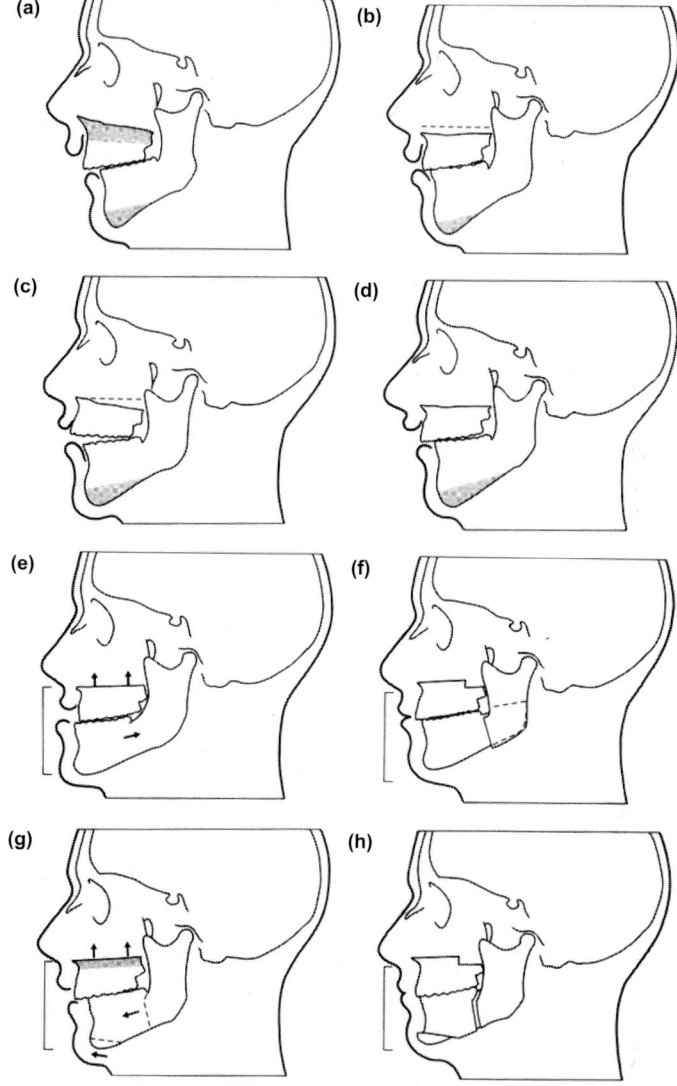

Figure 10.24 The four basic varieties of a long face. The shaded areas indicate skeletal excess. Each form of vertical maxillary excess may co-exist with
a vertical chin excess. (**a**) Vertical maxillary excess. (**b**) A low maxilla. (**c**) A
tilted maxillary oclussal plane producing an anterior open bite. (**d**) A short

(*Continued*)

Each form of vertical maxillary excess may co-exist with vertical chin excess.

a) Vertical maxillary excess with vertical chin excess.
b) A low maxilla with plus vertical chin excess.
c) A postero-inferior tilted maxillary occlusal plane producing an anterior open bite (plus vertical chin excess).
d) A short upper lip simulates vertical maxillary excess which may be exaggerated by vertical chin excess.

The surgical management of VME cases is the reduction of maxillary height with a Le Fort I vertical impaction, which is determined by the upper lip-incisor relationship. It is essential to measure the unaesthetic tooth excess at rest with dividers and a ruler and record it in the planning notes. Remember any maxillary impaction will tend to shorten the upper lip by up to 25% and some overcorrection is therefore desirable

Treatment Planning

As maxillary elevation produces a forward rotation of the mandible it reduces chin depth. It is also necessary to decide whether the final occlusion and profile will be satisfactory or will also require a mandibular osteotomy. The two simple ways of making a decision are (a) by a planning tracing and (b) by precise model surgery using an anatomical articulator. The study models will also indicate

---

upper lip simulating vertical maxillary excess. All VME is treated by a Le Fort I impaction, which allows a forward autorotation of the mandible. This will eliminate minor degrees of vertical chin excess. (**e**) Here impaction creates a prognathous mandible requiring a push back. (**f**) (**g**) and (**h**) A forward mandibular movement with an augmentation genioplasty.

whether the dental arches match or require modification by orthodontic therapy or additional segmental surgery.

a) Draw the repositioned maxilla on the lateral skull tracing
and, with dividers, rotate from the lower incisor tip around the
centre of the condyle into the new occlusion. In this way it is possible to see if on autorotation, the mandible will

1. find a satisfactory anteroposterior occlusion (Figures 10.24a–
   10.24d),
2. require a setback because of an acquired prognathic relationship (Figures 10.24e and 10.24f), or
3. require a forward mandibular slide and genioplasty to improve
   the incisor relationship and profile (Figures 10.24g and 10.24h).

Minor discrepancies (< 3mm) in the postoperative occlusion can
be resolved by a forward or backward movement of the maxilla
which must be planned on the articulator to provide the appropriate
intermediate wafer. This will confine the surgery to one jaw.
However most cases need a mandibular osteotomy. P.T.O.

Figures 10.25a and 10.25b show a moderate degree of vertical
maxillary excess with incompetent upper lip and marked incisor
exposure. The maxillary impaction corrected the vertical height,
labial contact and autorotation improved the chin profile.

The combination of vertical maxillary excess with a vertical
chin excess requires careful consideration especially with a degree
of mandibular retrognathism.

The correction requires a Le Fort I elevation, together with a
mandibular advancement and a combination of vertical chin reduction
with an anterior advancement genioplasty (Figures 10.26a to 10.26h).

Vertical Chin Excess (VCE)

If this is not great and is associated with VME, treat the maxilla and
leave the chin alone as the forward autorotation of the mandible or

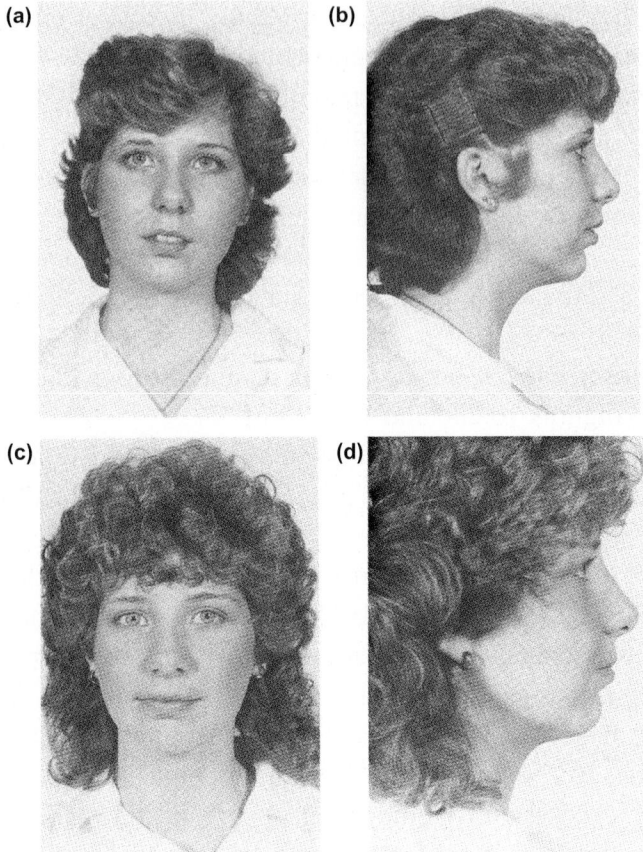

Figure 10.25   **(a)** and **(b)** Moderate vertical maxillary excess with incompetent long upper lip and marked incisor exposure. Maxillary impaction corrected the vertical height, labial contact and autorotation improved the chin profile.

an associated mandibular setback procedure invariably reduces the vertical chin profile.

If VCE is significant or is the principal cause of the long face, a wedge reduction genioplasty is the treatment of choice (Figure 10.27). Do warn all patients that the excess facial soft tissue may take 6–12 months to remodel after a large maxillary elevation.

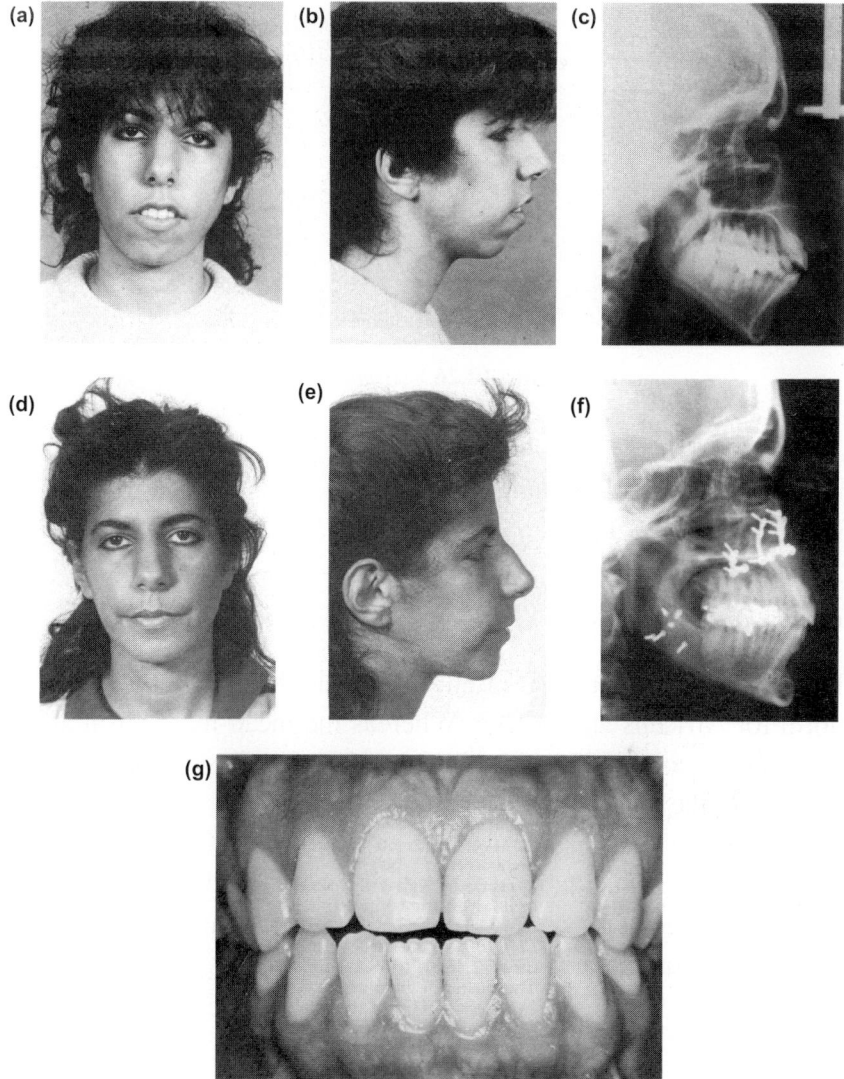

Figure 10.26 Vertical maxillary excess with a vertical chin excess but mandibular retrognathism. Hence the correction requires a Le Fort I elevation, together with a mandibular advancement and a vertical chin reduction but with an anterior augmentation genioplasty. **(a)** to **(c)** and **(g)** Preoperative. **(d)** to **(f)** and **(h)** Postoperative.

(h)

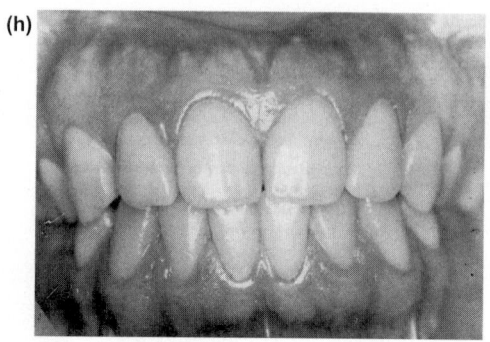

Figure 10.26   (*Continued*)

Long faces with an anterior open bite are discussed in the next section.

Bimaxillary Proclination

Bimaxillary proclination is often well within the acceptable aesthetic norm for Africans and Asians. Whereas the mean interincisal angle for Caucasians is 135°, this falls to 125° for these racial groups. Therefore the need for correction will not only depend on the cephalometric analysis but also the patient's aesthetic expectations.

The more problematic presentation is a bimaxillary proclination in combination with an anterior open bite and incompetent lips which is discussed later (see Figure 10.31).

Treatment

Where the dental bases are normally related and the vertical facial proportions acceptable, the treatment of choice is orthodontic retroclination with fixed appliance therapy closing any interincisal spacing. If the patient will not accept this, the alternative management consists of upper and lower anterior segmental osteotomies utilising space from the extraction of all four first premolars.

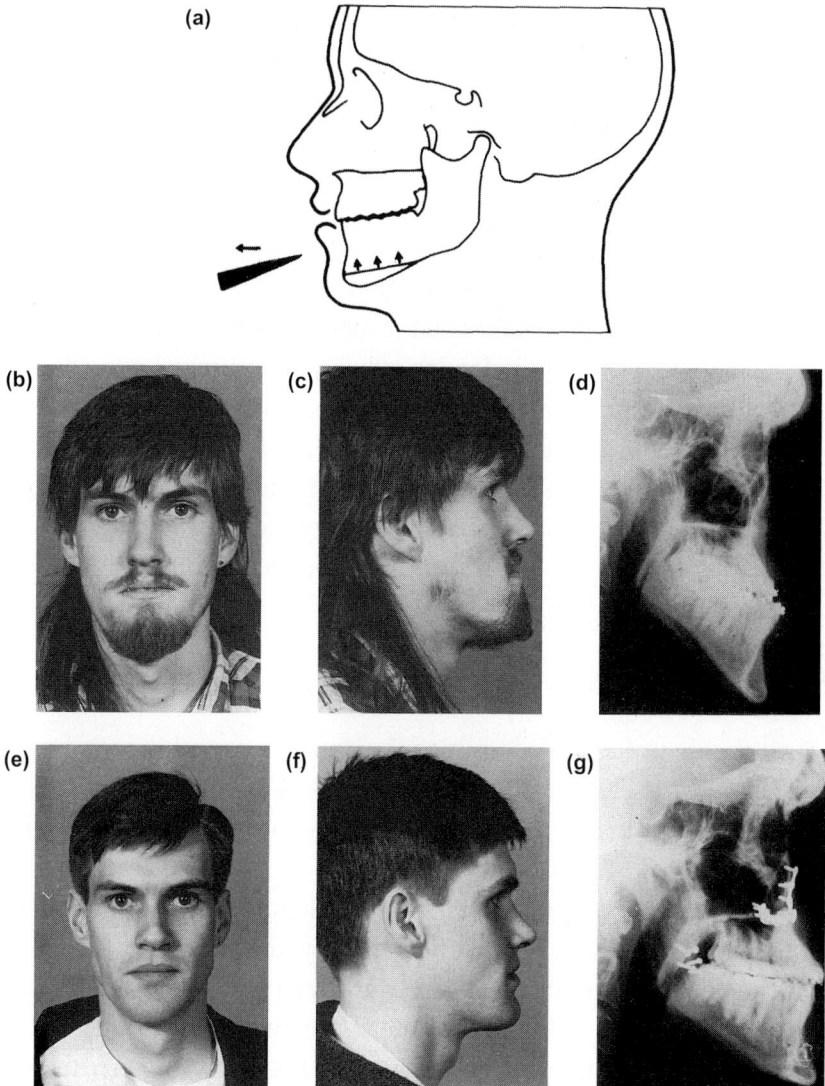

Figure 10.27 **(a)** Vertical chin excess is treated by a wedge reduction genioplasty preserving the lower border. **(b)** to **(d)** Preoperative vertical maxillary excess combined with a vertical chin excess which is camouflaged with a beard. The vertical chin excess was reduced by the removal of a wedge of bone, in addition to a mandibular pushback. The Le Fort I elevation corrected the vertical maxillary excess. **(e)** to **(g)** Postoperative.

If the deformity includes an anterior open bite this can be closed surgically but if related to an enlarged tongue, a tongue reduction is carried out at the same time (see Figure 10.31). Unfortunately the all-surgical solution may create two problems.

i)   Model surgery may show that with markedly proclined incisors the rotation required to correct the interincisal angle will produce distally inclined upper canines, and in the lower alveolus a step defect between the canines and second premolars. This is an obvious indication for orthodontics rather than a surgical correction.

ii) Anterior segmental osteotomies in patients with an increased facial height and an excessive upper incisor show can be very unsatisfactory. If there is initially an excess of dentoalveolar exposure on smiling, this will be exaggerated by segmental surgery without a Le Fort I upward impaction. This problem will be reviewed in the next section.

The Open Bite Deformity (Apertognathia)

Of all the dentofacial deformities the anterior open bite can be the most challenging. Relapse is well recognised but has become less of a problem with the Le Fort I osteotomy with its segmental modifications and rigid fixation.

Open bite is commonly classified as dental (acquired) or skeletal (congenital). This classification is not wholly reliable.

The dental open bite has been considered an acquired deformity because it primarily affects the anterior teeth and is usually attributed to childhood habits such as thumb sucking, with perpetuation of the gap by a tongue thrust to close an inadequate lip seal. However, not all so called dental open bites can be associated with such habits and not infrequently the incompetent lip seal is due to an increased lower facial height . In other words, the problem, although localised, can be a congenital skeletal deformity or rarely secondary to an enlarged tongue (see Figure 10.32). The principal diagnostic feature of the true acquired open bite is a normal maxillary-mandibular plane angle of $27 \pm 5°$.

The Skeletal Open Bite

The skeletal open bite has an increased maxillary-mandibular plane angle (>35°) and may be localised or extend posteriorly into the molar region (see Figure 10.33).

A similar deformity may arise from a loss of ramus height due to a variety of causes, including bilateral condylar fractures, degenerative arthopathies, idiopathic condylysis or following resorptive condylar remodelling in neuromuscular disturbances of the face.

There are two principal types of skeletal open bite with important surgical implications.

i)   Class II (Figure 10.28). Here the mandible appears to be rotated backwards and may be small. The maxillary occlusal plane is

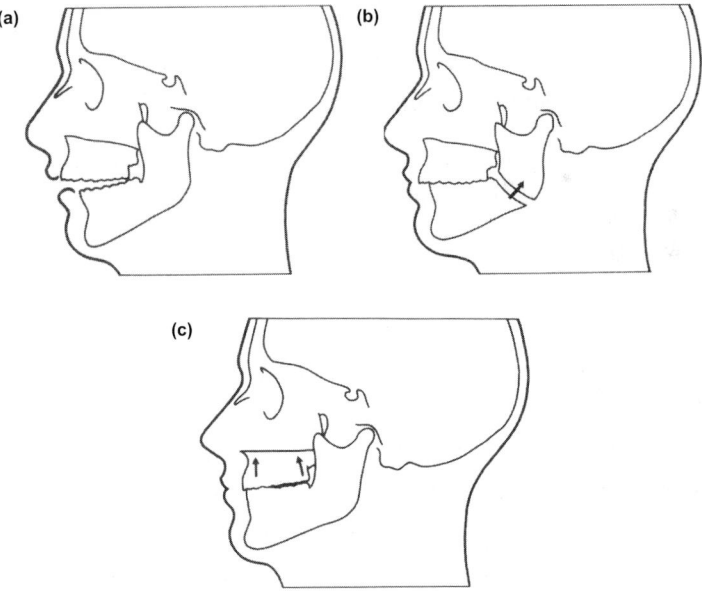

Figure 10.28   (**a**) Any attempt to correct a marked class I or class II anterior open bite with a ramus osteotomy which stretches the 'pterygomasseteric sling' will lead to a relapse. (**b**) The arrow indicates the strong musculofascial relapsing force. (**c**) A Le Fort I elevation with a posterior upward rotation allows the entire mandible to autorotate forwards and close the open bite within musculofascial constraints of the posterior facial height.

usually tilted upwards and forwards with an increased posterior superior dentoalveolar height. Some patients also appear to have a reduced anterior maxillary dentoalveolar height. The overall appearance is that of a skeletal Class II jaw relationship with a long lower face.

ii) Class III (Figure 10.29). Here the mandible is large with a normal maxilla. The posterior inferior facial height is in excess of 44% of the total posterior facial height. The overall appearance is a skeletal Class III with a long lower face.

Therefore a more useful open bite classification would be:

1. Dentoalveolar open bite: where the deformity is a localised dentoalveolar defect with normal facial proportions.

   a) Congenital.
   b) Acquired, e.g. sucking habits, alveolar trauma, enlarged tongue (including lymphangioma, haemangioma), and neuromuscular disturbances.

2. Skeletal open bite: where the dentoalveolar separation may be localised or extensive and is associated with an increased lower

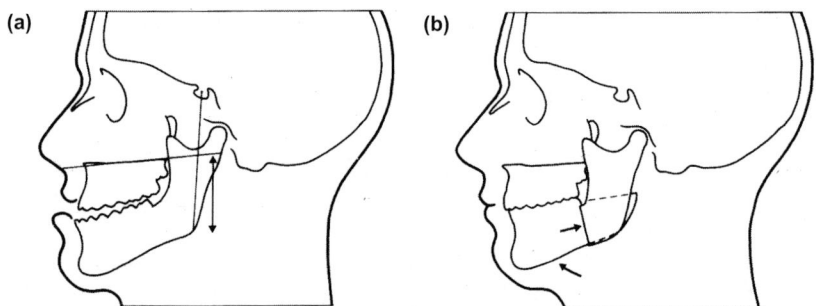

Figure 10.29 (a) and (b) The rare pure Class III open bite with a large ascending ramus may be corrected by a mandibular pushback procedure without relapse. Here, with the increased posterior inferior facial height (i.e. in excess of 44% of the total posterior facial height (S–Go) the pushback and rotation osteotomy do not stretch the "pterygomasseteric sling". See Case Figure 10.35 (p. 301).

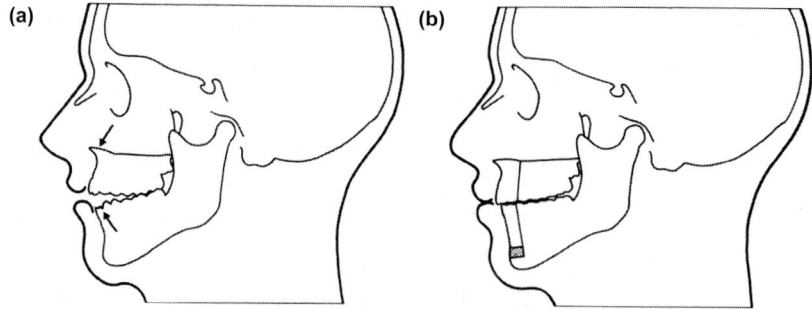

Figure 10.30 **(a)** and **(b)** An anterior (dentoalveolar) open bite with appropriate orthodontic preparation can be closed with bimaxillary anterior segmental osteotomies. The preoperative dentoalveolar open bite is treated by levelling of the upper incisors orthodontically and raising the lower incisors surgically. See Figure 10.31.

facial height and maxillary-mandibular plane angle. The two principal groups are:

(a) Congenital.

Class I, II or III.

(b) Acquired.

Bilateral condylar fractures, malunited untreated maxillary fractures, destructive arthopathies, idiopathic condylysis, condylar remodelling due to muscular dysfunction, acromegaly.

The Dento-Alveolar Open Bite

Treatment

Open bite deformities restricted to the anterior dentoalveolar segment with a normal facial height and proportions, can be successfully corrected with either orthodontics or segmental surgery, rotating the upper incisors downwards (Wassmund) and elevating the lower incisor segment (Kole) (Figure 10.31). However, this will only be successful if, on completion

a) the lip seal is competent and relaxed;

b)   there is no excessive display of the upper incisors especially on smiling; and

c)   the tongue is not enlarged.

The choice of surgery will be determined by the height of the gap and the length of the upper lip. Minor degrees of incisor open

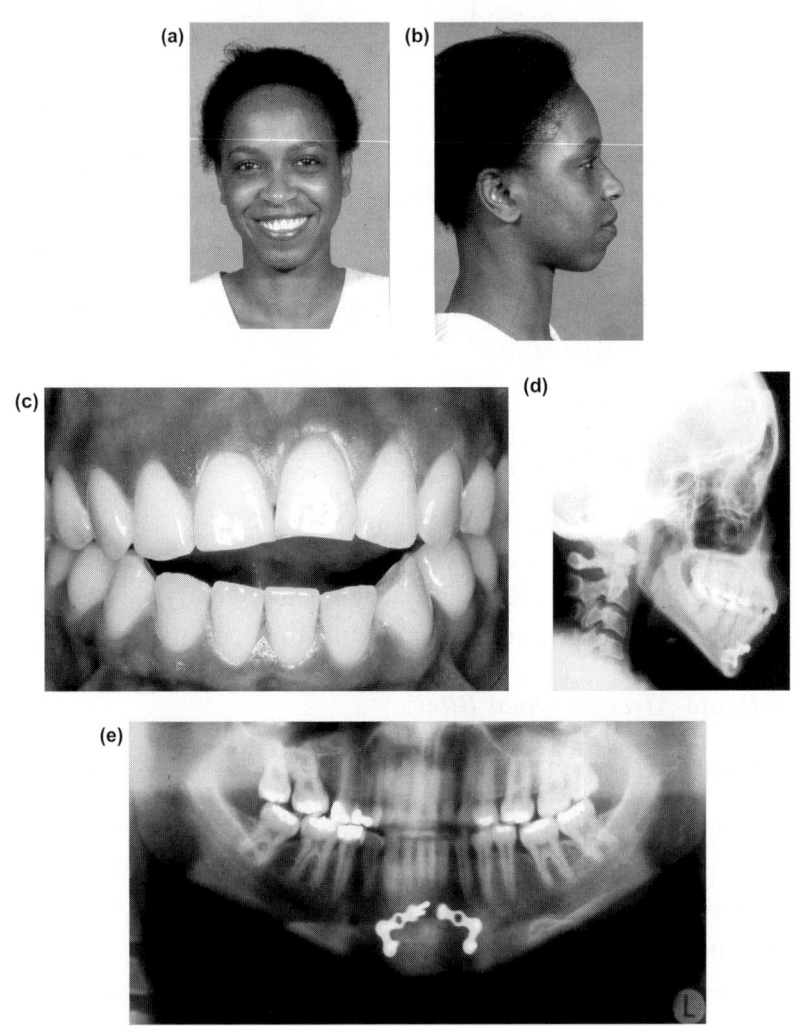

Figure 10.31   Dental anterior open bite treated with a combination of orthodontics and surgery.

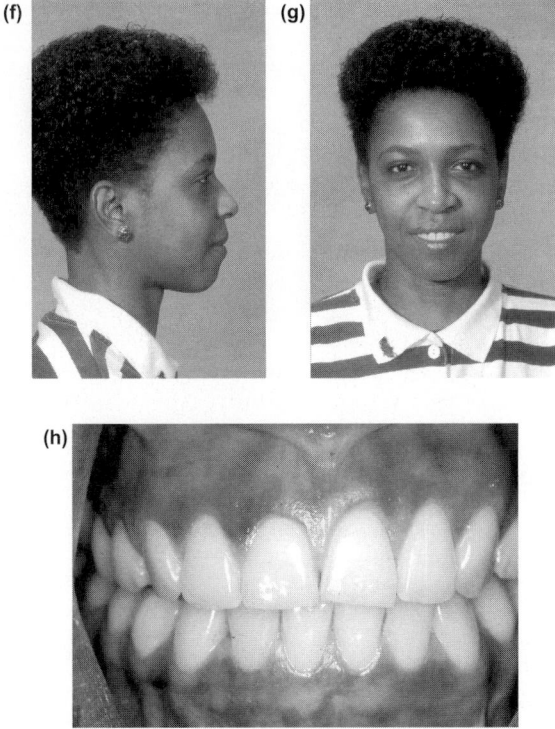

Figure 10.31 (*Continued*)

bite may be corrected with a maxillary anterior segmental osteotomy (Wassmund/Wunderer). Where the separation is larger it is necessary to close part of the gap with an additional lower segmental osteotomy (Kole) (Figure 10.31). The lower incisor segment may be rotated or elevated with an interpositional graft. The graft material may be rib or iliac crest, or an alloplastic material such as hydroxyapatite.

However be sure that

i)   its closure would not expose more than 4 mm of tooth below the upper lip margin and would therefore be better treated as a skeletal open bite incorporating a Le Fort I impaction.

ii) the patient does not require a tongue reduction, The treatment of a large tongue combined with an anterior open bite is shown in Figure 10.32.

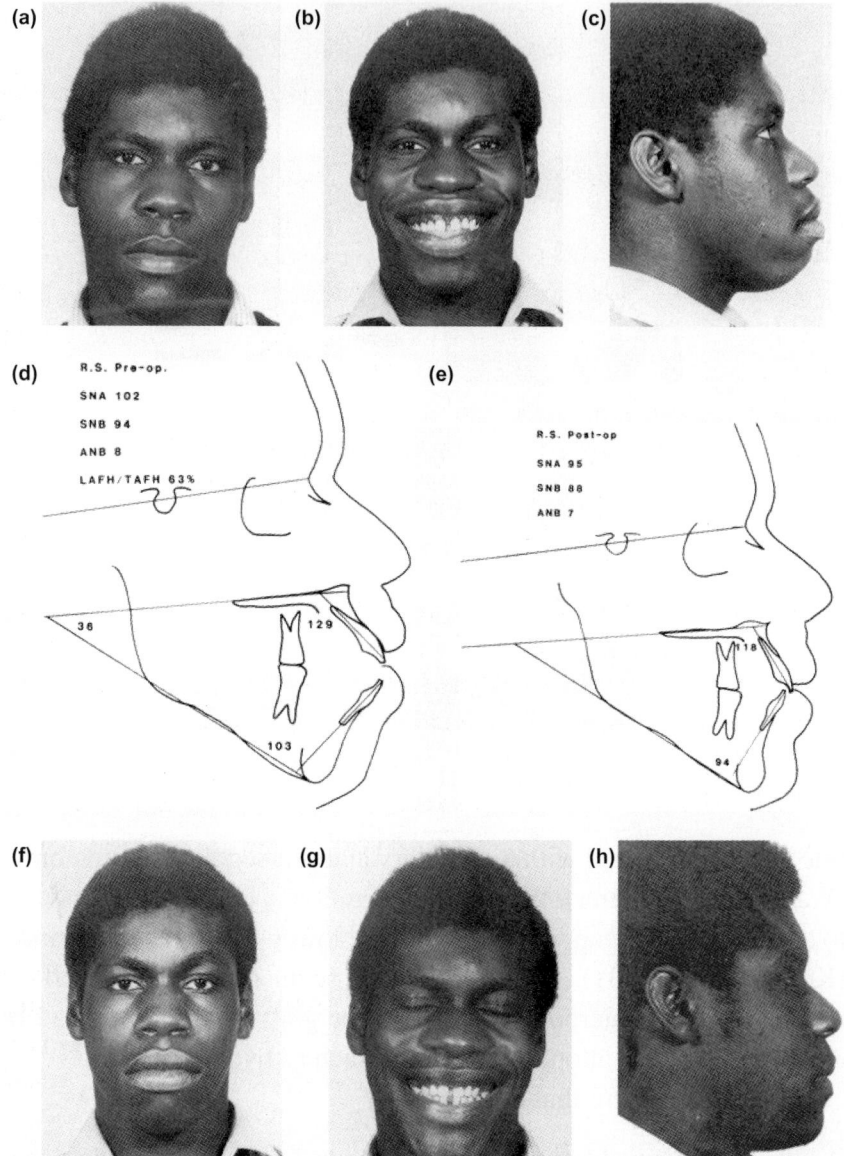

Figure 10.32   The combination of large tongue and anterior open bite treated by tongue reduction and segmental surgery. (**a**) to (**d**) Preoperative. (**b**) The tongue-incisor relationship with the molars in occlusion. (**f**) to (**h**) Post-operative.

The Skeletal Open Bite: Classes I and II

Attempts to treat these cases with operations on the mandible alone invariably gave rise to relapse, regardless of the procedure and the period of fixation (see Figures 10.28 and 10.32).

The anatomical problem is that of rotating a retroplaced mandible upwards and forwards around the fulcrum created by the second or third molar teeth. This overextends the pterygomasseteric musculofascial sling. Unfortunately no surgical ingenuity can beat this restraining force (Figure 10.33). If however the maxillary occlusal plane is normal, minor to moderate degrees of open bite can be treated with a sagittal split osteotomy and robust rigid fixation.

Treatment

The aims of the surgery are to produce a normal maxillary occlusal plane by reducing the posterior facial height with a Le Fort I impaction. This allows the mandible to rotate forwards and close the open bite. As always the starting point is the upper incisor-lip relationship. If it is satisfactory and the articulated study models show that the maxillary occlusal plane will occlude with the autorotated mandibular teeth, surgery may be limited to a Le Fort I osteotomy with removal of a posterior maxillary wedge This wedge will equal the anterior open bite as measured in millimetres between the incisal edges (Figure 10.34).

Where there is an element of vertical maxillary excess identified clinically by an increased anterior alveolus and incisor exposure, then a differential Le Fort I vertical impaction osteotomy designed to include the remove of bone both posteriorly and anteriorly, but with more from the back than front.

Variations

1.   Where both occlusal planes have exaggerated curves of Spee they will require flattening either orthodontically or surgically.

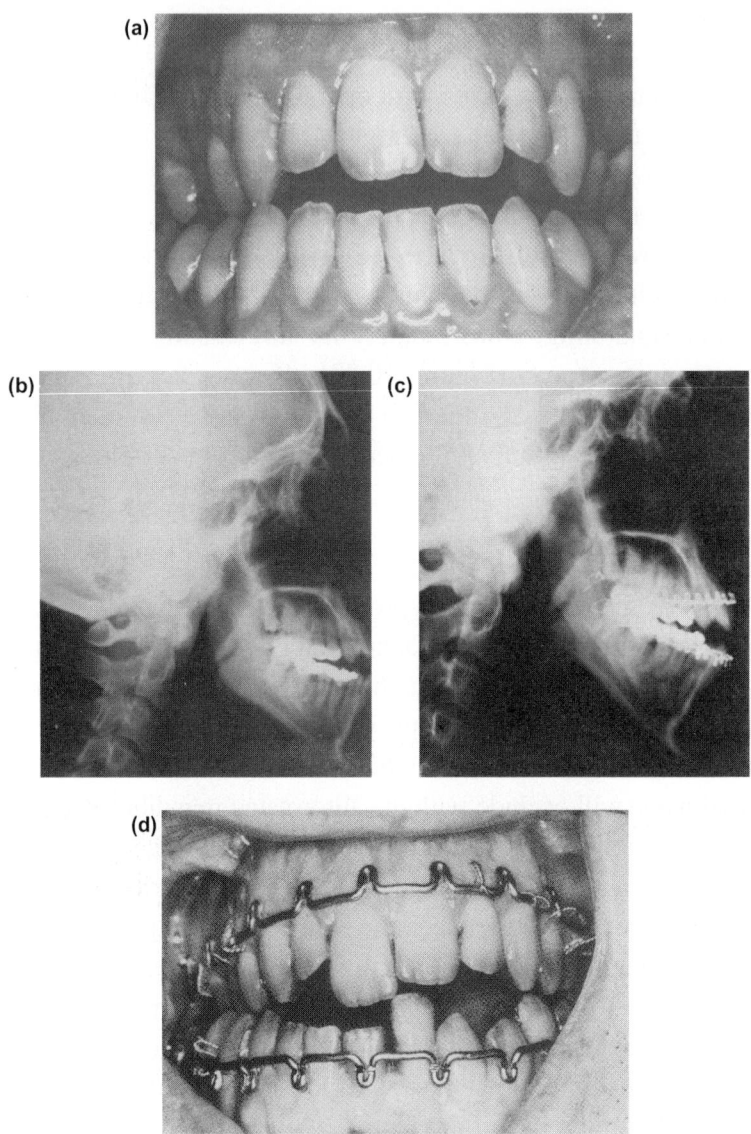

Figure 10.33   An attempt was made to close this skeletal Class I open bite **(a)** and **(b)** with a sagittal split osteotomy, interosseous wiring and arch bar inter-maxillary fixation. The postoperative illustrations **(c)** and **(d)** show the arch bars after the removal of the IMF. Note that the relapsing force was able to extrude several incisor teeth despite the intermaxillary fixation.

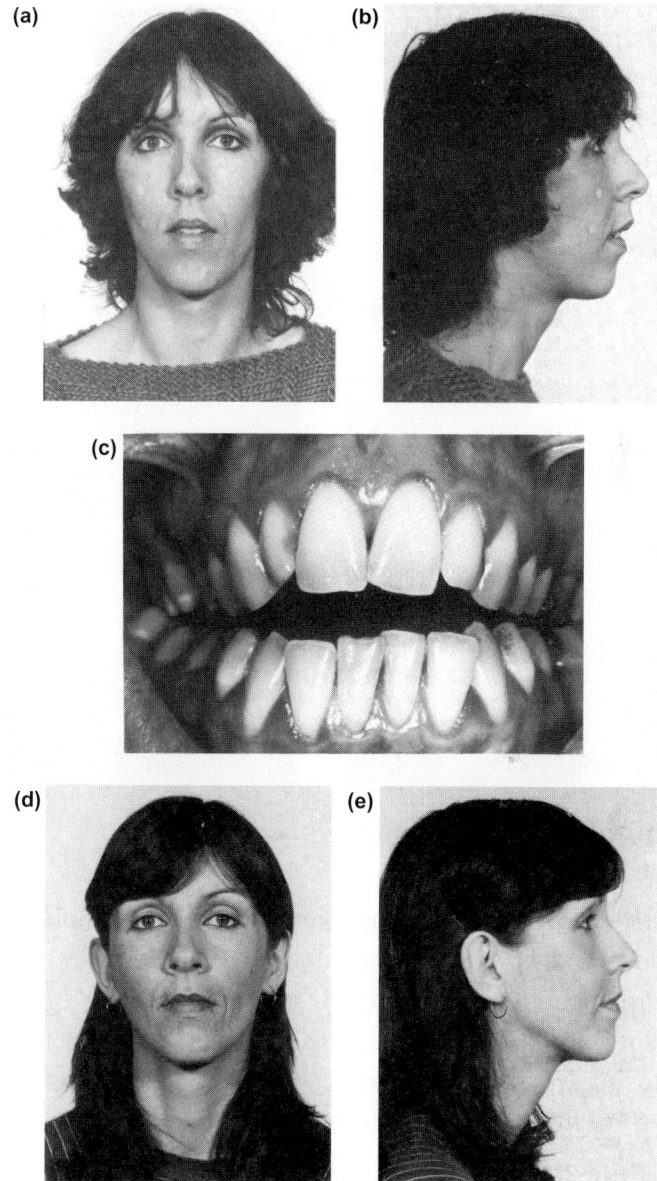

Figure 10.34   Long face with incompetent lips, narrow alar width and anterior open bite corrected with a posterior Le Fort I elevation. **(a)** to **(d)** Preoperative. **(e)** to **(h)** Postoperative.

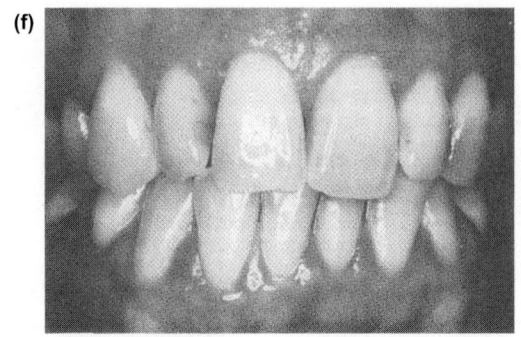

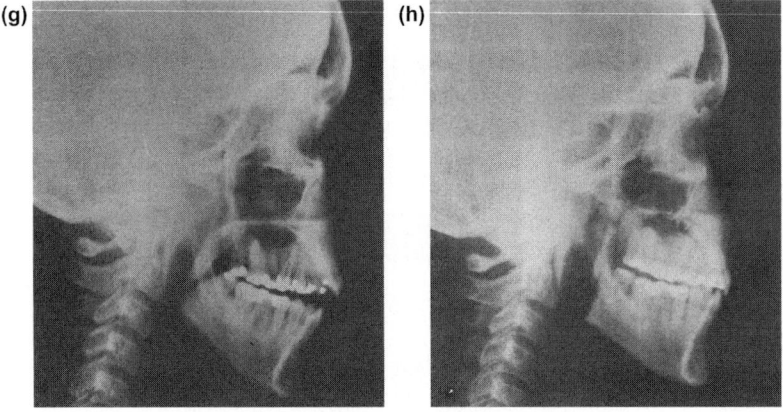

Figure 10.34   (*Continued*)

Orthodontic levelling of the maxillary and mandibular occlusal planes is done with fixed appliances, but in severe cases it is impossible to produce matching occlusal tables. In this case the incisor and canines are levelled independently of the buccal segments requiring segmental surgery to achieve flat interdigitating occlusal planes. The surgical protocol will be:

i)   In the maxilla, an anterior segmental section is carried out between the canine and premolars from above after the down-fracture. This allows a downward rotation of the incisor segment flattening the maxillary occlusal plane.

ii) The maxilla is then elevated as a whole.

iii) In the mandible a segmental elevation or anterior mandibulotomy may also be necessary (Figure 10.35).

2. The maxillary arch may have to be widened orthodontically or surgically to accommodate the lower dentition. In the latter case a midline section from above is required.

3. Where Class II retrognathism is marked, the maxillary elevation is carried out with a forward movement of the mandible by a sagittal split osteotomy with an augmentation genioplasty.

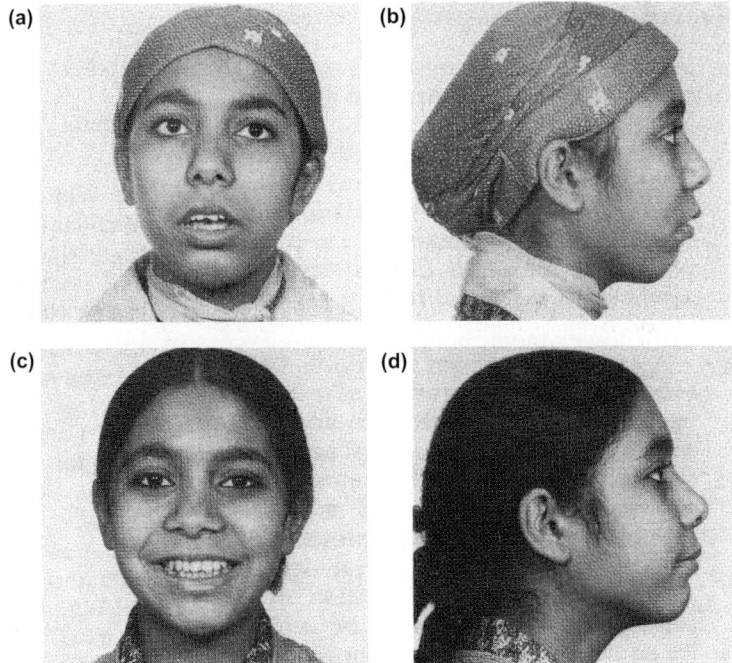

Figure 10.35 Orthodontic preparation was not possible for this patient with diphenyl hydantoin gingival hyperplasia, vertical maxillary excess, an anterior open bite and a marked curve of Spee. Therefore a Le Fort I elevation was combined with an anterior segmental osteotomy to level the occlusal plane and correct the incision lip relationship. The mandible autorotated to close the open bite. (a) to (c) Preoperative. (d) to (f) Postoperative.

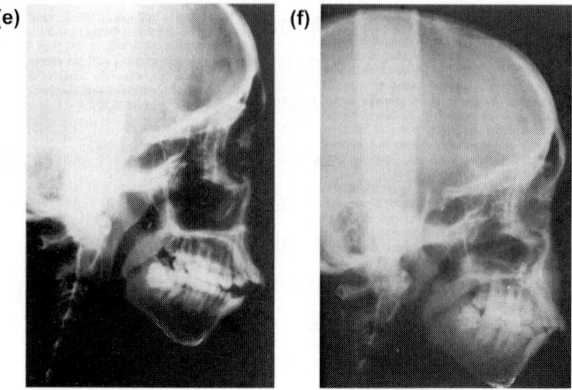

Figure 10.35   (*Continued*)

The Skeletal Open Bite Class III

Treatment

1. a)   Where there is no VME and the maxillary occlusal plane is normally inclined, but the mandibular ramus and body length are increased (which can be confirmed by the posterior lower facial height being in excess of 44% of the total posterior facial height), a sagittal split osteotomy is performed to displace the mandibular body upwards and backwards to occlude with the maxillary teeth (Figures 10.29 and 10.36). Bicortical screws or well placed buccal bone plates will provide end result stability.

    b)   Where there is an associated degree of maxillary retrusion this can be corrected by a Le Fort I forward movement which will reduce the open bite and mandibular setback.

2. In the more common, mixed case, consisting of a prognathous mandible with a VME, a Le Fort I elevation of the maxilla will be essential. This will increase the degree of mandibular prognathism and therefore the pushback (Figure 10.37).

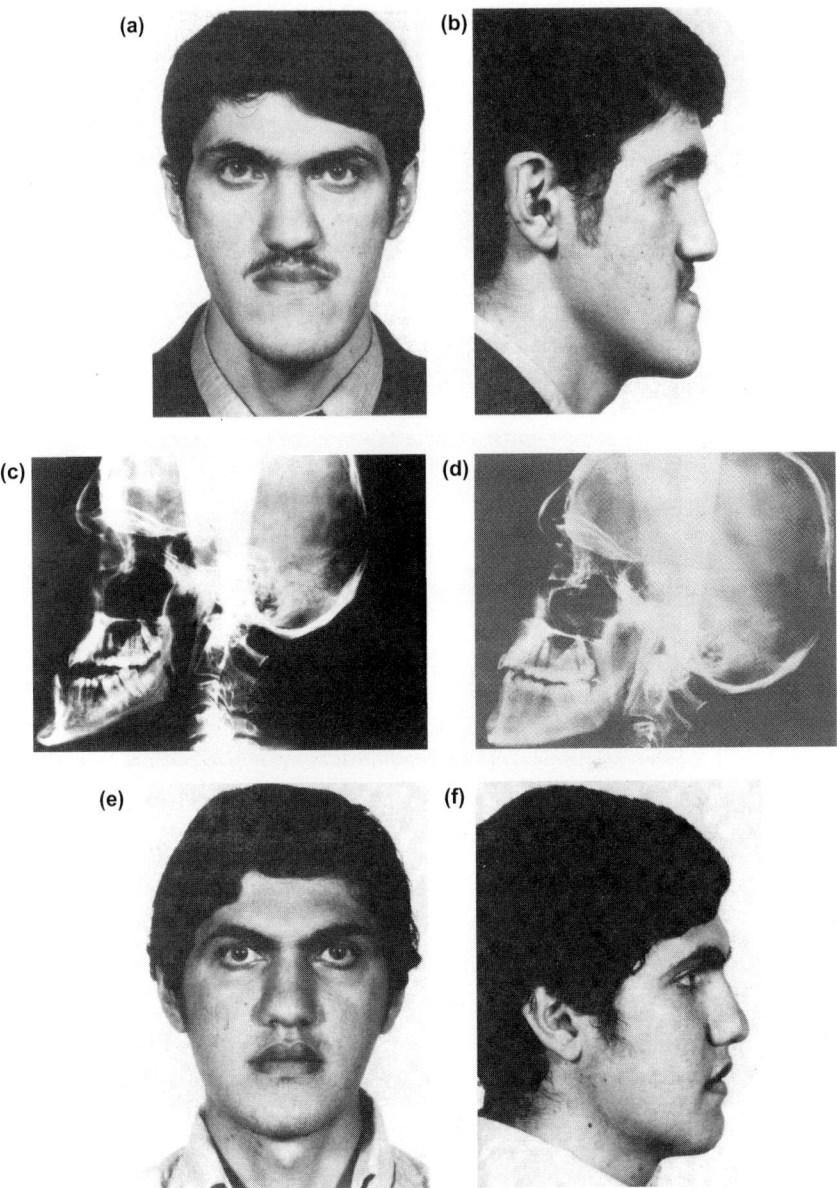

Figure 10.36 An non-decompensated Class III skeletal open bite which was treated only by a mandibular setback and trimming of the chin point. (**a**) to (**c**) Preoperative. (**d**) to (**f**) Postoperative.

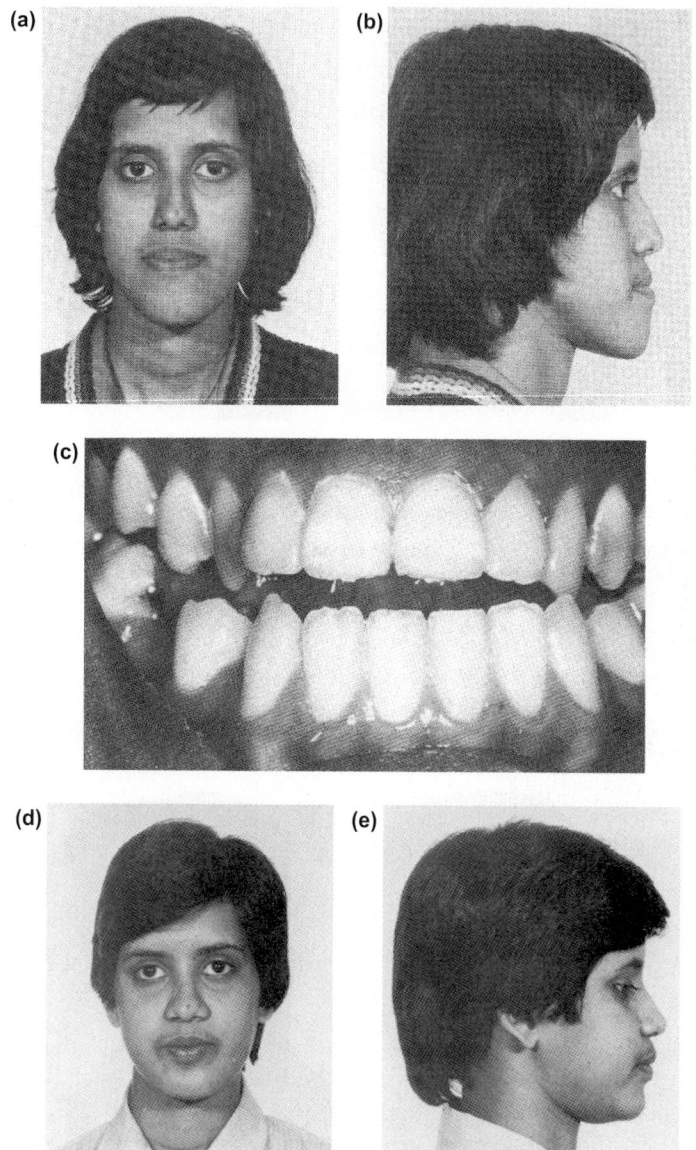

Figure 10.37 A non-decompensated combination of vertical maxillary excess, mandibular prognathism and an open bite **(a)** to **(d)**. This was corrected by a Le Fort I elevation and a mandibular setback **(e)** to **(h)**. Note the postoperative facial soft tissue excess which has remodelled over the subsequent 4 years; **(i)** shows the stable result 4 years later.

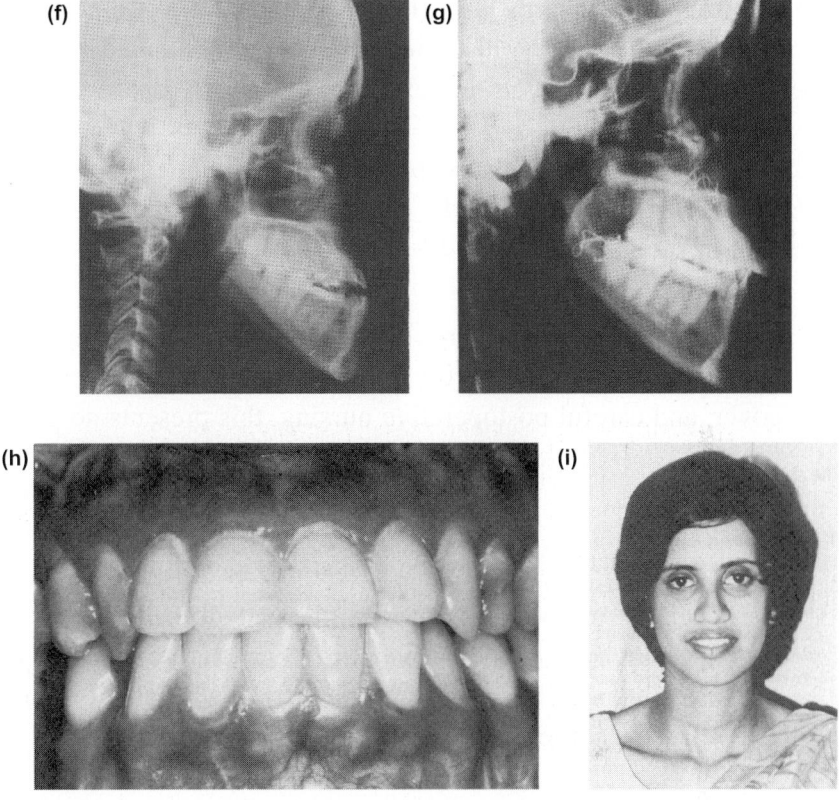

Figure 10.37   (*Continued*)

The Large Tongue

This is an area of some uncertainty. Most of the tongue lies in the oropharynx, where it is paradoxically called the posterior "third". The anterior two-thirds is a very adaptive and mobile organ which cannot be easily assessed anatomically or functionally. Tongue reduction was formerly carried out on theoretical grounds to prevent a relapse following the reduction in oral volume by a body ostectomy procedure for prognathism. The custom ceased with the introduction of the sagittal split osteotomy with its increased stability because it was assumed that the tongue moved backwards with the mandible. As tongue position is determined by the hyoid bone, which is not affected by this operation, surgical tongue reduction was correctly discarded for the wrong reason.

However, some patients do present with proclined incisors, a localised anterior open bite and a clinically large tongue. The management of such a case should be as follows:

1. Reduce the tongue at the same operation as the open bite segmental osteotomies. With careful haemostasis, antiodema steroidal cover, and careful postoperative nursing, this presents no great problem.

Or, if in doubt:

2. Carry out the osteotomies but warn the patient that if a relapse becomes obvious, particularly with recurrent proclination of the lower incisors, then a tongue reduction will be necessary. The relapse can then be corrected orthodontically.

The Short Face

This is uncommon in non-cleft patients and, as usual, can present in three forms:

1. Where the shortage is essentially in the lower face. This is the marked Class II division 1 mandible with a small anterior dentoalveolar height and an everted lower lip. The mid-face is normal or acceptable (Figure 10.8).
2. Where there is a decrease in middle facial height, occasionally with a small alveolar process and small teeth in both jaws (Figure 10.38). As cleft patients present with additional problems, they will be dealt with separately in Chapter 11.
3. A combination of both.

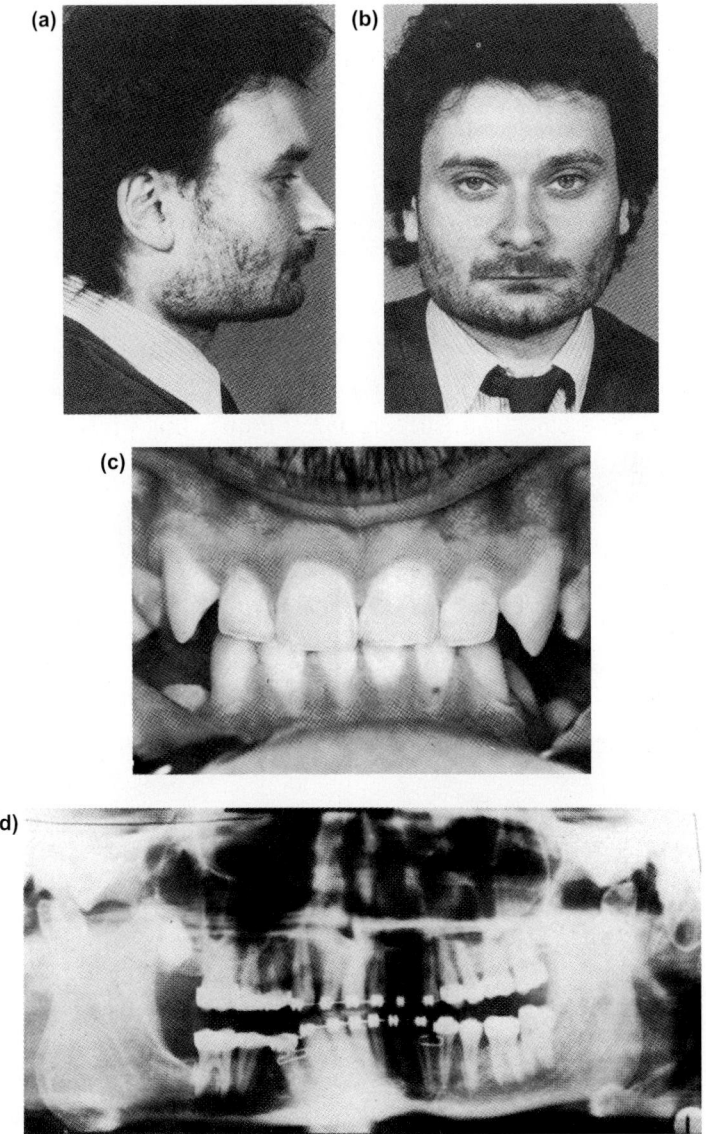

Figure 10.38   **(a)** to **(m)** A short face with vertical maxillary deficiency and also a marked lack of mandibular vertical height. This is an acquired developmental defect due to prolonged wearing of a Milwaukee brace to correct scoliosis in childhood. Preoperative **(a)** to **(d)**. Presurgical orthodontics levelled the incisor and buccal occlusal planes independently. The maxilla has been lowered by a Le Fort I

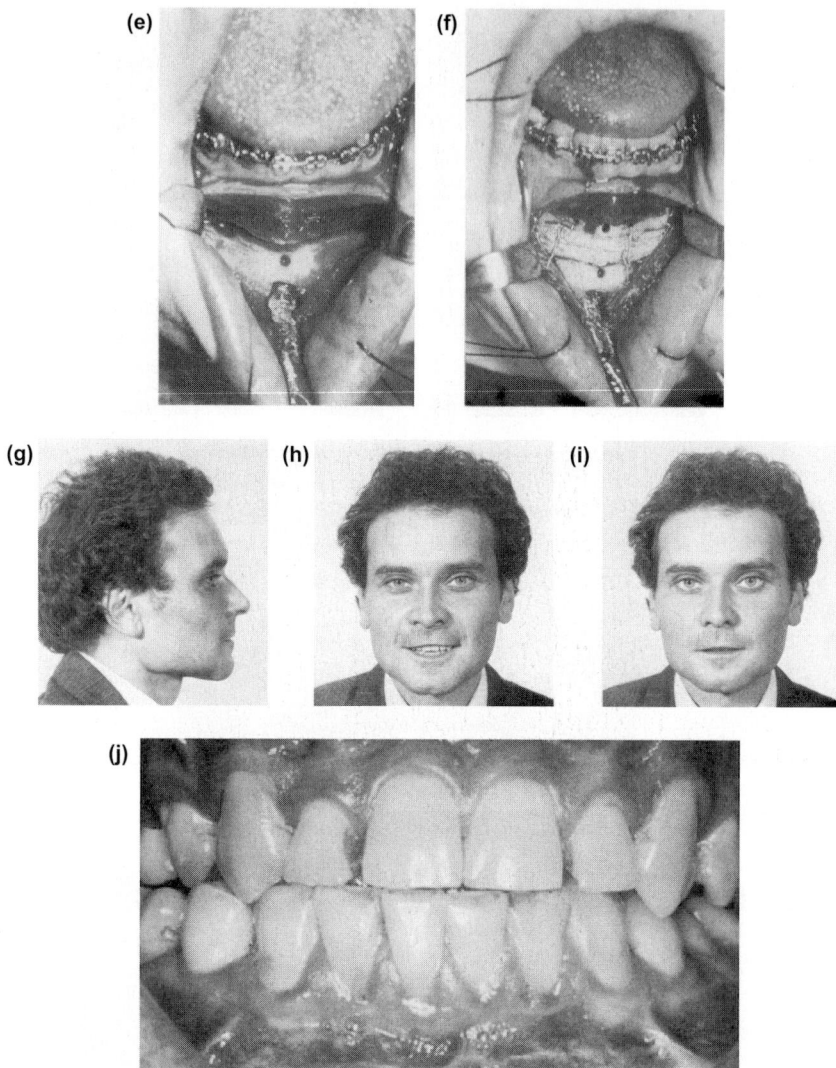

Figure 10.38 (*Continued*)   osteotomy with split rib interpositional grafts fixed with bone plates. The mandible has been advanced to correct the retrognathism. The underdeveloped anterior inferior dentoalveolar height has been corrected by a combination of a segmental mandibulotomy set down with a Proplast interpositional graft. The mandibulotomy also flattens the occlusal place (**e**) to (**i**). Genioplasty section before (**j**) and after insertion of a alloplast wedge (**k**). Preoperative (**l**) and postoperative (**m**) lateral skull radiographs.

(k)

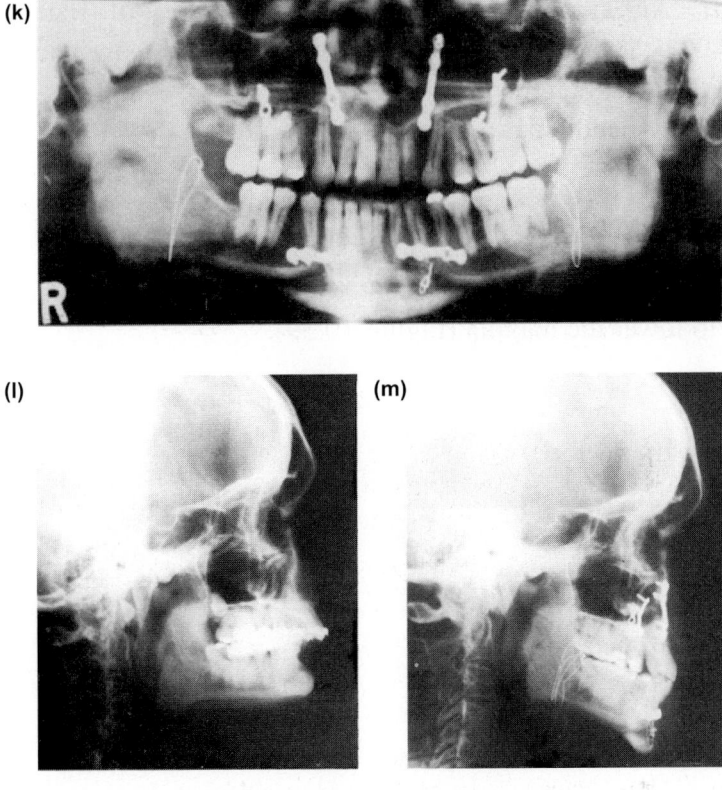

(l)   (m)

Figure 10.38 (*Continued*)

Treatment

1. Lower face deficiency

There is usually over-eruption of the incisors, producing a marked curve of Spee. Therefore the choice is between:

i) a) Preoperative orthodontic levelling of the occlusal plane.
    b) A mandibular advancement. Bone can also be inserted as a vertical augmentation sandwich genioplasty (Figure 10.38).
ii) a) Orthodontic levelling of the occlusal plane at two levels.

b) An anterior mandibulotomy which will flatten the occlusal plane and simultaneously increase the lower facial height.

c) A mandibular advancement (Figure 10.8).

2. Mid-face deficiency

Treatment is by a Le Fort I osteotomy with an interpositional bone graft to lower the maxilla (Figure 10.39).

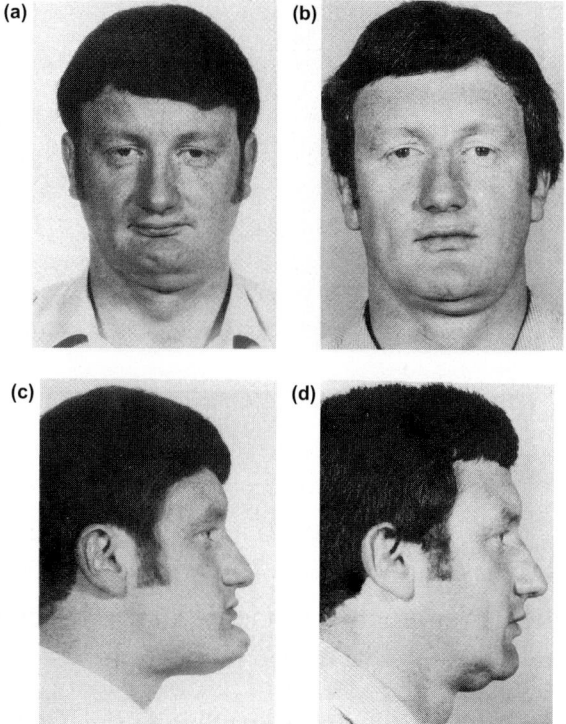

Figure 10.39 A short face due to a maxillary vertical deficiency with dentoalveolar hypoplasia. The maxilla was set down 1 cm with iliac crest interpositional bone grafts and the mandible repositioned with sagittal split osteotomy. **(a)** to **(c)** Preoperative. **(d)** to **(f)** Postoperative.

(e) (f)

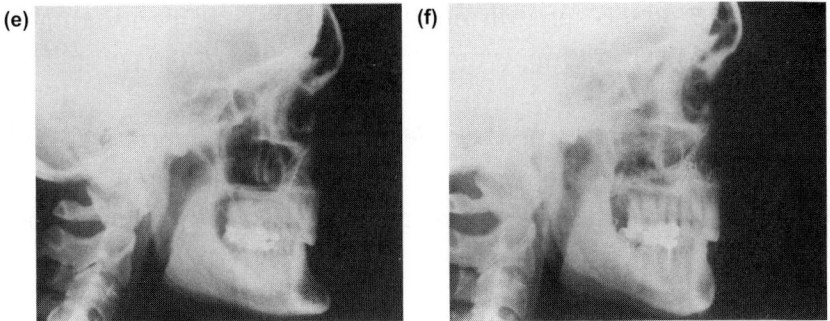

Figure 10.39 (*Continued*)

Preoperatively an estimate must be made of the required increase in facial height. This may be determined clinically by inserting wax wafers of increasing thickness between the teeth until the desired profile "in occlusion" with the lips at rest is achieved. Add 25% to give the immediate postoperative vertical separation of the jaws and height of the interpositional graft. This is measured and recorded.

Operative Procedure

1. The cuts of the sagittal split are made but not separated.
2. A Le Fort I osteotomy is carried out, with the maxilla well separated from the pterygoid plates. The maxilla is then wired temporarily to the unchanged mandible using an intermediate wafer.
3. Using dividers and ruler to confirm the planned separation (i.e. increased facial height) measured from the canine tips to the inner canthi, bone plates are screwed to the upper border of the maxillary osteotomy, and then the split rib or iliac crest cancellous bone blocks are wedged between the bone cuts and secured with screws. Face the medullary

surface of the split rib outwards against the periosteum to ensure the best opportunity for graft vascularisation (see Bone Grafts).

4. Intermaxillary fixation is released, the mandible is split and fixed using the final wafer.

5. The throat pack is removed and the nasopharynx and hypopharynx carefully aspirated.

Maxillary Asymmetry

Maxillary asymmetry may be:

i) Primary and associated with deformity of the whole facial skeleton. In mild disturbances it can be difficult to decide whether one side is reduced in height or the other increased. However, in primary deformities, in addition to the coronal tilt in the occlusal plane, there is usually a cant in the orbital plane.

ii) The late presentation of a secondary maxillary alveolar response to the lateral open bite in a unilateral mandibular hyperplasia. Fibrous dysplasia of the maxilla and slowly-growing benign tumours will also present in the same way.

Treatment

• Minor degrees of orbital asymmetry are acceptable and therefore the surgery only consists of levelling the occlusal plane by a Le Fort I osteotomy, removing bone on the long side.

• If the difference in height is split between the two sides the coronal ipsilateral upward rotation, creates a horizontal deficiency on the short side. This deficiency may be closed by inserting the removed bone fragments into the defect stabilised with screws and plates. A sagittal split or subsigmoid osteotomy will be required to rotate the mandible into occlusion with the repositioned maxilla (Figure 10.40).

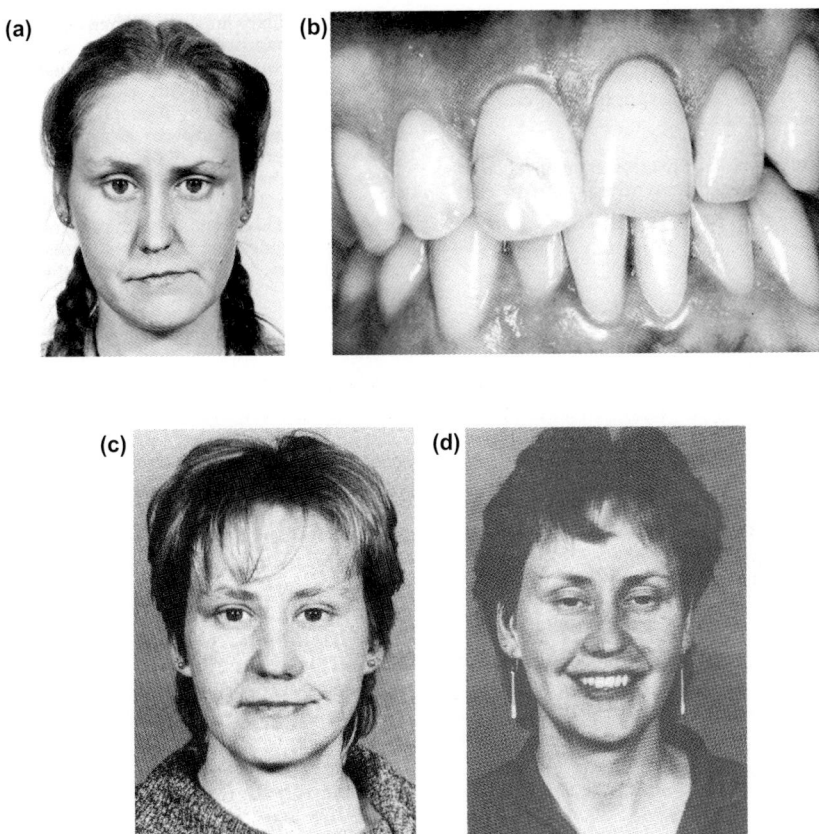

Figure 10.40 Maxillary asymmetry with a marked slope of the occlusal plane. This was corrected by bimaxillary osteotomies rotating the maxilla upwards on the right side, and bringing the mandible into occlusion with a bilateral sagittal split both jaws. A fillet of bone should be removed on the inner aspect of the right ascending ramus to allow it to rise in the coronal plane and occlude with the maxilla. **(a)** and **(b)** Preoperative. **(c)** and **(d)** Postoperative.

- With a unilateral maxillary fibrous dysplasia, a Le Fort I down-fracture allows the solid dysplastic tissue to be radically removed from orbital floor to antral floor, leaving the periosteum to regenerate the facial antral wall.

Encapsulated tumours, such as ossifying fibromas, may be removed in the same way.

11

Secondary Cleft Lip and Palate Deformities

Introduction

Cleft lip and palate deformities are the most common congenital deformities of the facial region. This chapter will focus on the secondary correction of cleft-related deformity.

The management of secondary deformity must involve the surgeon, orthodontist and speech pathologist working closely with the paediatrician, ear nose and throat surgeon, plastic surgeon, and clinical psychologist when appropriate.

The clinical problem depends on the type and severity of the cleft and on the type, extent and quality of the primary surgery and any revisions of these "primary procedures". Compromises between function, aesthetics and growth have to be made which determine the timing of surgery. For instance the timing of palate repair is a balance between enabling speech development and optimum facial growth. What ever the compromise the number of operations must be kept to the minimum.

Important Factors

1. The amount of tissue in the original embryological defect (Figure 11.1).

    Although structures may be displaced, the amount of soft tissue is not usually deficient in the unrepaired unilateral or

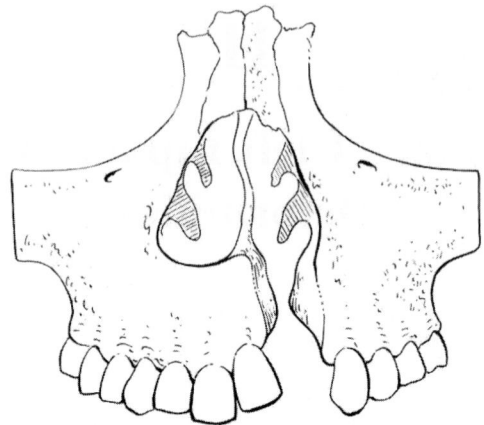

Figure 11.1   A complete cleft of the lip and palate extends through the alveolus in the region of the left lateral incisor with or without fistula extending into the nose.

bilateral cleft deformity (Figures 11.2a–11.2d). Impaired growth and development usually arise from subsequent surgery rather than inherent differences in growth potential. The exception is in some bilateral cases where the premaxilla and pro-labial segment can be relatively small before surgical intervention (Figures 11.3a and 11.3b). True aplasia of tissue is uncommon although can be seen in cases of mid line clefting.

2.   The nature and quality of the primary surgery.

Facial deformity will develop as a consequence of scar contraction following surgery especially in the palate (Figures 11.4a–11.4c).

Patients with similar clefts repaired in different ways may exhibit different patterns of facial growth. Figures 11.5a–11.5h illustrate two brothers, both with complete right side unilateral cleft lip and palate operated using different palatal techniques demonstrating different mid facial growth.

3.   Also important is the preservation of tissue. Tissue removal should be avoided whenever possible.

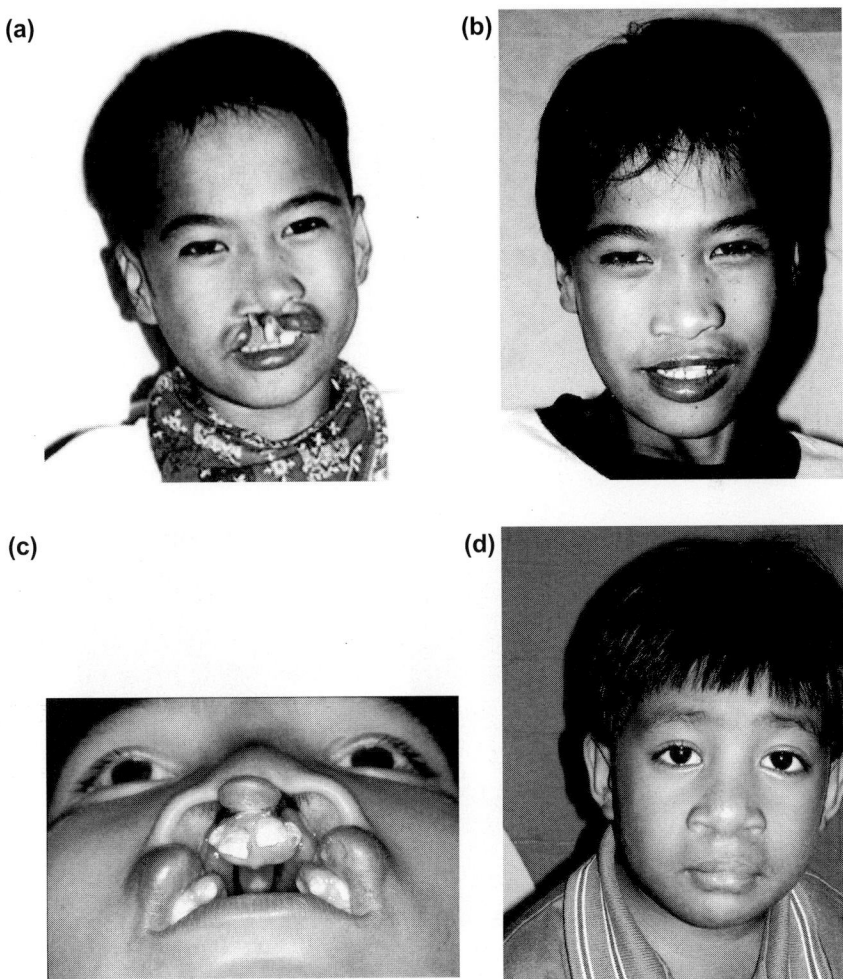

Figure 11.2 Soft tissues are not normally absent in the typical untreated unilateral or bilateral cleft (**a**), (**c**) preoperatively, and (**b**), (**d**) postoperatively.

The surgical correction of skeletal cleft deformity presents a greater challenge than most orthognathic procedures. A variety of programmes for treating these cases is possible. Unfortunately the selection of operation is usually dictated by the surgeon's preference rather than objectively compared data.

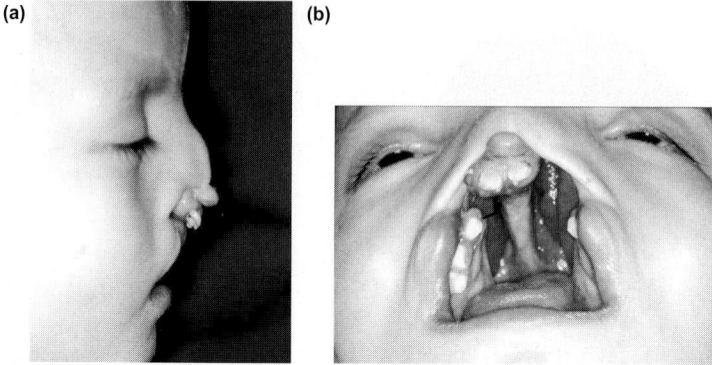

Figure 11.3 Hypoplasia may occur in bilateral cases — particularly of the premaxilla and prolabial segments.

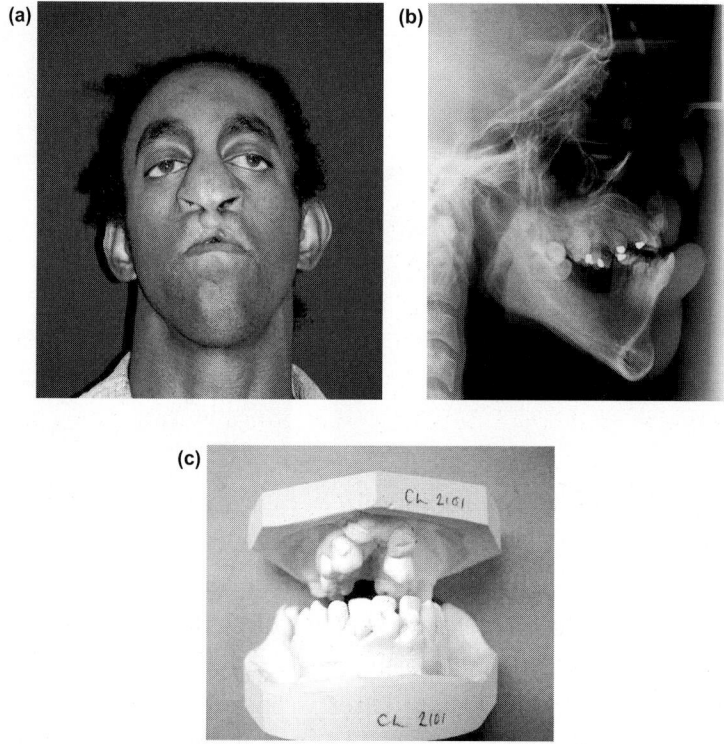

Figure 11.4 Surgery, particularly to the palate can cause secondary changes resulting in marked deformity of the mid-face.

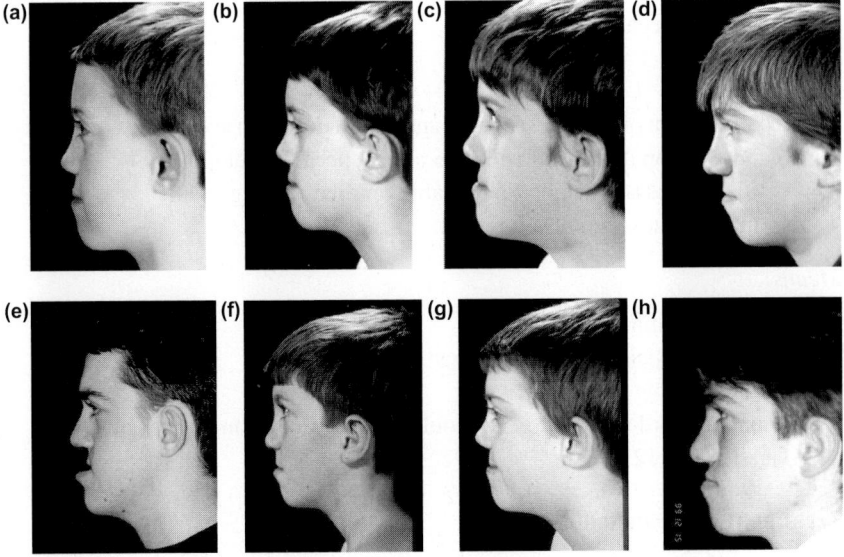

Figure 11.5 Surgically impaired growth potential can be impossible to predict as illustrated by these two brothers.

Surgical Instrumentation

Intra-oral access is possible with a Mushin dental prop but this can be distracting at crucial moments. A self-retaining gag such as a Featherstone is better, but for ultimate ease one should use a cleft palate gag such as the Kilner modification of the Dott or the Dingman, which also provides simultaneous retraction.

The choice of needles is crucial, and include the 5/8 25 mm (Denys Browne), a 16 mm slim blade needle or the small J shaped compound curved needle mounted with 4/0 or 5/0 Vicryl Rapide (Ethicon). Children do not like suture removal. Small needles demand a fine-tipped ratchet needle holder, e.g. Stille Converse, and very fine dissecting forceps, e.g. Adsons. Subperiosteal flap dissection within a cleft also requires a small

Table 11.1   Pathway of care

Early stages of treatment

Aims:

1. Reconstruction of the oral sphincter and restoration of an acceptable appearance.
2. Reconstruction of the soft palate to allow speech development.
3. Avoid unnecessary surgery and enable optimal facial growth.
4. Normal psychosocial development.

Means:

1. Lip repair within first 6 months.
2. Soft palate repair at one year of age.
3. Speech therapy.
4. Secondary hard palate surgery should be delayed as long as possible. Usually until 12 months.

Treatment in the mixed dentition

Aims:

1. Orthodontic alignment of the developing dentition.
2. Reconstruction of the alveolar cleft and dental arch form.
3. Oronasal fistula closure.
4. Restore normal symmetrical maxillary bony contour.
5. Stabilisation of the dentoalveolar segments.
6. Maintenance of a healthy adult dentition.

Means:

1. Orthodontics essential for surgery.
2. Alveolar reconstruction with bone grafting.
3. Segmental alveolar distraction osteogenesis where appropriate.
4. Fistula closure.
5. Preventative and restorative dental care.

Treatment in adolescence and early adulthood

Aims:

1. Correction of any disturbance of facial growth and skeletal imbalance.

(Continued)

Table 11.1   (*Continued*)

2. Reconstruction of nasal deformity.
3. Correction of any soft tissue deformity.
4. Correction of any occlusal disturbances.
5. Provision of an aesthetically pleasing smile.

Means:

1. Presurgical orthodontic treatment.
2. Malar maxillary distraction osteogenesis where appropriate.
3. Orthognathic surgery to correct secondary skeletal deformities.
4. Post-orthognathic orthodontics.
5. Residual fistula closure.
6. Dental reconstruction.
7. Definitive nose and lip correction.

sharp periosteal elevator such as the McDonald, Friers pattern or even a Mitchell's trimmer.

The Surgical Procedures

Establishment of bony continuity (bone grafting of the alveolar cleft).

- The optimum time for alveolar bone grafting is between 7 and 12 years, before the permanent canine on the cleft side erupts and when half to two thirds of its root has formed.
- At this age, anteroposterior and transverse maxillary growth is practically complete apart from the alveolar development of the erupting permanent teeth. Hence grafting at this time does not affect mid face growth but provides the all important bone support for the erupting canine.
- The bone also enables orthodontic positioning of the canine.
- Creates a one piece maxilla for orthognathic surgery.

- Provides stabilisation for any prosthetic replacement.
- It is also possible to simultaneously graft the alar base.

Prior to grafting, presurgical orthodontics will have expanded the maxillary arch to restore the arch form between the major and lesser segments. The teeth adjacent to the cleft will have been aligned providing there is sufficient bone around the roots and a good periodontal attachment to accommodate the alignment.

If the premaxillary segment has been surgically repositioned forwards or orthodontic arch expansion has been used to facilitate the grafting procedure, a retaining appliance is essential to prevent collapse before consolidation of the bone graft.

The Problems

- A unilateral alveolar defect.
- Anterior oronasal fistula.
- Alar-base asymmetry.

Surgical Treatment

1. Instruments should comprise a basic intraoral surgical set with the addition of a fine periosteal elevator, such as a McDonald, Frier or Mitchell's trimmer, and skin hooks. Access may be gained with a Dingman cleft palate or Featherstone gag.
2. The incision is made down to bone around the margin of the anterior fistula, except where the fistula lies high in the anterior vestibule beneath the upper lip. At this point there is no underlying bone and the incision is through mucosa only (Figures 11.6a–11.6d).

    Figure 11.6b shows how the narrow strip at the cervical margin of the tooth is sliced to create as wide a band of de-epithelialised tissue as possible.

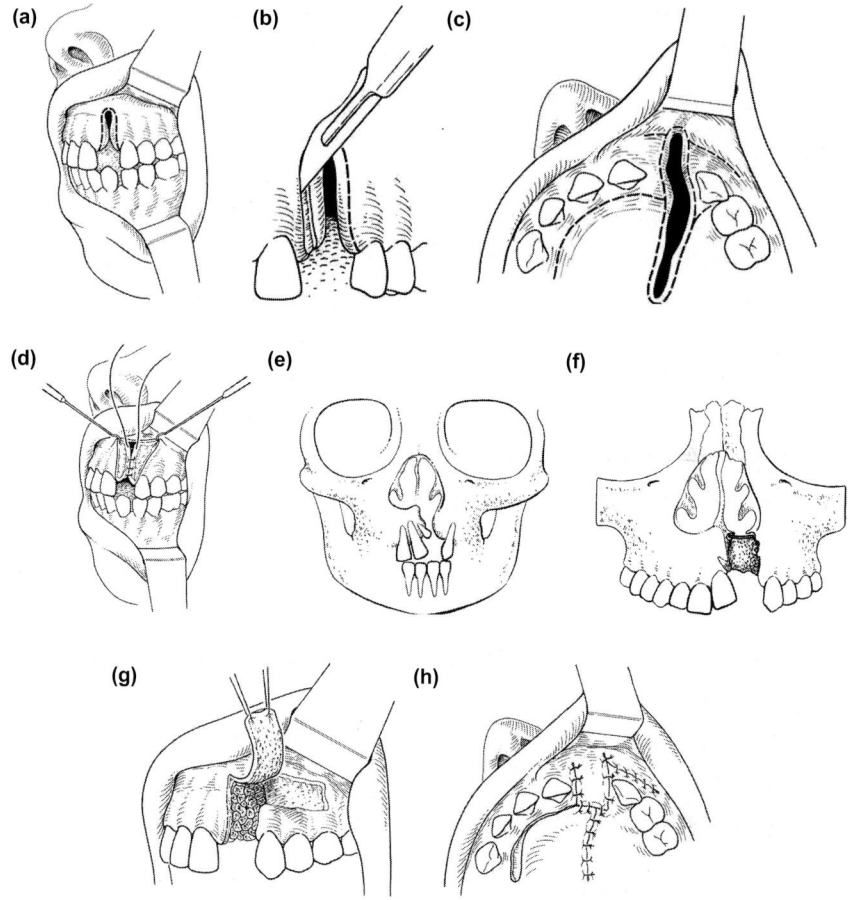

Figures 11.6 Alveolar bone grafting with simultaneous repair of oral and nasal mucosal layers. The rotator finger flap (**g** and **h**) is seldom used in current practice.

The initial incision can be extended safely along the buccal sulcus overlying the lesser segment unless a segmental osteotomy is required.

If the fistula or alveolar defect extends into the palate a palatal flap will need to be raised (Figure 11.6c).

Subperiosteal dissection is directed into the fistula and the liberated soft tissues are pushed up towards the nasal cavity.

Much of this tissue becomes redundant and can be cut away leaving just sufficient to form a nasal layer.

3. Where the soft tissues bridge the cleft, i.e. in the buccal sulcus and behind on the palate, two layers are created by sharp dissection.

4. If the fistula is wide enough the nasal layer can be closed with resorbable sutures on a very small needle (Figure 11.6d). If the bone defect is too narrow to insert a suture in the nasal layer (Figure 11.6e), a piece of oxidised cellulose (Surgicel, Ethicon Ltd, Edinburgh, UK) or acellular submucosal matrix can be inserted to seal the nasal surface of the cleft (Figure 11.6f). Any supernumerary teeth are extracted and cancellous bone chips are packed into the whole defect.

5. Cancellous bone chips are obtained from the iliac crest and packed firmly into the bone cleft. A substantial amount may be required as it is particularly important to pack bone up under the lateral part of the alar cartilage to create a nasal sill (Figure 11.6g).

6. An oral defect remains at the site of the original incision. These margins cannot be brought together as they are largely attached gingiva.

7. A mucogingival transposition flap pedicled superiorly in the sulcus is raised and mobilised by dividing the inelastic periosteum with a sharp blade. When rotated into position it leaves a bare area of buccal alveolus distally, which will epithelialise spontaneously. This technique is most useful after bone grafting in the patient with a mixed dentition. In these cases the oral defect is narrow and the transposition flap is taken from the gingival margins of the deciduous molars, which are usually extracted at the same time (Figures 11.7a–11.7c).

8. The flap is rotated over the bone graft and sutured to the margins of the fistula with 5/0 Vicryl on a 16 mm slim blade needle. This must be done meticulously with multiple fine sutures to produce a watertight edge-to-edge closure (Figure 11.6h).

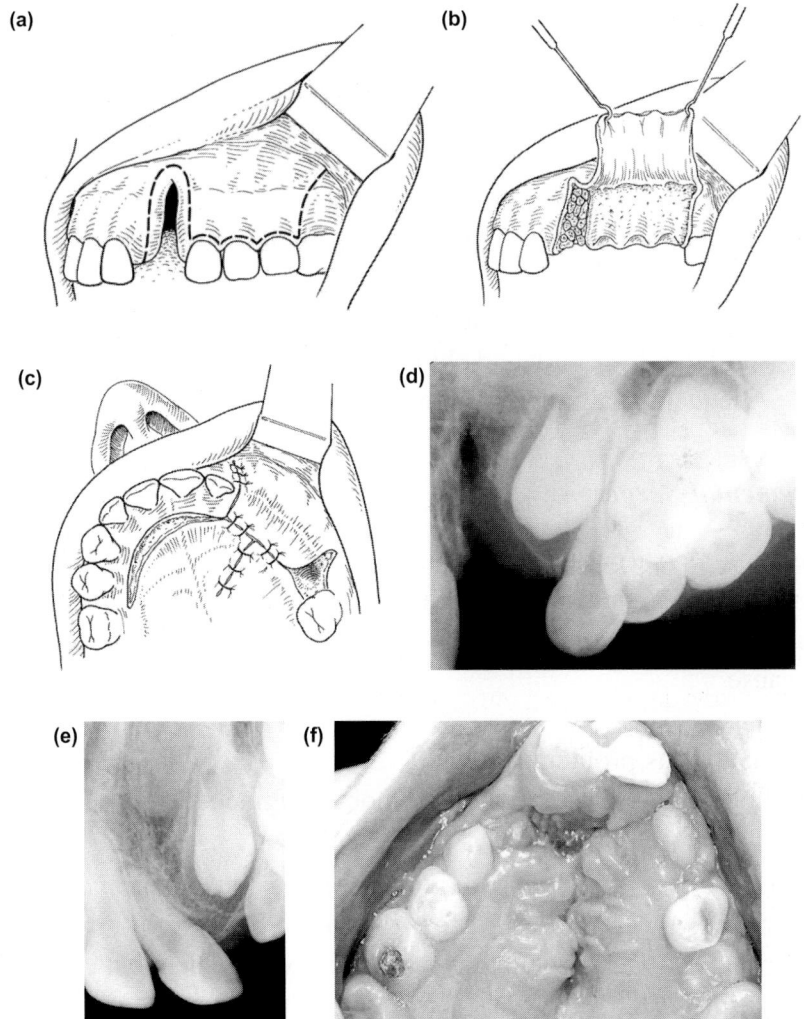

Figure 11.7   (**c**) Raising and rotating a buccal transposition flat. (**d**) Ungrafted cleft. (**e** and **f**) Canine erupting through consolidated bone graft.

9. The palatal flap from the greater segment is not always required in small defects.
10. Figures 11.7d–11.7f show the alveolar defect before and after grafting and the erupting canine.

Postoperatively

Intraoral bone grafts in cleft patients require meticulous postoperative care. The following precautions are recommended:

1. Preoperative intravenous antibiotics should be administered and then postoperative prophylactic antibiotics given orally for 5 days.
2. Maintain scrupulous oral hygiene. The patient is given a semi-solid diet by mouth and chlorhexidine gluconate mouthwashes.
3. Adequate analgesia for both oral and donor sites.

Segmental Surgery

Segmental surgery is now rarely required at the time of alveolar bone grafting, as orthodontic preparation or distraction osteogenesis will usually align the segments. It should be avoided because

a) fixation is problematic and
b) bone grafts do not unite with mobile segments.

However, the local dentoalveolar relationship may be improved by combining the alveolar bone graft with an osteotomy to the lesser segment or premaxilla. The most common indications are:

1. Adequate vertical and anterior growth of the greater alveolar segment but vertical deficiency of the lesser segment. This may be associated with dental arch collapse and recession with asymmetry of the nasal base.
2. The fistula is too large to close for bone grafting, and soft tissue coverage is not possible.

3. Orthodontic expansion of the arch has not been possible as the lesser segment may be trapped palatally.
4. Distraction osteogenesis is not available.

The Problems

- A unilateral alveolar defect.
- Anterior fistula and nasal base asymmetry.
- Deficient vertical growth of the lesser segment and collapse of the maxillary dental arch.

The Surgical Treatment

- Osteotomy to reposition the lesser segment.
- Bone graft to the alveolar defect and osteotomy site.
- Closure of the anterior oronasal fistula.

1. The initial incision is made around the intraoral margin of the fistula, as before. A horizontal sulcus incision can be made at this stage to improve access but this incision should now be made along the line of the greater segment (Figure 11.8a).
2. The lesser segment osteotomy is carried out at the LeFort I level from the buccal side by inserting a suitably protected bur or the narrow blade of a reciprocating power saw. The horizontal cut is carried through until the blade action can be palpated beneath the attached palatal mucosa (Figure 11.8b).
3. The lesser segment is still not free posteriorly. In cleft patients the anatomy of the tuberosity-pterygoid plate junction is frequently distorted and the bone may be very dense in this area. In order to free the segment, a 1 cm mucosal incision is made behind the tuberosity and a 7 or 10 mm thin osteotome directed vertically (Figure 11.8c).

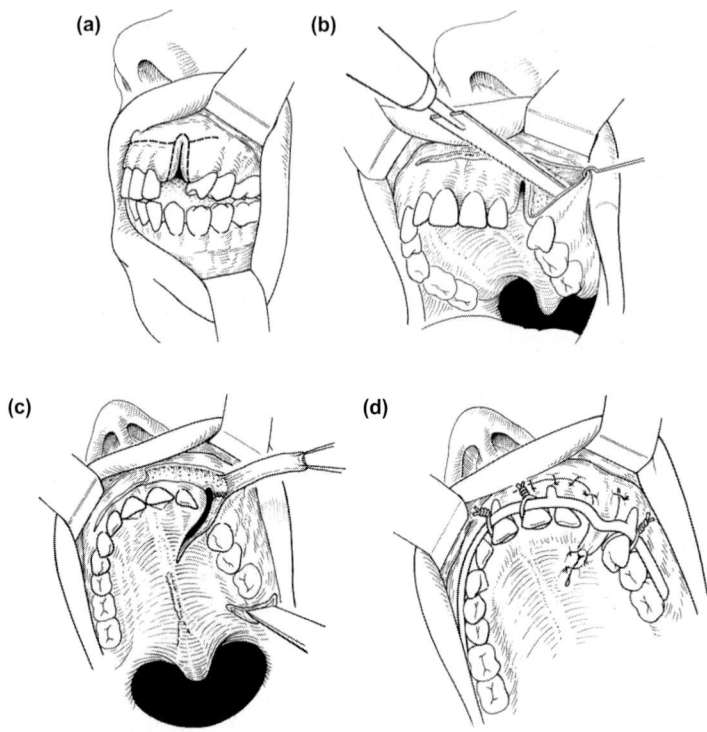

Figure 11.8 Lesser segment of alveolar osteotomy at the time of alveolar bone grafting.

4.   The freed lesser segment is now further mobilised by blunt dissection until it can be aligned according to the preoperative plan.
5.   If the dental arch is expanded to any extent it will open up the cleft of the hard palate. This can only be made good by lifting and rotating the mucoperiosteum covering the palatal aspect of the greater segment and suturing it to the freshened edge of the palatal mucosa covering the lesser segment. The palatal mucosa covering the lesser segment should remain attached to maximise the blood supply to the segment. In practice, nasal layer closure is not found to be a problem, even after surgical expansion of the maxillary arch.

6. Cancellous bone chips and sheets of cancellous bone obtained from the iliac crest or by trephining the tibia, are used to fill the alveolar defect and to pack the osteotomy site on the lesser segment.

7. The lesser osteotomised segment is immobilised by attachment to the greater segment using a preformed arch bar (Figure 11.8d) ligated with 0.35 mm prestretched soft stainless steel wire.

8. There remains the oral mucosal defect on the buccal and alveolar aspect of the cleft. It is not advisable to raise an anteriorly based finger flap or buccal mucogingival transposition flap if above changes are made as suggested, this should be removed because this would compromise the buccal mucosal attachment to the osteotomised segment. The vestibular finger flap is therefore based posteriorly and raised from the mucosa and submucosa of the buccal sulcus between the anterior part of the greater segment and the lip, as shown in Figures 11.8c and 11.8d.

9. Suturing and postoperative care are as already described above.

Bilateral Clefts (Figure 11.9)

Orthognathic surgery for bilateral clefts is very difficult and should only be attempted by experienced surgeons. Three presentations will be considered. However all cases are complicated by:

 i) scarring of the prolabium indicating poor vascularity,
 ii) multiple previous operations,
iii) a large anterior palatal fistulae extending bilaterally through the alveolus, and
iv) marked asymmetry.

Presentation 1 — The Problems

•   Large anterior palatal fistulae extending bilaterally through the alveolus.

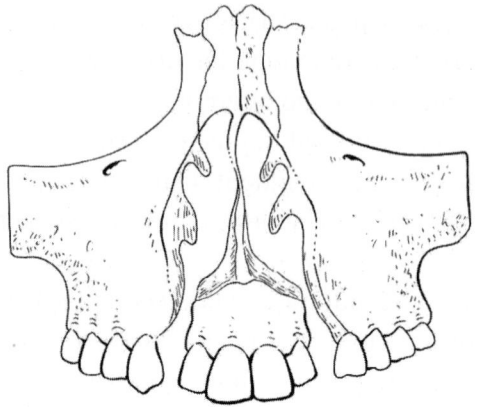

Figure 11.9   Care must be taken not to compromise the blood supply of the pre-maxillary segment in bilateral cleft cases.

- Recession of the nasal tip.
- Shortening of the columella.
- Symmetrical flaring of the alar bases.

The Surgical Treatment

Closure of the anterior fistulae with bone grafts to the alveolar defects.

- Reconstruction of the nasal sills providing bony support to the alar bases.
- Lengthening of the columella, and forward repositioning of the alar cartilages with narrowing of the nasal tip.
- Rotation of the alar bases inwards towards the mid line.
- Narrowing of the nasal bridge (see Rhinoplasty).

1. Orthodontic expansion of the maxillary arch must precede surgery. Rapid maxillary expansion may be employed if the scarred palatal tissues are later mobilised surgically.
2. If the maxillary arch alignment and forward development is adequate, surgical dissection of the anterior fistulae and alveolar

defects can proceed as in the unilateral case, duplicating the surgery for each of the two clefts (see previously).

3. Teeth in the premaxillary segment adjacent to the cleft alveolus on each side may be found to be denuded of bone. This applies particularly to any remaining lateral incisors. In order to achieve a successful bone graft such teeth must be removed.

4. It is difficult to raise a healthy mucoperiosteal flap from the palatal aspect of the premaxillary segment which can be sutured to the scarred palatal mucosa behind and the buccal flaps which are rotated inwards to cover the bone graft.

   It is therefore better to confine the autogenous grafts to the higher and buccal parts of the alveolar defect and to make no attempt to achieve a bridge of bone across the anterior part of the hard palate.

Presentation 2 — The Problems

*   Retroposition of the premaxilla with collapse of the maxillary arch, but satisfactory vertical growth of the bilateral posterior segments.
*   Nasal deformity as above, but more severe.

The Surgical Treatment

*   Osteotomy of the premaxilla in severe cases.
*   Bone graft to the alveolar defects with closure of anterior fistulae.
*   Rhinoplasty.

1. If the orthodontic expansion is satisfactory and produces a satisfactory alignment of each segment, surgical closure of the anterior fistula can proceed as in point 1 above.

2. Frequently, expansion of the lateral segments is achieved but the premaxilla remains retroposed (Figure 11.10a). In this case,

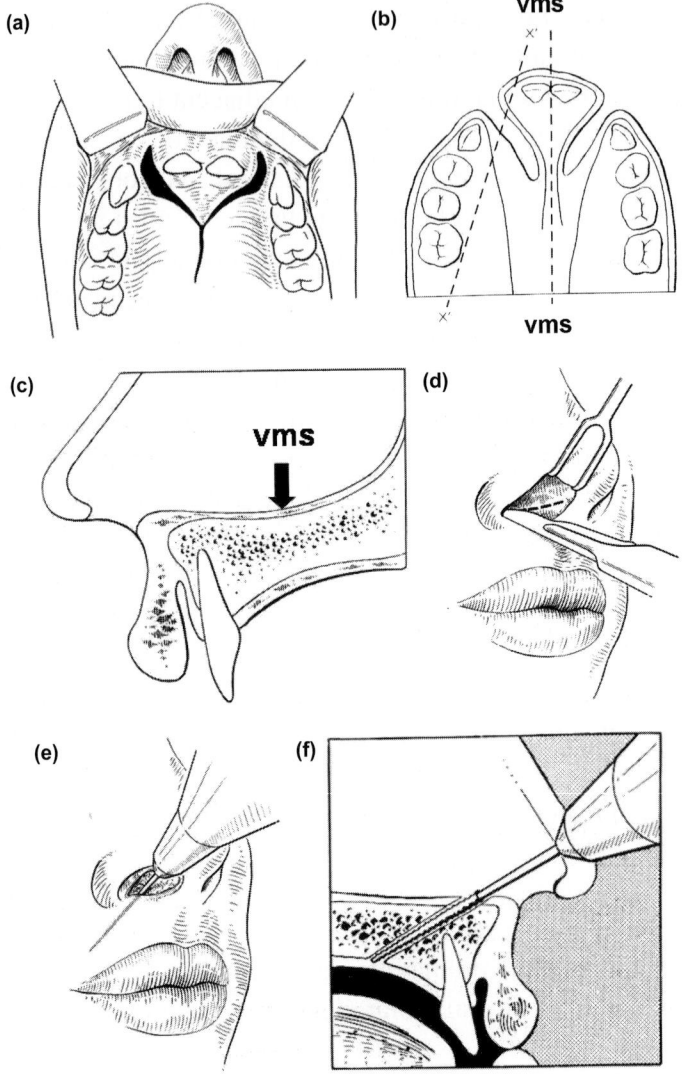

Figure 11.10   Osteotomy of the retroposed premaxillary segement in the bilateral case by sectioning of the vomerine-premaxillary spur (vms). Once displaced forwards the mucosa is carefully raised to provide cleft closure (**g–l**).

an osteotomy of the premaxilla alone is necessary at the time of the alveolar grafting.

3.   Retropositioning of the premaxilla also prevents surgical dissection of the clefts from a buccal approach. The premaxilla is

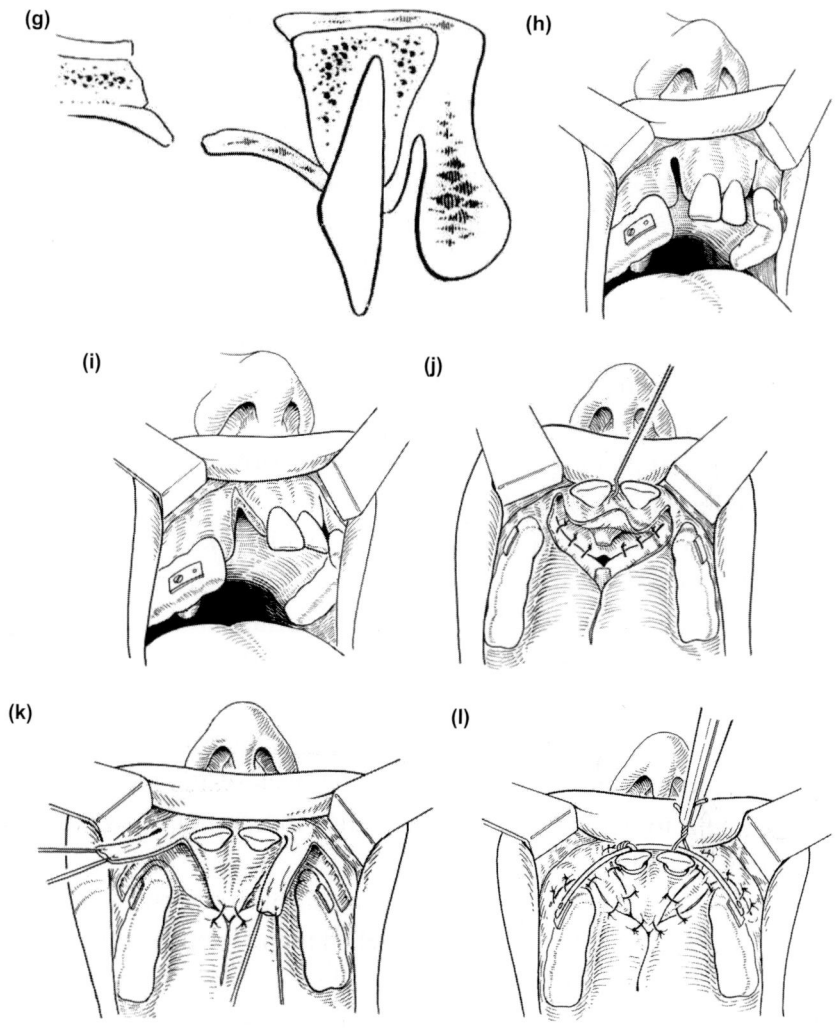

Figures 11.10 (*Continued*)

held back by a solid spur of bone extending forward from the anterior part of the base of the vomer, the vomerine-premaxillary spur, VMS (Figure 11.10b). Figure 11.10c shows the sagittal section of a bilateral cleft to illustrate the vomerine-premaxillary spur of bone. This spur may have a cartilaginous section behind the premaxilla in some cases but is too dense to be fractured by manipulation alone.

4.   The surgical exposure of this spur of bone can be achieved via the nose. Horizontal incisions are made in the nasal mucosa overlying the anterior part of the base of the septum (Figures 11.10d and 11.10e).

   The mucosa is raised by sharp dissection on each side of the septal base in a downwards and backwards direction towards the oral cavity just behind the premaxilla. In this way the vomerine-premaxillary spur is dissected free of its overlying mucoperiosteal cover without penetrating the mucosa on the nasal and oral aspect. The spur is cut with a surgical fissure bur at which point the premaxilla can be swung forwards, opening up the cleft on each side with its mucoperiosteum still attached (Figures 11.10h and 11.10i).

5.   Dissection of each side of the cleft can now take place as in the unilateral case and bone grafts inserted. Note the preservation of the mucosa on the back of the premaxillary segment to assist palatal closure together with the anteriorly based vestibular flaps (Figures 11.10j to 11.10l).

6.   Figure 11.10j illustrates the amount of palatal mucosal which needs to be carefully raised from the back of the premaxillary segment to achieve oral closure after the premaxilla has been repositioned.

7.   The premaxilla is immobilised by means of a preformed arch bar. Cap splints may be previously applied to the lateral segments but the premaxilla itself is best retained by gentle 0.35 mm ligatures to a preformed arch bar screwed to locking plates on each of the two cap splints on the lateral segments (Figure 11.10l).

8.   Rhinoplasty is carried out as a secondary procedure.

Presentation 3 — The Problems

•   A retropositioned premaxilla with a collapsed maxillary arch.
•   Inadequate vertical growth of the lateral segments.

- Mid facial retrusion.
- Severe nasal tip recession.

The Surgical Treatment

This presentation would benefit from distraction osteogenesis. However if not available surgical correction can be performed in two stages separated by 6 weeks. It is impossible to carry out, with consistent success, segmental osteotomies, grafting of alveolar defects, closure of fistulae and total maxillary repositioning in one operation.

1. Orthodontic expansion of the lateral segments is usually required.
2. The premaxillary osteotomy and grafting is performed as in point 2 above. In this case it is frequently necessary to reposition the premaxilla upward to align with the lateral segments, in which case part of the nasal septum may have to be cut away to accommodate the segment.
3. A simultaneous segmental osteotomy of one or other lateral segment may be required to achieve satisfactory total arch alignment. If the lateral segments have been expanded orthodontically against resistance from the scarred palatal tissues, the palatal mucoperiosteum must be mobilised surgically at this stage to prevent relapse.
4. After at least 9 months, and preferably 1 year, a standard Le Fort I osteotomy with down-fracture can be undertaken in those cases where alveolar reconstruction has been successful. The repositioned maxilla no longer requires extraoral craniomaxillary fixation in addition to miniplate internal fixation.
5. Rhinoplasty is carried out after the maxilla has been shown to be stable for 1 year.

Lesser Segment Alveolar Distraction

Segmental alveolar distraction may overcome the technical difficulties of dividing and fixing small osteotomy segments. By slowly moving the lesser segment at one millimetre per day towards the cleft, the size of the alveolar and dental gap is reduced. This decreases the size of both the graft and the flaps raised to close the fistula. It may even eliminate the need for an autogenous bone graft.

- Segmental distraction is only possible in young patients with erupted teeth on which brackets and tubes can be applied to fit a rigid wire to guide the distraction forward and around the arch form.
- Care must be taken to preserve the vascular supply to the osteotomised bony fragment and so a tunnelling approach is used buccally and palatally in order to perform the osteotomy cuts.
- The segment of alveolus chosen to be distracted will determine the site of the interdental osteotomy cut.
- This site requires the provision of space by the orthodontist, and a rigid archwire is fitted before surgery to guide the distraction.

The Surgical Preparation for Distraction

1. A horizontal incision is made through the buccal mucosa and the flap is raised to provide access for the horizontal segmental cut and a vertical interdental cut which is started buccally with a fine surgical bur (Figures 11.11a and 11.11b). Interdental space has been made orthodontically. The adjacent palatal mucoperiosteum is also raised with a fine elevator such as a Frier or a MacDonald exposing only sufficient bone to make the equivalent vertical cut through the palatal alveolus.

2. The palatal horizontal cut is now made by a tunnelling approach through the anterior cleft margin with a periosteal elevator (Figure 11.11a) and then the distal interproximal bone is divided with a fine osteotome.

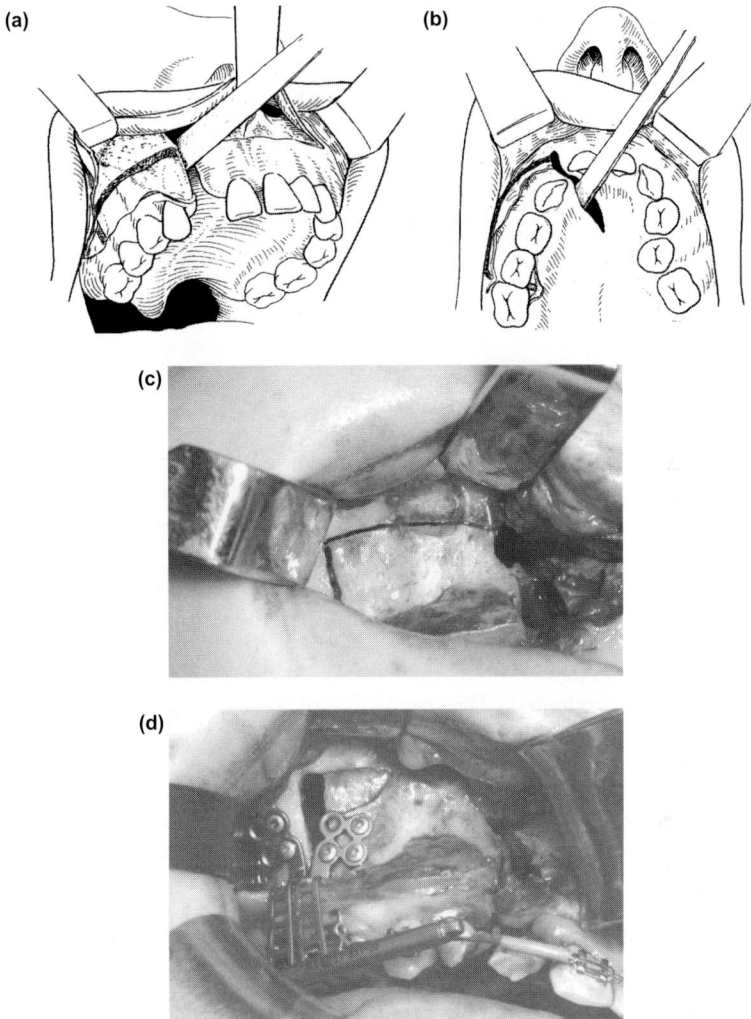

Figure 11.11   Segmental alveolar distraction.

3. The distractor is placed buccally across the vertical osteotomy site. The clover leaf plate on each side of the division is secured with three 5 mm screws and a trial distraction is carried out to ensure the fragment moves easily and the 3-dimensional vectors are correct (Figure 11.11d).

(e)

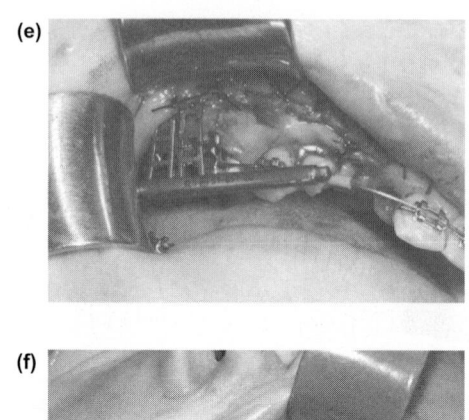

(f)

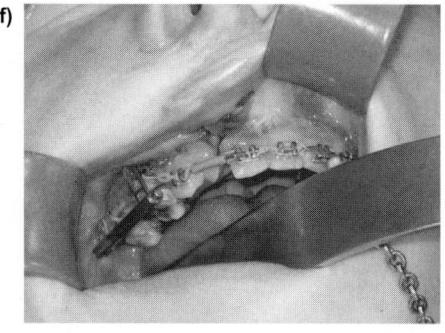

Figure 11.11   (*Continued*) The completion of segmental alveolar distraction.

4. The wound is sutured without the need for relieving incisions. Postoperative care is as stated above.
5. The distractor is activated after 5 days to achieve 0.5–1.0 mm a day guided by the rigid arch wire within tubes attached to each tooth on the segment to ensure controlled forward movement. On completion of the distraction, as seen in Figures 11.11d–11.11f, a consolidation phase of 4–6 weeks is required to ensure maturation of the callus.
6. The distractor is then removed under an general anaesthetic and a gingivoperiosteoplasty is performed as for an alveolar bone graft to complete the closure. Bone grafting is rarely required as the alveolar cleft has been closed as a function of the osteodistraction.

Residual Fistulae

Small Fistulae

A double-layered closure is the most reliable technique, as is described in the alveolar bone grafting section. Figures 11.12a and 11.2b show a rotation flap based on the posterior palatal vessels, which must be patent. Reflection of the flap and skeletalising the exposed vessels gives a more manoeuvrable island flap.

The Surgical Treatment (Figures 11.12a to 11.12d)

1. Outline the fistula with a pen and the adjacent contralateral pedicled flap.
2. Infiltrate with a local anaesthetic containing vasoconstrictor.

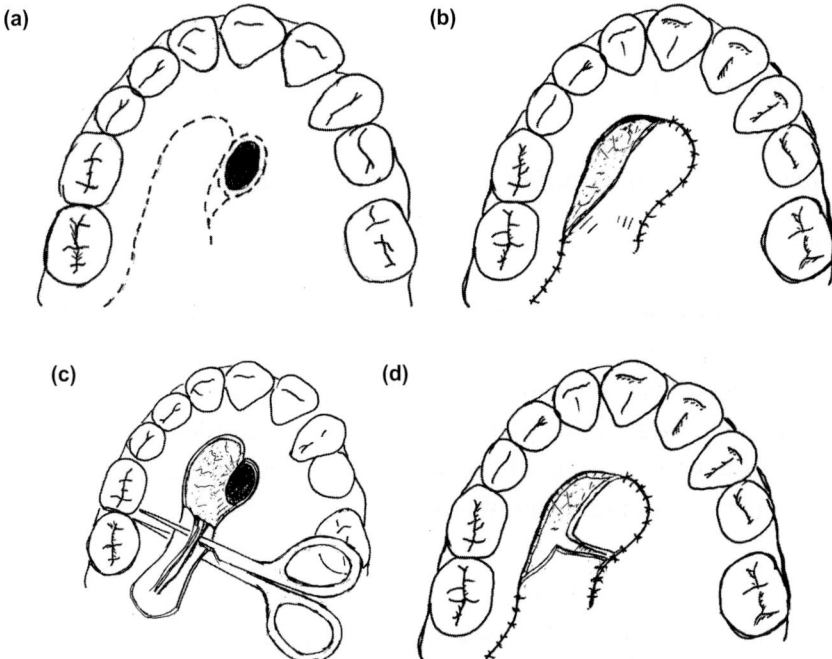

Figure 11.12 Closure of a small residual palatal fistula.

3. Incise the margin of the fistula and undermine and elevate the inner fistula margin tissue into the nose sufficiently to close with a purse string suture using a small J shaped needle.
4. Incise the outline of the pedicled flap down to bone and elevate back to the posterior palatine foramen.
5. Separate the vessels visible on the under surface from the overlying submucosa with fine scissors, carefully and widely. If they have been thrombosed due to previous surgery go to point 8.
6. Cut the thick mucosal pedicle leaving the island flap attached by its palatine vessels.
7. Rotate the island flap over the lined fistula and suture with interrupted 4/0 vicryl sutures. The bare area should be covered with a ribbon gauze and Whiteheads varnish pack sutured around the margins and over-sewn for stability.
8. If the vessels are not readily separable, rotate the broad based pedicled flap (Figure 11.12b) suture and pack the bare area.

A pedicled sliding flap is shown in Figures 11.13a to 11.13c.

Closure of Large Fistulae in Cases Presenting Late

The Problem

Large defects of the anterior hard palate require a different strategy. They result from the expansion and advancement of grossly collapsed maxillary dental arches. Large fistulae also exist in some older patients due to the pattern of surgery practised 40 years ago or more. Such large oronasal communications become a major problem when full dentures are worn.

The Surgical Treatment

1. Unilateral or bilateral segmental alveolar distraction slowly closes the dental and alveolar gap and will generate bone in the alveolar region (see above) but if not available a flap will be required.

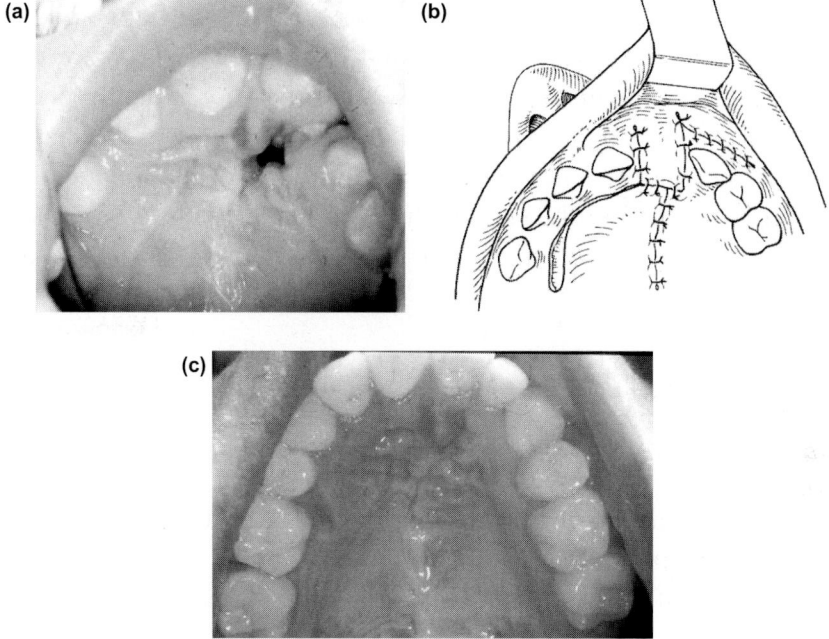

Figure 11.13   Large palatal fistula closure.

2. Tongue flaps.

    •   The tongue has an extremely good blood supply and has been extensively used for reconstruction of large palatal fistulae.

    •   Reconstruction is performed in two stages. The second stage to divide the pedicle and inset the flap may be 10–14 days from the initial procedure.

    •   The use of lingual mucosa over the alveolus is an unfavourable environment for tooth eruption and long term maintenance of periodontal health.

Lateral tongue flaps are reliable axial flaps and tend to be well tolerated and stable, despite tongue movements during the transfer stage.

Anterior-based dorsal tongue flaps are random flaps and are less well tolerated during the period of transfer as they are distorted by movements of the tongue. This may occasionally prejudice the blood supply. However, they provide an ideally shaped tissue transfer and leave little or no deformity of the tongue. The width is made slightly greater than the defect with two to three millimetres of muscle included with the mucosa to ensure the blood supply.

The Surgical Treatment

The Lateral Tongue Flap

1. The tongue margin is injected with 1:200,000 adrenaline in 0.5% Bupivacaine. Hypotensive anaesthesia is used if available. A 2/0 black silk mattress stay suture through the tip facilitates access.
2. The flap is incised comprising the lateral one-third of the tongue based posteriorly, but excluding the tip (Figure 11.14a).
3. A marginal flap of palatal mucosa is raised from the recipient site area to facilitate suturing and to increase the area of contact (Figure 11.14b). The free tip of the tongue flap is then sutured with 5/0 vicryl to the anterolateral lip of the fistula. The margin of the flap is firmly sutured to the adjacent palatal mucosa. It is better to close a left-sided fistula with a right-hand tongue flap, and *vice versa*, as it is found in practice that the flap lies more naturally when so arranged.
4. The tongue flap remains with its dual attachment for 14 days, at which point a further anaesthetic is administered. An inexperienced anaesthetist may find difficulty in intubating a patient with a tongue flap attached to the anterior palate because of the obvious problems associated with the insertion of a laryngoscope. To avoid this problem, the base of the flap can be severed

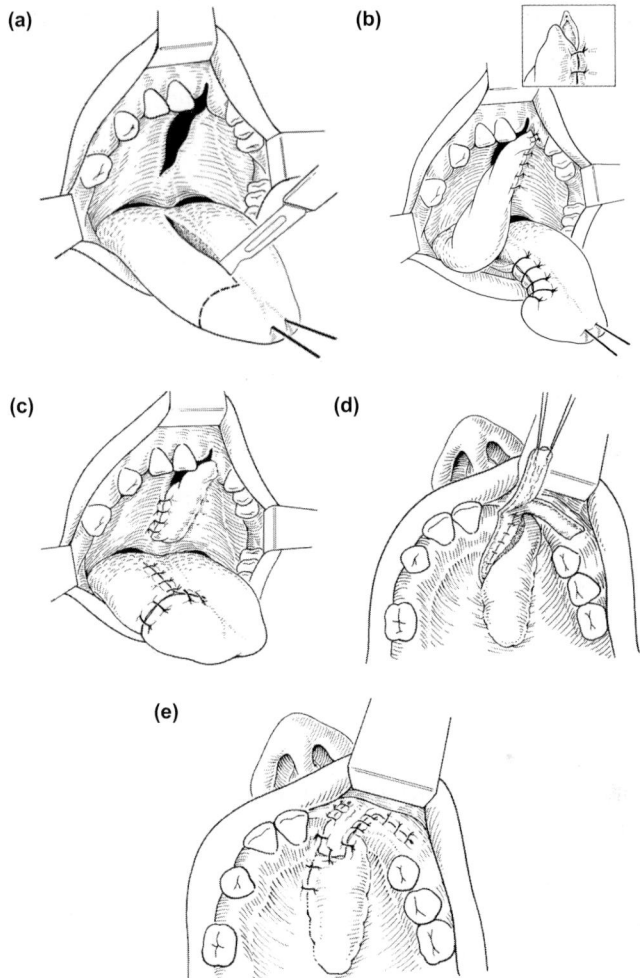

Figures 11.14 The lateral tongue flap used to close a palatal fitula.

under local anaesthetic prior to the induction of general anaesthesia but in practice this is rarely necessary.

5. After division, the tongue flap free edges are sutured to palatal mucosa round as much of the fistula as possible (Figure 11.14c). The flap will be used as a split tube but it is usually impractical

to form a sutured nasal layer at this stage. As long as the transferred flap can be attached completely to one side of the fistula, the nasal surface can be left until later. The flap remnant attached to the tongue is fashioned to fit back into the side of the tongue. Tongue shape can usually be restored almost to normal.

6. As it is rarely possible to complete the closure of a large oronasal fistula when the tongue flap is first separated, 2–3 further weeks later the remaining free edge of the fistula is separated into the oral and nasal layers. The tongue flap is split along its free margin and its nasal surface used to complete the nasal layer. The oral mucosal defect is closed, partly by the oral surface of the tongue flap and partly by a vestibular flap, as shown in Figures 11.14d and 11.14e. Separation of an oral and nasal layer means that a bone graft can be inserted at this stage if necessary.

7. The completed flap tends to be somewhat bulky, however carefully it has been trimmed. If it is intended to be used as a denture-bearing area, it may be thinned later.

The Anterior Based Dorsal Tongue Flap

1. The tongue is held forward with two lateral 2/0 black silk stay sutures. The flap is marked with ink and the site injected with local anaesthetic and a vasoconstrictor (Figure 11.15a).

   As the mucosa and submucosal muscle is profusely supplied with a rich vascular plexus, especially at the tip of the tongue, the base of the flap does not have to overly the proximal blood supply. The anterior base provides a flap that is easy to insert but restricts the tongue's movements during the transfer stage.

2. The posterior and lateral margins of the fistula are incised with a No. 11 blade and raised with Mitchell's trimmer to provide a shelf-like flap. This stage helps to estimate the width and length of the flap. A base of 3 cm allows a flap of 5 or 6 cm in length.

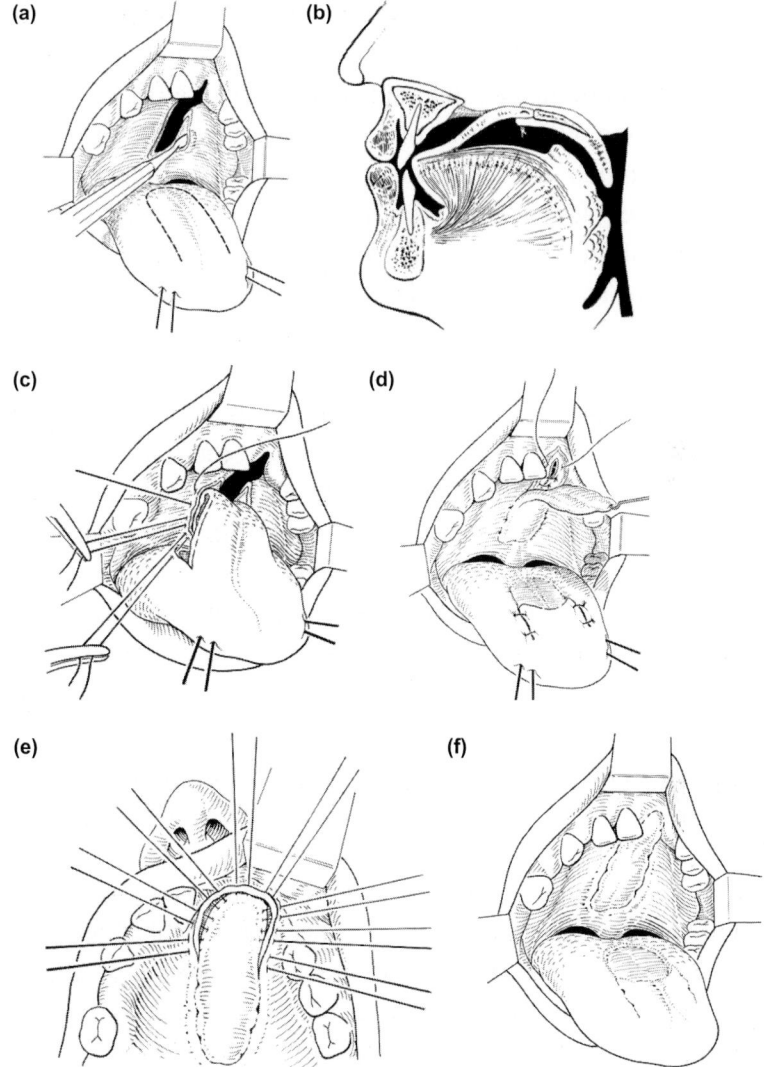

Figures 11.15   The anteriorly based dorsal tongue — stage 1 (**a–c**) and stage 2 (**d–f**).

The tongue flap is incised to a depth of 4 mm to include an undersurface of submucosal muscle, and is then carefully dissected free. Bleeding points on the donor site are sealed with bipolar diathermy to ensure only localised coagulation.

3.   The tongue flap is set into the palatal mucosa shelf margins, with the raw submucosal surfaces in contact and the papillated lingual mucosa facing upward towards the nose (Figure 11.15b). This is done with a series of 5/0 vicryl mattress sutures. These are left untied and clamped with mosquito forceps to allow freedom of access until the maximum number of sutures is inserted (Figure 11.15c). They are now carefully tied with a triple knot and cut short. There is no need to close the nasal layer at this stage.
4.   The flap may be rested by inserting loose intermaxillary tie wires through eyelets around the teeth in upper and lower dental arches.
5.   Three weeks later the base is divided and the flap (with its raw surface now re-epithelialised) trimmed and set in anteriorly in the same way as was the tip (Figure 11.15d). If the anaesthetist anticipates difficulty in intubation, the flap can be incised under local anaesthetic just prior to the intubation procedure. Ideally this should be done in the operating theatre. Excess flap is sutured back on to the de-epithelialised donor site, which heals spontaneously with minimal defect (Figures 11.15e and 11.15f).
6.   If a cancellous bone graft is inserted, the nasal mucosal layer is raised and closed with 4/0 vicryl (Ethicon Ltd, Edinburgh, UK).

Note: This technique, which provides an easy and reliable means of inserting the flap margin, is possible because of the rapid epithelialisation of the raw muscle on the undersurface of the flap. Furthermore, it takes on the normal mucosal character instead of remaining a patch of tongue on the palate.

Extraoral Flaps

If intraoral tissue is not sufficient for the largest fistulae a microvascular transfer of a free radial skin flap or free radial fascial flap can be combined with local mucosal turn-over flaps to close the nasal layer together with bone to fill any bony defects of the alveolus and hard palate.

Residual Oronasal Fistulas in the Soft Palate

Oronasal fistulas in the soft palate require correction if there is a loss of oral pressure during speech. The best approach in the presence of poor speech is a complete re-repair of the soft palate. This improves the function of the velopharyngeal mechanism and speech improves as a consequence.

Residual Nasolabial Fistulae

If left until alveolar bone grafting there will be less overall scarring. Presurgical orthodontic expansion gives good access to the whole cleft. The fistula is excised and good nasal layer should be reconstructed as described above in the alveolar bone graft section. The interpositional bone graft improves the success of the closure.

Orthodontic Considerations

The objectives of presurgical orthodontic treatment for the cleft patient are not the same as non-cleft patients. The most obvious differences are;

i)   Management of the dental gap in the cleft region.

   In the unilateral case with a full dentition on the non-cleft side, closure of the space in the cleft gap may not be aesthetic, whereas in the bilateral case where both maxillary lateral incisors are missing, a satisfactory aesthetic result can be achieved by bilaterally closing the space. However, closure of the spaces will change tooth contacts and may make intercuspation difficult to achieve.

   Orthodontic alignment following the alveolar bone graft will optimise the bone support for the teeth. It also aligns the tooth roots to produce the best possible incisor and canine crown angulation thereby facilitating a range of restorative options for replacing the missing lateral incisor.

ii) Transverse dento-alveolar collapse.

Achieving sufficient maxillary expansion and transverse stability is a great challenge. Orthodontic expansion of the dental arch must be within a reasonable expectation of stability. Dental relapse disturbs the surgical result in both the antero-posterior and lateral dimensions. Permanent transverse retention may be needed to overcome rigid palatal scarring.

With significant transverse deficiency surgical widening at the time of the maxillary advance may be considered but a posterior cross-bite is preferable to the creation of a fistula or losing segments due to ischaemic necrosis.

Orthognathic Surgery

Orthognathic correction should be delayed until facial skeletal growth is complete. Other congenital defects, such as congenital heart disease must be identified early.

Specific Problems in Cleft Patients

- The Class III skeletal problem affects the paranasal, nasal, infraorbital, and zygomatic regions in the anteroposterior and lateral planes, and may even cause exorbitism with poor eyelid support.
- The associated malocclusion frequently includes anterior open bites and posterior cross bites which impair eating, speech and the long-term health of the teeth and their supporting bone.
- The deformity also impairs nasal breathing and drainage, olfaction and hearing.
- Dental development may also be delayed in both arches but is most evident in the cleft segment and may compromise the presurgical orthodontics.

- The repaired alveolar cleft is a potential site for fracture at the time of the down-fracture.
- If the maxillary alveolus has not been reconstructed, alignment of the alveolus can be incorporated into the orthognathic procedure. However it complicates the planning of the surgery and increases the potential morbidity. Segmental osteotomies are less stable than one-piece maxillary osteotomies.
- Previous surgery produces scarring of the labial and buccal vestibule, the palate and behind the maxillary tuberosities. This presents problems with the surgical incisions, mobilisation and postoperative closure of the surgical wound.
- A pharyngeal flap may make advancement of the maxilla difficult and will need to be divided. The patient has to be informed well in advance.
- Earlier distraction osteogenesis is an option for management of the maxilla if the patient has gross skeletal deformity (see later).

Preparation of the Patient for Surgery

The preparation of the patient and parents starts earlier than in the non-cleft population. Families with cleft lip and palate children get considerable support from self-help organisations. Despite this these deformities have profound psychological effects and the support of a clinical psychologist is often helpful.

Dental Care and Preparation

Oral hygiene instruction, dietary advice, periodontal and restorative treatment should be initiated before pre-surgical orthodontic preparation. The early loss of teeth has catastrophic consequences for any future orthodontic, orthognathic and restorative dental treatment.

Treatment Planning

The basic facial and orthognathic evaluation is the same as the non-cleft case with important refinements.

a)   Lip-incisor relationship.

As in the non-cleft case, the lip to maxillary incisor relationship is extremely important. The major surgical moves are predominantly in the maxilla and with a tight, previously scarred upper lip, small skeletal moves have a pronounced effect on the incisor exposure. Surgical and orthodontic changes in incisor angulation will have a similar effect.

b)   Asymmetries.

Both dental and skeletal asymmetries are dominant features, often with compensatory asymmetries in the mandible. Where possible, preoperative orthodontic management will make the surgical correction technically easier. If dental asymmetries are to be corrected after surgery, space will need to be maintained.

c)   Preoperative speech assessment and counselling.

Ideally all cleft patients should have a full preoperative speech assessment with nasoendoscopy and videofluoroscopy. The patient with adequate velopharyngeal function preoperatively generally maintains function, unless the maxillary advance is large. Patients with borderline velopharyngeal function are at risk of developing hypernasality postoperatively. These patients need to be identified and followed up for evaluation and corrective treatment.

The Choice of Operation

Maxillary Hypoplasia

- The LeFort I osteotomy will give acceptable results at the occlusal level with antero-posterior advancement and vertical lengthening.
- Transverse maxillary widening can be accomplished by a paramedian osteotomy of the hard palate on the non-cleft side within the constraints discussed above.
- Patients with severe hypoplasia of the infraorbital and malar regions can be improved by the high LeFort I level osteotomy. Graft augmentation either at the same time or as a secondary procedure combined with a rhinoplasty may be necessary.
- The modified LeFort II or Kufner LeFort III osteotomy, do not give accurate control of movement in asymmetrical cases.
- Nasal airway obstruction may arise from a deviated nasal septum narrowing of the nares, hypertrophied turbinates, nasal polyps and posterior choanal constriction from sub-periosteal bone and asymmetrical vomer flaps.
- Pharyngeal obstruction can be caused by hypertrophied adenoidal tissue or pharyngeal flaps.
- The management of these problems is an essential part of the orthognathic procedure. Paradoxically the adenoid mass may contribute to velopharyngeal function and its removal may precipitate velopharyngeal inadequacy.

Implications for the Mandible and/or Chin

- Although many cleft patients may also have a latent mandibular hypoplasia, there is invariably a relative mandibular prognathism. Functional, aesthetic and surgical considerations may need a mandibular setback. The maxillary surgical limitations are severe palatal scarring, borderline velopharyngeal insufficiency or a tight inferiorly based pharyngoplasty flap.

- During maxillary advancement and inferior positioning, the anterior maxilla is differentially positioned more inferiorly. This will produce a posterior open bite deformity unless a mandibular ramus procedure is undertaken simultaneously. Differential down grafting of the anterior maxilla also results in a counter clockwise rotation of the mandible which may make the chin retrogenic. This can be corrected by a simultaneous augmentation genioplasty.

Maxillary Advancement in the Previously Bone Grafted Maxilla

At the time of orthognathic surgery all oro-nasal fistulae should have been closed and the dentoalveolar arcade should be intact. Presurgical orthodontics will have aligned and coordinated the dental arches. In these ideal circumstances the osteotomy technique is similar to a non-cleft patient undergoing maxillary surgery. However, infection, bone and soft tissue necrosis, delayed healing, loss of teeth and relapse all occur with greater frequency.

Special Considerations — The Osteotomy Cuts
and the Down-Fracture

- In most cases a standard vestibular incision taken higher in the labial sulcus gives good access posteriorly and ensures a good vascular supply buccally. Care must be taken to preserve the parotid duct.
- Subperiosteal dissection is carried out with elevation of the soft tissues to the infraorbital nerves superiorly and to the pterygomaxillary fissures on both sides. The nasal mucosa is elevated bilaterally from the nasal floor.
- In bilateral cases, where the blood supply to the premaxillary region is compromised due to gross scarring from previous surgery, a full labial incision and down fracture may be unwise and a tunnelling approach is preferable from a small vertical incision

in the mid line to give access to the premaxillary bone to enable full mobilisation of the maxilla.

Ancillary Surgical Manoeuvres

Segmental Maxillary Surgery

- If vertical steps are present in the maxillary arch, orthodontic segmental levelling is undertaken and the maxilla expanded prior to surgery. However with severe displacement and gross arch collapse this may not be achievable. Segmental distraction osteogenesis may be an appropriate alternative.
- Although surgically moving segments vertically avoids intrusive and extrusive orthodontic mechanics and may be more stable long term it is the most difficult of the three options.
- Surgical expansion, segmental alignment and levelling require interdental osteotomy cuts for which a minimum of a 3 mm of interdental space needs to opened by the orthodontist by tipping the roots away from the osteotomy site or bodily opening up a gap prior to surgery. Endodontic and periodontal complications will follow without careful presurgical planning.
- The palatal and interdental cuts are performed from above, following the down-fracture. A limited vertical tunnelling approach laterally facilitates access to the buccal cortical plate which is divided with a fine bur but the interdental cut is completed with a narrow 5 mm Osteotome. Ideally orthodontic bands rather than bonded brackets should be placed on the teeth adjacent to the interdental osteotomy site as bonded appliances do not withstand the forces needed to mobilise the maxilla in segmental cleft surgery.
- A large rectangular arch wire with surgical hooks should be wired to the orthodontic bands to aid fixation. A heavy supplemental arch wire fitted into distal tubes is required to help locate and stabilise the occlusal relations of the segments, with

the help of a wafer in addition to the bone plate osteosynthesis. This can be a chrome cobalt or a high impact acrylic intermediate wafer. The wafer can be left *in situ* for two weeks postoperatively to supplement the fixation.

Airway Considerations

- Whilst the maxilla is down fractured contouring of the inner aspects of the nose can be achieved easily and time should be taken to bur out any bony excesses in the nostril on the cleft side.
- Asymmetries in the piriform region can be corrected which may interfere with the repositioning of the maxilla or distort the nose. The mucosa of the nostril floor can also be repaired at this stage.
- With a unilateral cleft the septum is usually deviated towards the non-cleft side inferiorly with a bowing towards the cleft side. A septoplasty may be necessary to correct the aesthetic and functional problems. The subnasal approach after the down-fracture provides excellent access to the cartilaginous septum, the vomer and the perpendicular plate of the ethmoids.
- Partial or complete inferior turbinectomies may be indicated if they are enlarged and cause nasal obstruction. Submucosal turbinectomies can be performed under direct vision through an incision in the nasal mucoperiosteum.
- Antral and nasal polyps can be removed at the time of down fracture.
- Pharyngeal flaps raise additional concerns for the anaesthetist and surgeon. The pharyngeal flap that has a broad base or small portals may make intubation difficult and restrict the nasal airway postoperatively. The flap will need to be divided several weeks preoperatively and the patient's speech and language reassessed postoperatively. Inferiorly based flaps may restrict

maxillary advancement but at the time of down fracture access to the flap is relatively good and the flap may be lengthened. Superiorly based flaps are less restrictive on maxillary advancement and can also be lengthened at the time of maxillary advancement. Soft palate re-repair or a repeat pharyngeal flap should be considered carefully as they may further impair the maxillary vascular supply.

- Bone grafting — cortico-cancellous bone grafts should be used to fill the voids created by any inferior positioning of the maxilla as this will improve the stability of the osteotomy postoperatively. Bone grafts should also be shaped and placed to address any specific cosmetic deficiencies and asymmetries. These bone grafts can be tailored to meet the individual requirements of the patient and rigidly fixed to the surface of the maxilla and zygomas with mini screws or wire.
- Mucosal asymmetries of the lip may be corrected by using asymmetric V to Y closures of the labial mucosa. Final lip correction should be left until postsurgical orthodontic refinement of the occlusion including any minor changes in the incisor position, or cosmetic dental treatment have been completed.

Postoperative Manoeuvres

Intermaxillary elastics to orthodontic archwires may be used to assist in providing proprioceptive input in guiding the jaws into occlusion but should not be used in an attempt to recover a situation where the skeletal elements are incorrectly related. The prolonged use of elastic traction should be avoided as there is a risk of a bony non-union of the maxilla.

As a prophylactic measure, extraoral elastic traction using a face mask can be used in patients who are considered particularly at risk of relapse either due to scarring or who have had large surgical moves anteriorly and inferiorly. The value of this is uncertain (Figures 11.16a and 11.16b).

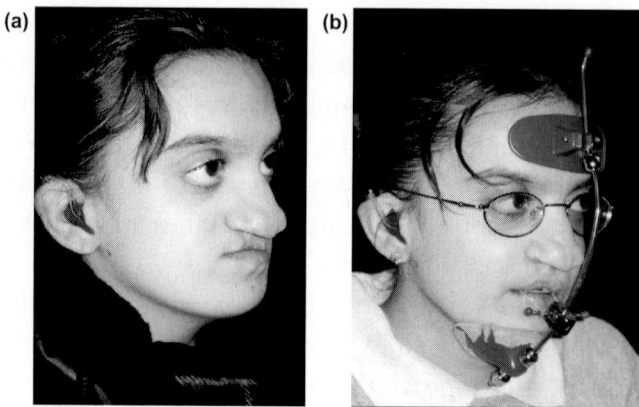

Figures 11.16   After maxillary surgical advancement, extraoral elastic traction support may be useful in a patient at risk of relapse.

Effects on Speech

Maxillary advancement increases the velopharyngeal distance so that postoperatively, patients are at risk of developing velopharyngeal incompetence. The soft palate mechanism in non-cleft patients has considerable reserve capacity and can adapt to an increase in length. The repaired cleft soft palate does not have this capacity to adapt especially after major advances. The patient with borderline velopharyngeal incompetence preoperatively is likely to develop worsening of their speech postoperatively.

Lip and Nose Changes with Maxillary Surgery (See also the Rhinoplasty Chapter)

- Mismanagement of the soft tissues during closure of the labial vestibular incision may cause shortening and thinning of the upper lip.

    The V to Y closure of a maxillary vestibule incision may increase the vermilion show in patients with a thin upper lip.

- Maxillary advancement widens the alar base, increases the projection and elevation of the nasal tip and the width of the nares.

  Various surgical manoeuvres can be used to prevent these unwelcome side effects. These include an alar base cinch suture, recontouring the bony piriform aperture either by trimming and/or asymmetric bone grafting and alar base resections.

Achieving Stability

Stability after orthognathic surgery is unpredictable due to scarring. The factors that increase stability include:

- Meticulous orthodontic preparation and quality of the occlusion achieved.
- Avoiding segmental procedures and unfavourable surgical moves.
- Surgical overcorrection where possible. The cleft maxilla usually requires a least a 9 mm advancement.
- Ensuring that all adhesions are divided so that the maxilla can be advanced passively into the planned position. If this is not possible then a compromise position must be planned and if necessary incorporate a mandibular setback.
- Alveolar bone grafting.
- Bone grafting for inferior repositioning of the maxilla.
- Internal rigid fixation for all moves.

Skeletal Relapse

Most relapse occurs within the first few months. Where the relapse is significant, the options depend upon the occlusal relationship. If the occlusion has compensated for the skeletal relapse, then masking procedures such as onlay bone grafts may be an option.

If the occlusion cannot be recovered through postoperative ortho-dontics, then further skeletal surgery must be considered but with no guarantee that the osteotomy will not relapse again. Maxillary dis-traction may be a reasonable option in the management of relapse.

Dentoalveolar Relapse

Transverse dentoalveolar relapse is a problem following large ortho-dontic or surgical palatal expansions. Such patients may require per-manent palatal retention. However it is better to accept a planned posterior cross bite than put the maxilla in an unstable position, as relapse at one site may undermine the stability of the whole maxilla.

Mid Face Distraction Osteogenesis

Indications

For the majority of patients, conventional orthognathic surgery gives excellent results that are stable and aesthetically pleasing. However there are some situations when distraction should be considered:

Severe Maxillary Deficiency and Complex
Three-Dimensional Deficiency

- With gross maxillary hypoplasia and a severe degree of scarring, the degree of advancement may be beyond the expected limits of stability of a conventional osteotomy. Distraction of the maxilla is preferable to a surgical compromise such as a mandibular setback.
- If the deformity is complex particularly in the upper mid face then a higher level osteotomy with distraction often gives a bet-ter result than a modified LeFort I with masking onlay bone grafts or modified LeFort II and LeFort III osteotomies that are difficult to perform and can give unsightly steps particularly over the radix of the nose.

- Slow expansion of the maxilla may produce a more stable increase in the width of the maxilla and face than surgical repositioning or presurgical orthodontics.
- Relapse surgery for distraction is less than a repeat osteotomy and full mobilisation with down fracture is not needed. One is less likely to run into poor vasculature problems in the re-operation site. By slowly advancing the maxilla the resistant forces may be overcome more easily.

Stability and Effects on Speech

Some claim that distraction produces less disturbance of speech with reduced incidence of velopharyngeal incompetence. The potential advantage of an increase in soft tissue following distraction also is helpful for the closure of large fistulae.

Disadvantages

- The procedure takes longer than conventional surgery and involves at least two stages.
- The control of the movement vectors in maxillary distraction is difficult and less precise than an osteotomy.
- Simultaneous mandibular procedures may be necessary and must be coordinated with the maxillary distraction to overcome a prolonged period without a functioning occlusion.

Method and Choice of Distraction Device

- The surgery is similar to conventional orthognathic surgery but instead of the maxilla being placed into the surgical wafer at the end of the procedure and fixed with plates, a distractor is applied.
- The choice of distractor is determined by the desired direction and distance the maxilla needs to be moved.

Internal Distractors

Are partially buried and give excellent control over vectors, but require

- adequate bone on both sides of the osteotomy cuts to fix them,
- extensive sub-periosteal stripping that may impair new bone formation, and
- a patient with good manual dexterity to turn the appliance either inside the mouth or externally in the temple region.

Extra-Oral Distractors

Are easier to activate, but

- give less control over the vectors of distraction,
- do not control the posterior maxilla well, and
- require a frame that is a disadvantage particularly if in place for the duration of the stabilisation phase.

LeFort I Distraction (Figures 11.17a–11.17e)

LeFort I distraction is performed by carrying out a standard or modified higher level LeFort I osteotomy cuts. If any of the previously described ancillary manoeuvres are needed then a maxillary down-fracture is incorporated into the procedure before the distractor is applied. External distractors are connected to the maxilla either with cap splints, or pre-formed arch bars, or directly to plates fixed to the bone or both. This depends on the desired moves and the need to control vectors during the distraction procedure. Controlling the vector can be difficult as often the distractor position is determined by the lip and nose and a compromise may have to be made.

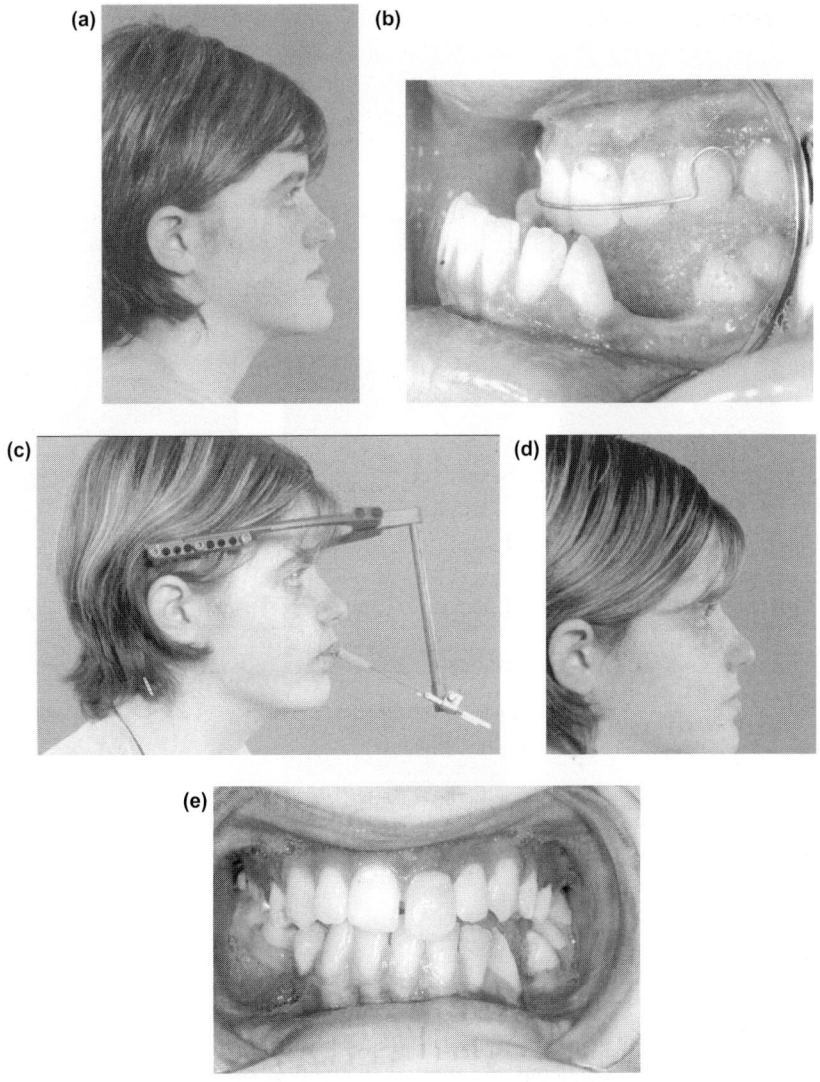

Figure 11.17 An external distraction frame used for maxillary advancement.

LeFort II Distraction (Figures 11.18a–11.18g)

For patients with severe maxillary hypoplasia a higher level of distraction is needed to improve the mid face aesthetics. This may need to be performed in combination with a mandibular sagittal split

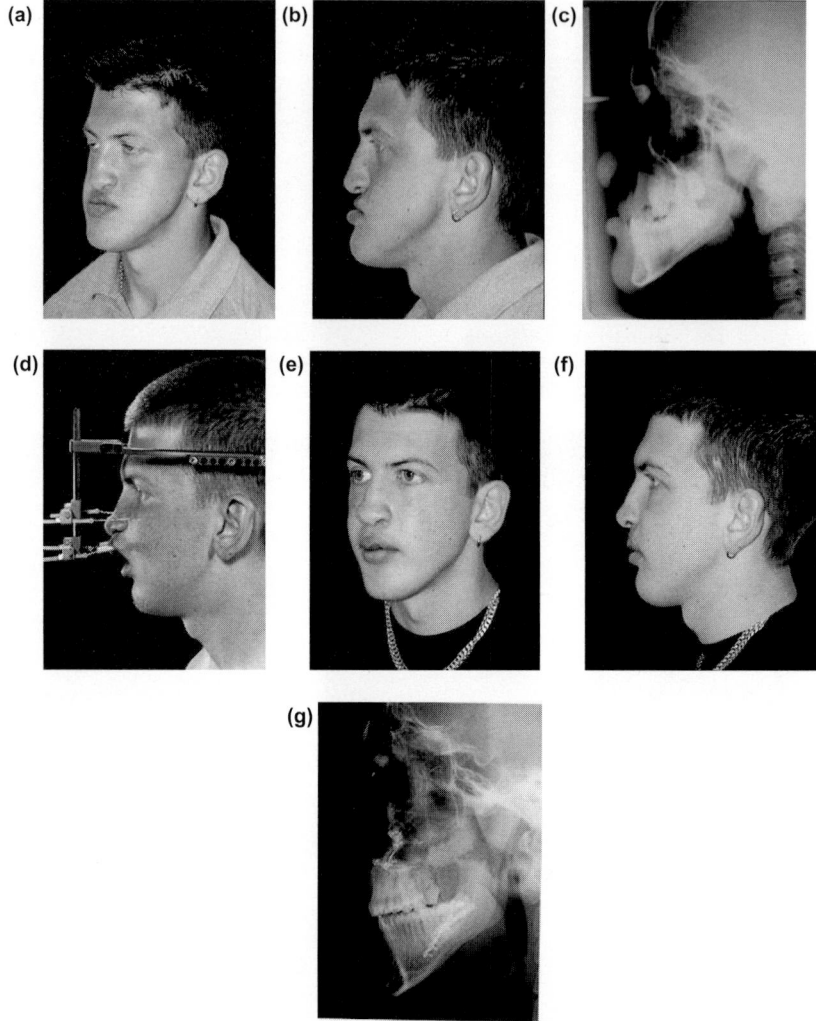

Figure 11.18 Simulataneous differential distraction of the maxilla at two or more levels may produce a better balanced facial contour.

osteotomy to improve the mandibular plane angle and to allow for the elongation of the maxilla in the vertical dimension. Further wires are attached to the hypoplastic malar bones to guide their distraction forwards. Slow distraction at this level seems to give a better shape to the nose than a standard LeFort II advancement that would normally require bone grafting and which can lead to steps and irregularities.

LeFort III (Kufner) Distraction

If there is significant orbital rim hypoplasia then distraction at the LeFort III level may be useful, particularly as bone grafts in this area are difficult to contour and produce disappointing results in the short term and are notoriously unstable in the long term.

12

Rhinoplasty Surgery

Introduction

Rhinoplasty surgery forms a vital part of the functional and aesthetic management of congenital or traumatic deformities of the facial skeleton. This chapter will cover important aspects of

- nasal anatomy,
- assessment of the deformity,
- surgical planning, and
- operative procedures.

It is essential that the reader refers to a comprehensive or specialist texts for detailed aspects of the surgery.

The nose is a complex structure cantilevered on the mid face. Its complex role embraces the senses of smell and taste, respiration, aesthetics and sex and so rhinoplasty surgery requires careful consideration. All mid face orthognathic surgery will affect the nose to a degree. LeFort I operation impactions broaden the alar width, and with inadequate trimming of the nasal septum they will lead to septal buckling and obstruction or deviation of the nasal tip. Advancements will raise the nasal tip and straighten out profile curvatures. For these reasons it is undesirable to do a rhinoplasty before, during or within 6 months of a mid face osteotomy.

Anatomy

It is important to understand the complex nasal anatomy which is made difficult by the nomenclature. The upper border of many structures is designated cephalic (headwise) and the lower border caudal (tailwise). The anterior surface of the nose is dorsal and posterior structures are posterior. Unfotunately some terms have been introduced in relation to the supine anaesthetised patient, so that what might be considered as anterior and posterior nasal sites are described as "high" and "low".

Figures 12.1 and 12.2 show the anatomical subunits of the nose, which is conveniently divided in thirds. The upper third consists of the bony pyramid, made up of the nasal bones with their articulation to the ascending processes of the maxilla and the bony septum. The paired upper lateral cartilages insert just under the caudal (lower) end of the nasal bones and their fusion with the midline cartilaginous septum in a "T" type configuration forms the middle third ("vault") (Figure 12.2). The attachment of the caudal aspect of the upper lateral

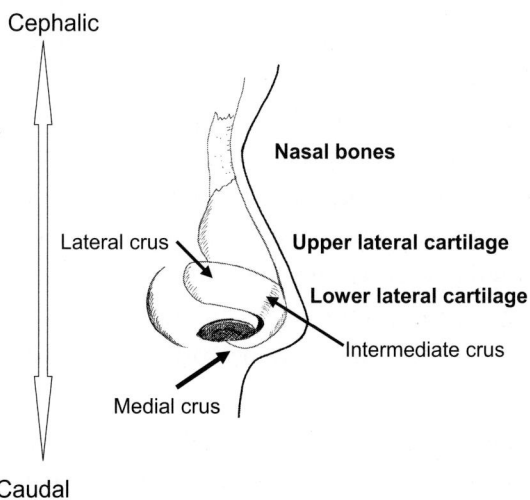

Figure 12.1   External anatomy of nose (lateral view).

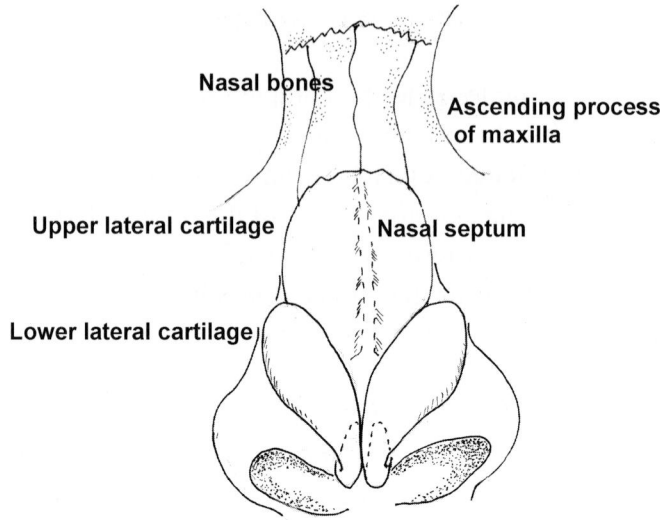

Figure 12.2   External anatomy of nose (frontal view).

cartilage to the cephalic (upper) aspect of lower lateral cartilages forms the boundary to the lower third of the nose and is referred to as the scroll attachment. The paired lower laterals, sometimes called the alar cartilages, form the a prominent part of the lateral surface of many noses and the nasal tip, They are divided into the lateral, intermediate and medial crurae — or processes (Figures 12.3a and 12.3b). The intermediate crurae form the "domes" and are the tip defining points of the nose.

The medial crura curve medially and backwards and their terminal processes, the so-called footplates abut against the border of the caudal aspect of the nasal septum and form the cartilaginous columella.

The columella with its cartilage and skin provide the external (caudal) border of the septum from the tip to the nasolabial angle. The outer margin of the nares are the soft tissue alar lobules that are devoid of cartilage.

The overlying superficial musculoaponeurotic system (SMAS) of the nose is a complex layer which provides a rich vascular supply covering to the underlying skeleton and is derived from the superior labial and facial arteries and corresponding venous and lymphatic

(a) **Lower lateral cartilage**

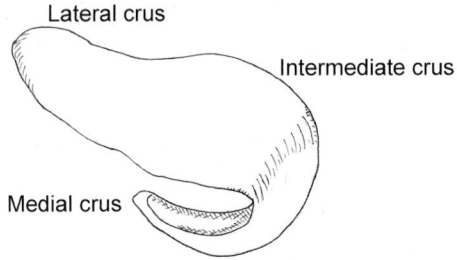

(b) **Lower lateral cartilages**

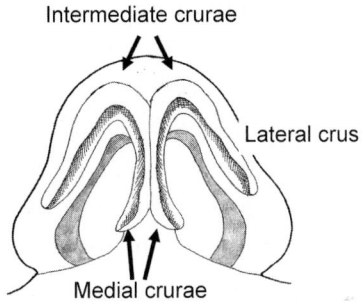

Figure 12.3 **(a)** and **(b)** Lower lateral cartilage anatomy.

vessels accompanying these. Its intrinsic aponeurotic muscles have elevator, depressor, compressor and dilator functions which contribute to olfaction and facial expression.

The external anatomy of the nose is readily studied in any crowded place.

Assessment

History

A detailed history covering the functional and aesthetic aspects of the nose is mandatory.

To assess function, the patient is asked specifically regarding the presence and duration of nasal obstruction, sinus disease and allergic type symptoms. It is important to document prior medical and surgical treatments and their efficacy in treating any functional or aesthetic complaints.

A detailed history of traumatic injuries to the nose and surrounding facial skeleton is essential especially if operated on, and an indication of the pretraumatic appearance of the nose is helpful. It is particularly important to gauge the patient's specific concerns about the appearance of each subsection of the nose with direct questioning. A generalised vague reference to a dislike of the overall look of the nose or any suggestion that the surgeon should decide where the problems lie is to be discouraged and may be suggestive of a dysmorphic disorder (see Chapter 6). The patient's thoughts about the overall improvement desired are sought and realistic expectations estimated. A general medical history should screen the patient for bleeding disorders, cardiovascular and respiratory disease and importantly a psychiatric history.

Examination

A detailed examination of the internal and external aspects of the nose is performed. Anterior rhinoscopy to detail mucosal, caudal septal and turbinate deformities is supplemented with an endoscopic evaluation of the posterior nasal cavity and middle meatal areas to exclude infective or obstructive sinonasal disease. The internal nasal valve area which is bounded by the upper lateral cartilage, inferior turbinate, nasal septum and nasal floor is specifically examined and any high septal deformity noted. This is the narrowest part of the nasal airway and significant internal nasal valve collapse can be demonstrated by Cottle's test (Figure 12.4) in which the airway improves when the cheek adjacent to the mid third of the nose, i.e. the upper lateral cartilage is pulled laterally.

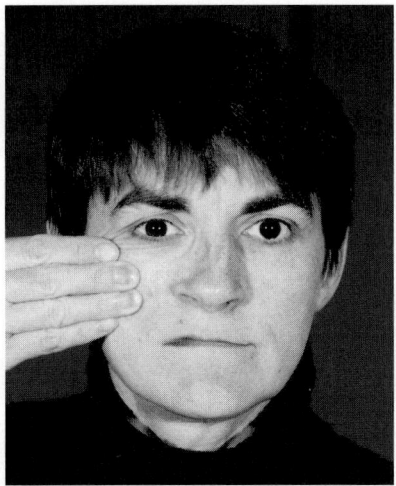

Figure 12.4 Demonstration of Cottle's test.

The importance of the balance of the nose to other aspects of the face is important. Assessment of this relationship should form the initial part of the external examination process. The patient's ethnic characteristics must also be considered. Facial and nasal asymmetries are documented and detailed to the patient.

The skin-soft tissue envelope is important and is critical in predicting postoperative changes. Thinner skin may show minor postoperative irregularities whilst very thick skin can hide any corrections made.

An initial evaluation of the underlying skeletal aspects of the nose considers three fundamental parameters: length (nasion to tip), projection of the dorsum and rotation of the nasal tip. Detailed examination should then document deformities in relation to these factors.

External deformity is most easily assessed and documented in nasal thirds. The frontal, lateral, oblique and basal views (Figures 12.5a–12.5g) are all separately visualised.

- The upper bony pyramid is examined for deviation, irregularity and the extent of any dorsal hump. The width of the base of the

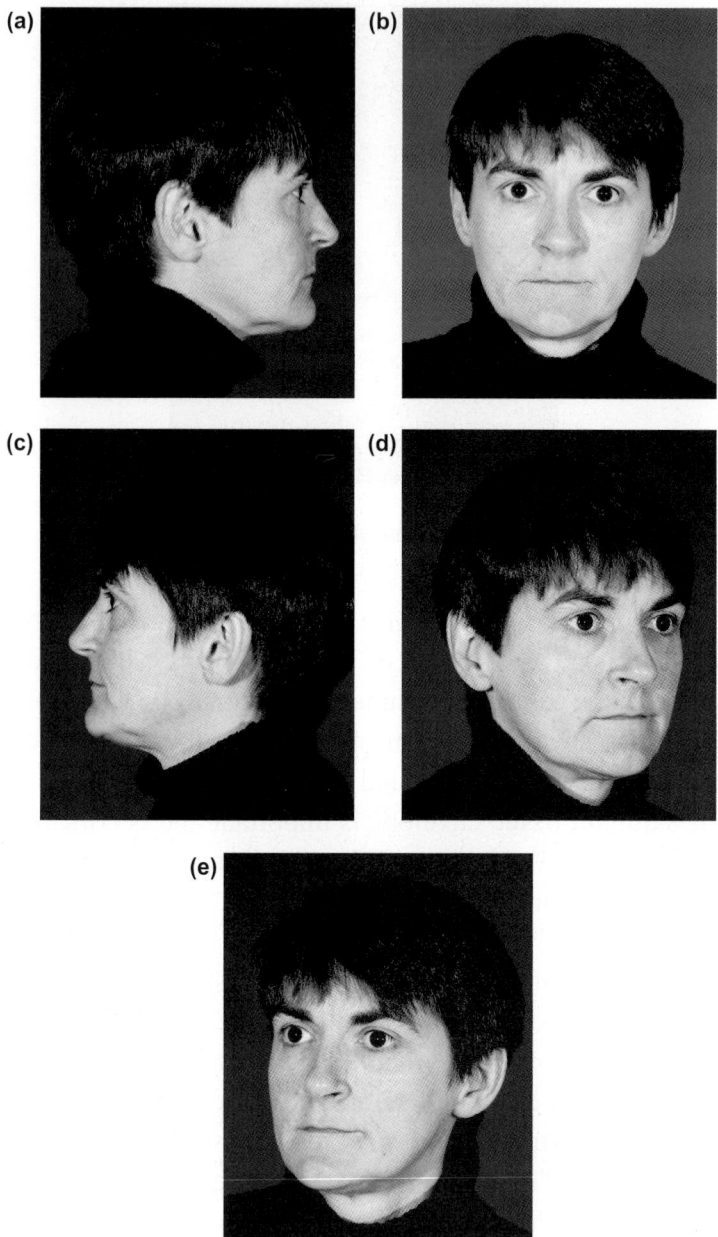

Figure 12.5   **(a)–(g)** Standard photography views.

(f)

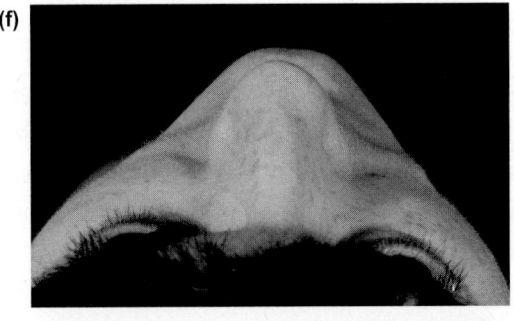

(g)

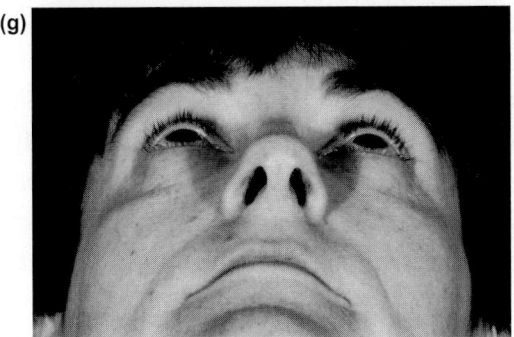

Figure 12.5 (*Continued*)

dorsal pyramid is determined and the dorsum palpated to ensure there is no "open roof" type deformity.

- Similar deformities are sought in the mid third of the nose which is cartilaginous. In this area, an assessment of any externally visible collapse in the nasal valve area is made by inspection and Cottle's test.

- The lower third nasal tip region, which is made up of the lower lateral cartilages is assessed for asymmetry, bulbosity, projection and rotation. A judgement regarding the width of the alar base in relation to the facial proportions is made. The alar width should match the normal intercanthal distance.

Documentation

Documentation of all aspects of the examination is critical for clinical and medicolegal purposes. A rhinoplasty assessment form can be very useful in this regard. It ensures all the areas of the evaluation are considered methodically and can be used for standardising the assessment for all patients.

The patient's expectations and all discussion points are clearly noted. A surgical plan is formulated to correct the specific deformities. It is essential to ensure the patient is given realistic expectations for the outcome of intended surgery, and limitations together with potential complications are discussed. It is very important to ensure that improvement is indeed likely and a risk benefit profile needs to be detailed to the patient prior to obtaining consent and carefully noted.

The surgical approach, be it endonasal or external, should be discussed with the patient and incisions outlined and documented.

Photography and Computer Imaging

Preoperative photography is an absolute requirement for analysis and medicolegal purposes. Standard view photographs form a useful way of communicating deformities and potential changes to the patient. They assist in operative planning and are invaluable for reference during surgery. In combination with postoperative images, they allow self- and peer-reviewed assessment of results.

Standardisation is critical both from the views taken and lighting and background conditions. Digital SLR photography has now largely taken over from 35 mm film and the new technology lends itself well to computer archiving and digital imaging. A standard neutral background such a pale grey, or green or blue is used and ideally a soft exposure is achieved using a flash unit and umbrellas placed equidistant from the patient and camera. The camera should be two metres from the subject and an appropriate zoom used to compose the image using the portrait outline. An overhead lamp, a

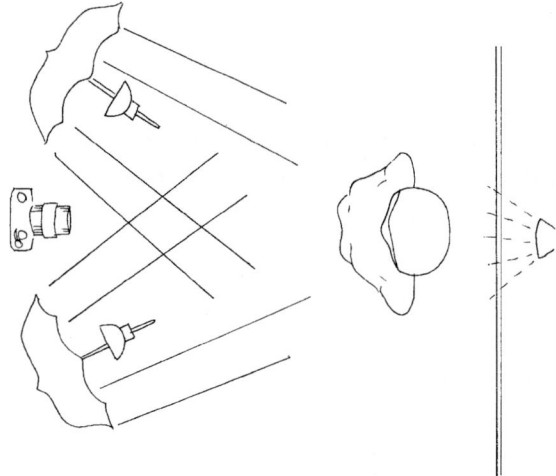

Figure 12.6   Photography setup.

"kicker" above the patients head can help eliminate unwanted shadows (Figure 12.6).

The standard views are as follows (Figures 12.5a–12.5g):

1. Straight frontal view. The patient looks directly into the camera with the eyeline in a horizontal plane.
2. Lateral view. The patients Frankfort plane should be horizontal. This view assesses dorsal profile and is critical in assessing the three basic parameters of length, projection and rotation of the nose. The nose-chin relationship is also clearly demonstrated. A separate lateral view with the patient smiling may outline dynamic movement in the nasal tip.
3. Oblique views. These views are at taken at 45 degrees to the frontal views and can outline asymmetries and contours.
4. Basal view. This view is taken looking up the nose and focuses on the nasal tip detailing asymmetry and deformity.
5. "Birds eye" view. This view is taken from the top of the patient looking down the nose. It can be useful in showing the subtleties of deviation of the nose.

Digital imaging has evolved greatly over the past few years and simple morphing is possible with inexpensive photo-imaging software. More complex programmes are, readily available with or without archiving capability and have purpose made user interfaces and more advanced digital manipulation of the images. With rhinoplasty surgery, they can be very useful in showing patients potential changes and postoperative outcomes. This is most useful in detailing profile changes in the lateral view but with some experience frontal views can be morphed to show potential width reduction and refinement in the nasal tip. Dedicated programmes have measurement abilities and so can be extremely helpful in operative planning. It is important not to convey unrealistic changes to the patient — this will be a source of dissatisfaction afterwards. As a rule a slight underestimation of the postoperative result is generally favourable. Most surgeons choose not to give printed images to the patient of the predicted changes but if you do so, a printed waiver should make clear that the image is only an indication of the likely result.

Surgical Approaches

As a general rule, it is best to limit surgical tissue dissection to a minimum to reduce the risk of vascular compromise of the skin-soft tissue envelope. In this way, additional scarring is prevented and healing is more predictable. Limited dissection also makes it easier to judge the underlying structural components and position of placed underlying grafts.

There are two basic approaches to the nasal skeleton:

  i)   the endonasal or closed approach and
 ii)   the external or open approach.

The advantages and disadvantages of each are much debated and many authors advocate one method to the exclusion of the

other. Each offers benefits in specific situations and should be within the repertoire of a rhinoplasty surgeon.

The least traumatic method of dissection to achieve the specific goal should be used and as such the endonasal approach is favoured for all simple cases unless a better result using the open technique.

Endonasal Approach

The endonasal approach only requires incisions within the nose with no visible external scars (Figures 12.8–12.10). Minimal soft tissue dissection is needed, making this method favourable for less marked deformities and is ideal for correcting bony dorsal irregularities. Its benefits lie in the limited soft tissue disruption allowing early and predictable healing due to the comparatively reduced scar tissue formation. Its main limitations are the restricted exposure of the underlying nasal skeletal elements. The endonasal approach can further be divided into delivery and non-delivery approaches dependent on whether the lower lateral cartilages are fully delivered. With delivery the cartilage is exposed and withdrawn from its overlying subcutaneous layer. The incisions required for these are detailed later.

External Approach

The external approach requires a mid-columellar skin incision which is joined to bilateral marginal incisions (Figure 12.11). More soft tissue dissection is required but provides an unparalleled view of the nasal structures, facilitating diagnosis and correction by bimanual tissue handling. Other benefits include binocular vision for the surgeon, control of bleeding with diathermy, precise placement and suturing of struts, battens, shield and spreader grafts. This approach also offers a definite teaching advantage although this should not be thought of as an indication for its use. The external approach is favoured for most major reconstructive rhinoplasty and revision surgery, particularly where the nasal tip needs addressing. Recent incision refinements and surgical technique have overcome some of the earlier criticisms of a columellar scar, delay in resolution of the supratip skin oedema, loss of tip projection and extra operating time. However with this approach, it may be difficult to assess the supra-tip area and the desired tip projection due to the lack of traction of the soft tissue prior to closure of the columella incision. Specific indications for the external approach in rhinoplasty include:

- congenital deformities such as the "cleft lip nose",
- extensive revision surgery,
- severe nasal trauma,
- the markedly deviated nose,
- marked tip deformities, and
- situations where assessment of the exact pathology is difficult.

Extended applications of the external approach enable greater exploitation of the nasal skeleton and the advantages this affords. It has been advocated for nasoseptal perforation repair, access to the nasal dorsum for treatment of nasal dermoids and even as an approach to hypophysectomy.

Operative Techniques

Anaesthesia

Rhinoplasty surgery is usually performed under general anaesthesia although local anaesthetic and sedation are also possible. The face is prepared with an aqueous detergent and draped to reveal the eyes, the corneas are simply protected with lacrilube ointment. The intranasal mucosal cavity is prepared preoperatively with a (10%) cocaine vasoconstrictor solution. Local anaesthesia with a vasoconstrictor is then injected to further minimise intraoperative bleeding. A dental syringe and needle are used with a 2% lidocaine and

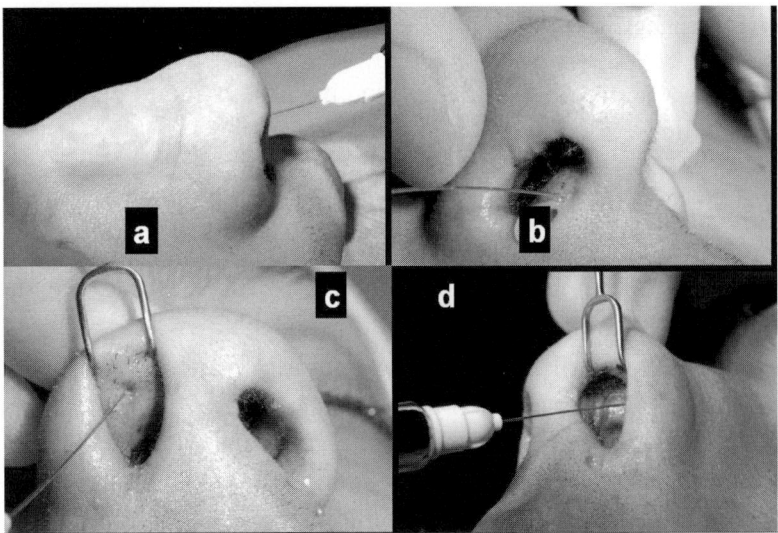

Figure 12.7 **(a)–(d)** Local infiltration technique for rhinoplasty.

1:80,000 adrenaline cartridge. The injection sites are as follows (Figures 12.7a–12.7d):

a) along lateral wall of nose through intercartilaginous area,
b) base of the columella and collumellar region if the external approach is used,
c) vestibular and non-vestibular aspects of the lower lateral carti-lages (the alar cartilages),
d) caudal septal cartilage area, and
e) alar bases if reduction planned (*not shown*).

Injection over the immediate dorsum is best avoided as the resultant swelling can make assessment of this area difficult. Lateral nose depot injections can be massaged upwards into the dorsal area to reduce bleeding when the skin-soft tissue envelope is being elevated. Leaving adequate time for the anaesthesia to take effect is critical in exploiting its haemostatic advantage.

Incisions

Elevation of the skin and soft tissue envelope is facilitated by various incisions.

1. *Intercartilaginous*

The intercartilaginous incision (Figures 12.8a–12.8c) is the most commonly used in endonasal rhinoplasty. It allows direct access to the mid and upper thirds of the nose but affords no exposure of the tip cartilages. It is often used in combination with other incisions if tip surgery needs to be performed.

The incision is made in the area separating the upper and lower lateral cartilages. A small linear hollow is seen intranasally demarcating the area between the caudal border of the upper lateral and the cephalic border of the lower lateral cartilages. It is usually seen and easily palpable when the alar margin is retracted upwards and everted using a two-pronged skin hook (Figure 12.8a).

- An incision is made into this hollow laterally (Figure 12.8b) and the blade is then turned forwards and medially along the intercartilaginous junction and onto the caudal septum to make a transfixion incision below the caudal cartilaginous septum, i.e. the incision passes through the membranous septum between the medial crura and the caudal septum.
- It is important to ensure this transfixion incision does not extend more than half way along the columella as further extension risks dividing the medial crural attachment to the caudal septum. This is one of the major tip support mechanisms, and division may result in postoperative tip ptosis. Conversely, an extended full transfixion incision can be utilised as a manoeuvre for deprojection of the tip if required.
- With retraction of the lower lateral cartilage, the overlying skin-soft tissue envelope can be gently elevated off the cartilaginous

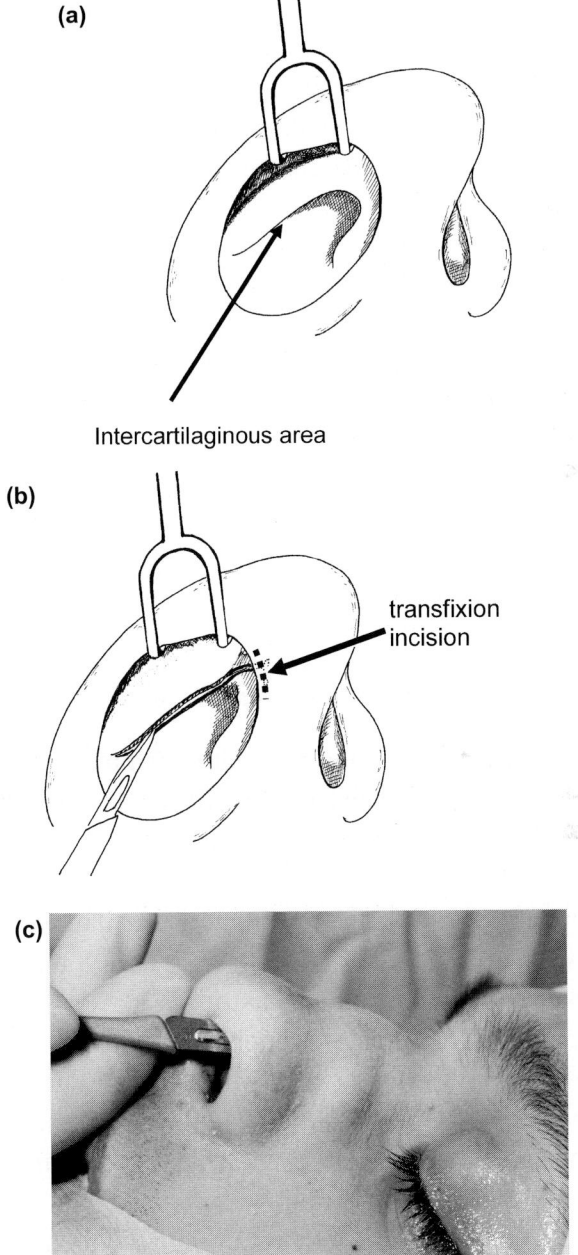

(a)

Intercartilaginous area

(b)

transfixion
incision

(c)

Figure 12.8 (a)–(c) Intercartilaginous incision technique.

dorsum of the upper lateral cartilages by sharp dissection upwards using a sawing motion with a No. 15 blade in a supraperichondral plane (Figure 12.8c).

- After the cartilaginous vault is freed of overlying tissue, an incision is made into the caudal end of the periosteum of the nasal bony pyramid.
- The periosteum and its overlying procerus muscle can then be elevated using the side of a Joseph elevator. Such elevation needs extend only far enough laterally to gain access to a dorsal hump.
- The intercartilaginous incision approach does not expose the lower lateral cartilages although retrograde exposure of the cephalic border may allow volume reduction of this area.

Whilst these incisions are mucosal and as such should heal very well, it is the author's preference to close these with fast absorbing sutures (4.0 Vicryl Rapide — Ethicon).

2. *Cartilage Splitting (Intracartilaginous, Transcartilaginous)*

The cartilage splitting incision facilitates volume reduction of the cephalic border of the lower lateral cartilages. It is frequently performed in addition to reduction of the dorsum.

- The cephalic border of the lower lateral cartilage is identified in the vestibular region and a length of at least 8 mm of cartilage is marked to be left as an intact strip.
- An incision is then made through the vestibular skin which is then freed from the lower lateral cartilage (Figure 12.9a).
- The cephalic edge of the cartilage requiring excision is exposed and incised at the appropriate level as determined by the amount of cartilage to be removed.
- The incised cephalic part of the cartilage can then be freed from the overlying soft tissue and skin and removed ensuring symmetrical amounts are taken.

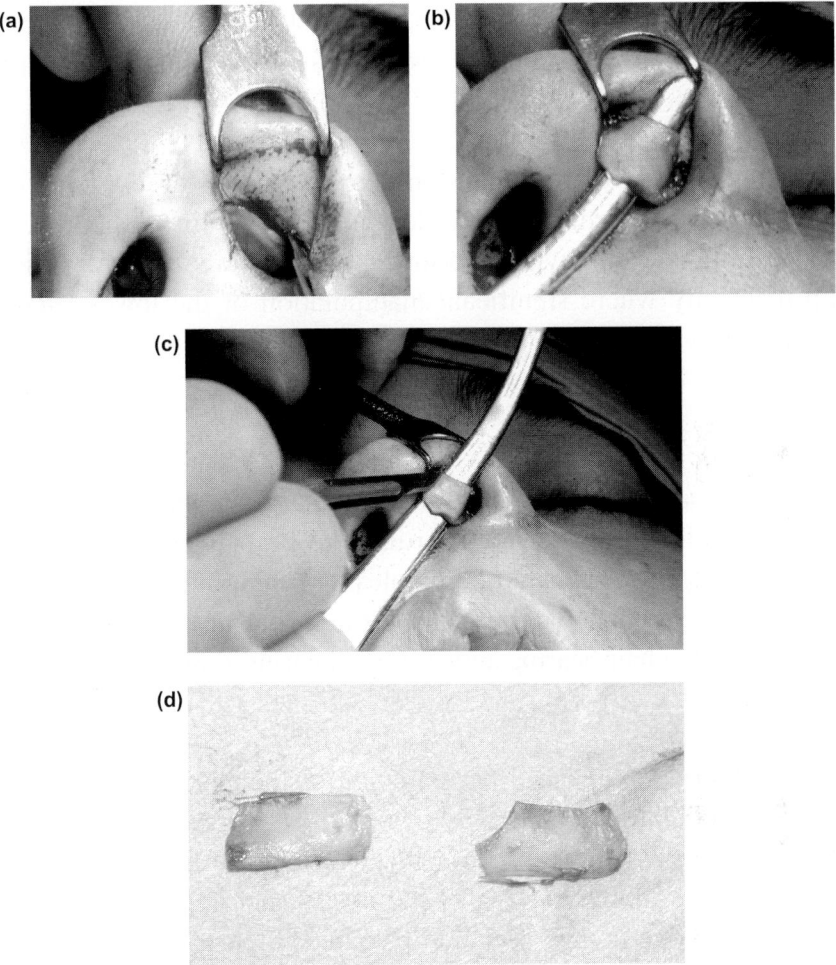

Figure 12.9   (a)–(d) Cephalic resection of the lower lateral cartilages via the cartilage splitting incision. (b) The entire cartilage mobilised from which a strip (c) from the cephalic border is incised leaving continuity, and then excised (d).

- Exposure of the nasal dorsum can then proceed as before.
- An alternative way of removing the cephalic border can be done when performing both the intercartilaginous and cartilage splitting incisions. A bipedicled chondrocutaneous

flap is delivered and can be "bucket handled" into the nasal cavity allowing accurate resection of the cephalic cartilage (Figures 12.9b–12.9d).

The cartilage splitting incision does not allow full exposure of the lower lateral cartilages and is deemed a "non-delivery" approach. As such this incision will not allow adequate correction of a major tip deformity where significant manipulation of the lower lateral cartilages is required.

3. *Marginal Incision*

The marginal incision follows the caudal margin of the lower lateral cartilages allowing the whole cartilage to be delivered and is the choice in dealing with more complex tip abnormalities using an endonasal approach. This margin is often, but not always, at the junction of the hair bearing and non-hair bearing skin in the vestibular area.

- Exposure is enhanced by retraction of the alar margin with a wide double-pronged skin hook and pressure with the middle finger on the upper margin of the alar lobule allowing eversion of the vestibular surface of the nostril. An impression of the caudal edge is then seen and palpated (Figure 12.10a) and an incision is then made through vestibular skin.
- Dissection proceeds using sharp Iris scissors in the supraperichondrial plane on the non vestibular side (Figure 12.10b). The dissection extends to the cephalic border of the cartilage and when combined with an intercartilaginous incision allows full exposure of the whole alar cartilage (Figure 12.10c).
- The cartilages can now be inspected and modified in any required way. Marginal incisions are closed with multiple fine absorbable sutures.

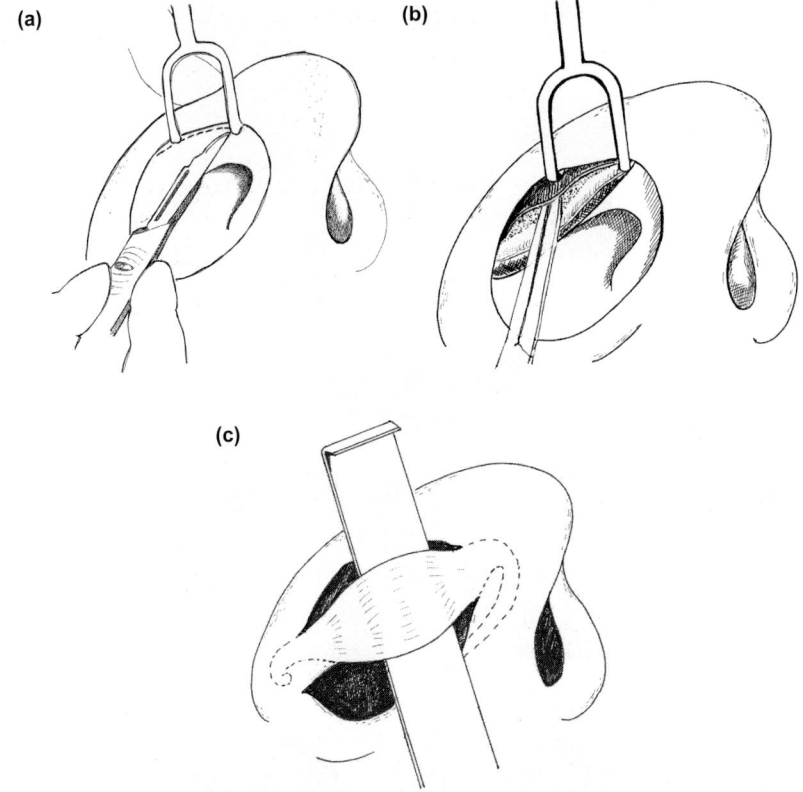

Figure 12.10   (a)–(c) Marginal incision to fully expose and deliver lower lateral cartilages.

4. *External Approach*

Whilst many variations of the columella incision have been advocated, the broken transcolumellar inverted V incision is most commonly used and the author's preferred configuration.

- The incision is made in the mid columella region overlying the medial crural footplates to ensure adequate support on closure thus preventing a depressed scar (see Figure 12.11a).

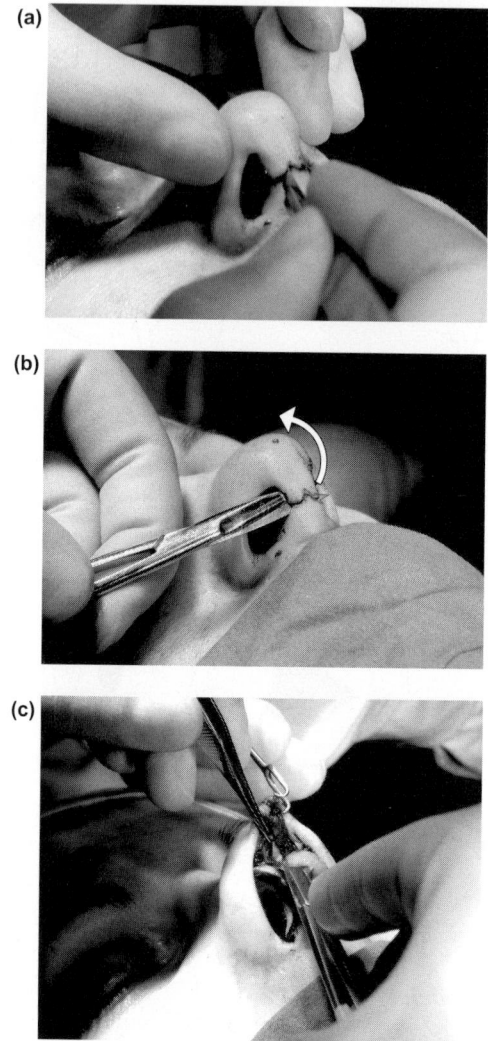

Figure 12.11 **(a)–(c)** External approach technique.

- It is essential to protect the integrity of the caudal end of the medial crura just beneath the incision to prevent postoperative notching in this area. This may be done by initially making only relatively superficial incisions inside the columellar margin which extend laterally to enable reflection to expose the tip.

- These marginal vestibular extensions of the transcollumella incisions are placed 2 mm inside the vestibule and joined by careful undermining of the columella skin with sharp Iris scissors. The scissors can then be used as a guard upon which the transcolumella incision is completed (Figure 12.11b).

- It is relatively easy to identify the caudal end of each of the medial crura and use this as a guide in extending the marginal incision more laterally using angled Converse/Walter scissors with a spreading movement (Figure 12.11c). These hug the caudal surface of the cartilage and cut the overlying soft tissue.

- To obtain adequate exposure of the nasal skeleton, the marginal incision should be extended laterally at least halfway along the lateral crus. Although the major tip support mechanisms are respected in the external approach, the disruption of the skin-soft tissue envelope overlying the lower lateral cartilages and the division of the medial intercrural ligamentous fibrous tissue leads to loss of some of the minor tip support mechanisms. Some ptosis of the nasal tip should therefore be anticipated in all cases.

- The columella incision is closed with five separate 6.0 nylon simple sutures. Eversion of the skin edges ensures favourable healing and vertical mattress sutures may be needed to ensure this. The initial closure of the incision is in the midline at the apex of the inverted V. If there is any risk of tension, a subcutaneous PDS suture is used in addition to the skin sutures. The marginal incisions are closed with fine rapidly absorbing sutures.

The Operative Sequence

The sequence of surgical correction in septorhinoplasty is widely debated. Some advocate correcting any nasal tip abnormality first, prior to addressing the dorsal deformity. The advantage stated is that trying to achieve dorsal correction to match the form of the nasal tip is easier than *vice versa*. Further, as the external nasal splint is applied shortly after corrective osteotomies, this reduces the ecchymosis and swelling that inevitably follows. Conversely it can be argued that the more aggressive methods of dorsal reduction and osteotomies are better performed prior to the fine nasal tip work. Whichever sequence used, it is generally accepted that septal correction should precede any correction of external deformity and that alar base corrections are performed as the final part of the operation.

1. *Septal Surgery (Figure 12.12a)*

Septoplasty surgery is not detailed in this chapter but forms an essential and difficult part of the correction of the traumatic and functionally impaired nose. Whilst bony restoration of the dorsum may improve the upper third aesthetics, septal surgery (essentially the quadrilateral septal cartilage) is important in allowing the cartilaginous dorsum to be re-aligned.

- Caudal septal deformities can displace the leading edge of the septum from behind the columella into the nasal airway, giving rise to nasal obstruction in this area (Figure 12.12b).
- The caudal septum also provides a firm support for the columella and trauma or surgical overresection of the caudal septum may lead to columellar retraction.
- Traumatic injuries may cause fractures within the quadrilateral cartilage of the septum leading to functional problems as well as loss of support in the supratip area — the "saddle" nose. A similar appearance may occur after a traumatic septal haematoma and abscess where there is necrosis of the cartilage.
- Over-resection of cartilage during septoplasty itself may also predispose to this deformity.

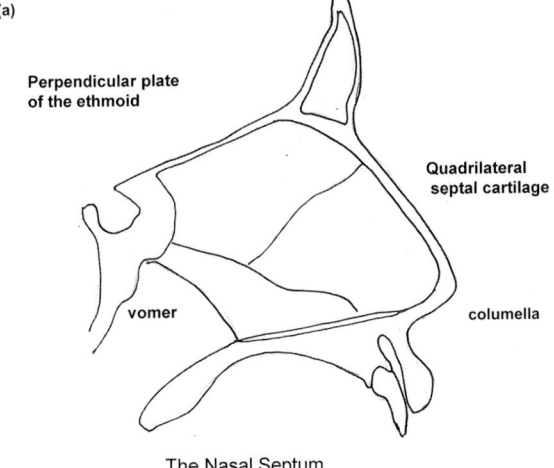

Figure 12.12 (a) Anatomy of the nasal septum. (b) Dislocated nasal septum leading to functional and cosmetic deformity.

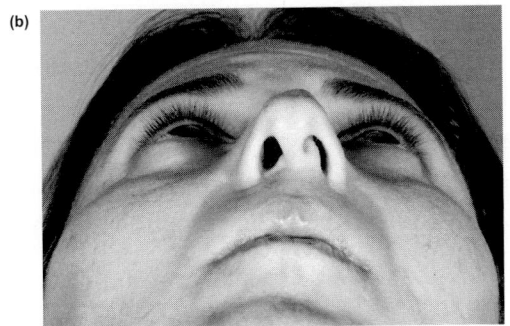

- Harvesting of the quadrilateral cartilage is often required for grafting purposes. However it is important to leave substantial support for the dorsum in the form of an L shaped dorsal and caudal septal butress at least 10 mm wide.
- The rhinoplasty surgeon is required to be able to perform standard septoplasty techniques to achieve predictable functional and aesthetically pleasing results.

Correction of the Osseocartilaginous Dorsum

1. *Hump Reduction*

It is important to judge the extent of resection required from the dorsum prior to local infiltration and elevation of the skin-soft tissue envelope. Attention should be given to the difference in thickness of this envelope at various aspects of the dorsum, it being thinnest at the rhinion, the lowest and most prominent point of the internasal suture. The dorsal hump consists of a bony and cartilaginous component. Endonasal approaches give more restricted views of this area but exposure is maximised by placing an Aufricht retractor along the dorsum under the skin and soft tissues (Figure 12.13).

External rhinoplasty exposure of the upper third of the nose may allow more accurate diagnosis and precise correction, although lack of traction of the tissues makes judgement more difficult.

- The initial incision occurs through the cartilaginous dorsum at the decided level by cutting through the cartilage from cephalically at the osteocartilaginous junction downwards caudally (Figure 12.14a).

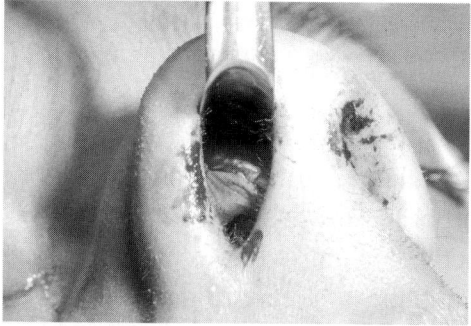

Figure 12.13   Aufricht retractor placed along dorsum of nose in endonasal approach.

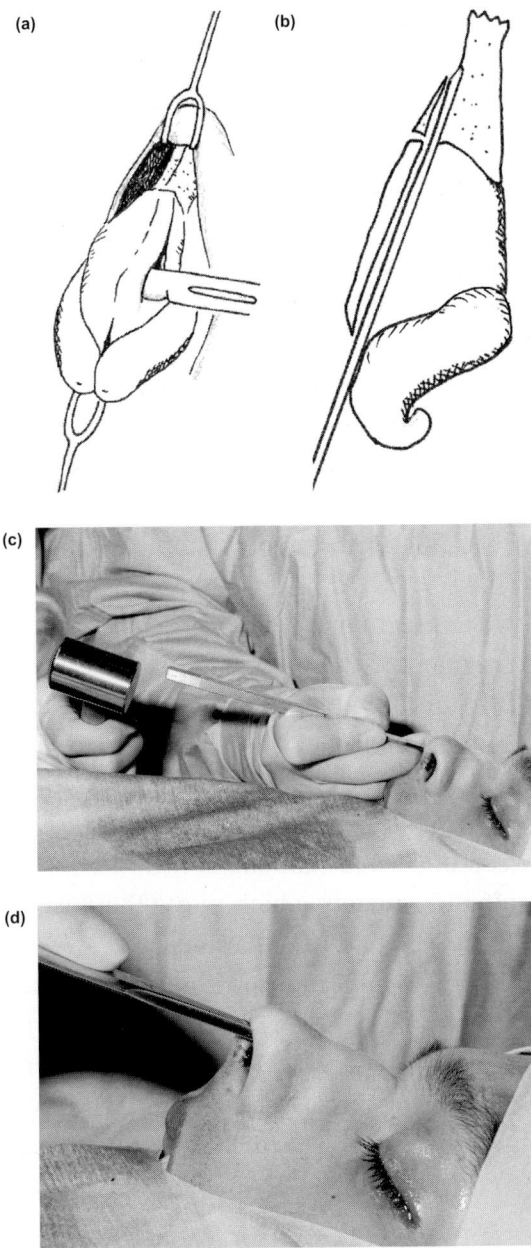

Figure 12.14   (a)–(d) Removal of dorsal hump.

- An osteotome can now be placed under the resected cartilage fragment with its edge facing the bone cephalic to this (Figure 12.14b). It is important at this stage to ensure the osteotome is held in a perfectly horizontal plane to ensure symmetrical bony removal (Figure 12.14c). The exception to this is when excising a bony hump in the presence of a bony pyramid deviation with nasal bones of unequal height. In this case the plane of the osteotome must be altered. An assistant performs a series of double taps with a mallet onto the osteotome to initially engage and then cut through the bone. If the soft tissues have been adequately mobilised, an en-bloc osteocartilaginous hump can be removed. This resected fragment is boat shaped and should consist of part of the nasal bones and the upper laterals/cartilaginous septum complex.

- Symmetry of resection of these structures is checked on the removed fragment. Coarse tungsten-carbide rasps can now be used to "fine tune" the dorsal resection to remove any significant excess bone and finer diamond rasps used to smooth any irregularities in the resected bone (Figure 12.14d).

- An important final step here is to turn the rasp upwards and gently sweep under the skin and soft tissue for removal of any small residual fragments which may otherwise be palpable or visible as postoperative irregularities.

- Rasping of the dorsum alone without using the osteotome is advocated by some surgeons. Due care is advised using this method as repeated use of a rasp may inadvertently traumatise the overlying skin, especially when thin, which can cause some persistent erythema. Bony reduction with powered instrumentation is a new and elegant alternative to the osteotome.

A common mistake is resection of the bony hump without appropriate reduction of the cartilaginous vault. This risks leaving a "pollybeak" deformity which can also occur secondary to soft

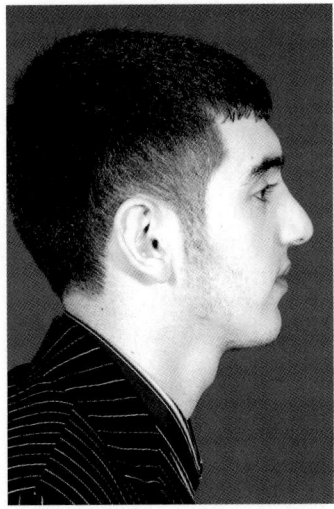

Figure 12.15 Pollybeak deformity in a revision rhinoplasty patient.

tissue scarring when the plane of dissection in this area is incorrect (Figure 12.15).

2. *Osteotomies*

Mobilisation of the bony vault is achieved by osteotomy. The bony pyramid may need

- re-alignment if deviated,
- narrowing at the base, or
- closure of the "open roof" that is an inevitable consequence of hump reduction.

Many aspects of the technique have been refined to produce predictable results with minimal ecchymosis and oedema.

- Local infiltration of the tissues lateral and medial to the bony vault with lidocaine and adrenaline is helpful in reducing bleeding. Microosteotomes are used and should be sharp and small (approximately 2–3 mm).

Medial osteotomy

The medial osteotomy extends from the caudal bony vault upwards in a slightly oblique fashion (Figure 12.16a).

- The osteotome is introduced intranasally and engaged into and advanced along the medial aspect of the nasal bone. A distinct note change is usually heard if the thicker frontal bone is reached. This medial fracture controls the site where a lateral bony back fracture occurs.

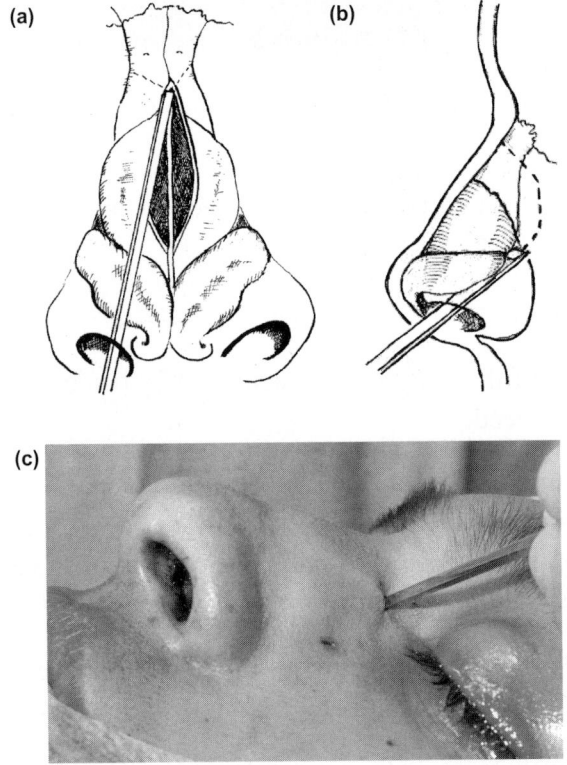

Figure 12.16 (a) Medial osteotomy. (b) Lateral endonasal "high-low-high" osteotomy. (c) Lateral percutaneous osteotomy.

Lateral osteotomy

The lateral osteotomy may be performed endonasally or percutaneously.

Endonasally;

- A stab incision is made intranasally in the mucosa overlying the pyriform aperture just above the attachment of the inferior turbinate to the lateral nasal wall.
- A thin guarded microosteotome is used, designed to preserve the medial periosteum and a laterally positioned guard allows palpation of the edge of the osteotome at all times. The so called high–low osteotomy refers to the supine patient where the upper nasal bone area is "high" and the lower bone is "low".
- The "high-low-high" osteotomy proceeds as follows: initially the osteotome is introduced *high* on the lateral wall of the pyriform aperture (Figure 12.16b). The osteotomy is extended down to and then *low* along the nasofacial groove. As it is extended upwards it is slowly curved from lateral to medially and ends *high* at the level of the medial canthus . This leaves a small triangle of bone at the base of the pyriform aperture which, if infractured, may lead to nasal blockage.

Extension of the lateral osteotomy beyond this level into the thicker nasofrontal bone risks a "rocker deformity" where infracture of the nasal bone causes protrusion at the superior fracture site. If a medial osteotomy has been performed, a controlled back fracture is achieved by twisting the osteotome medially.

The lateral osteotomy may also be performed percutaneously.

- Stab incisions are made through the skin at two points; midway between the medial canthus and the edge of the pyriform aperture low in the nasofacial groove and superiorly between the medial canthus and the top of the dorsum (Figure 12.16c).

- A sharp 2 mm microosteotome is introduced and a series of perforations are made low along the lateral nasal wall and a superior osteotomy is fashioned with perforations at the level of the medial canthus.
- Each perforation is made to go through the bone but not the medial periosteum. As the bone is perforated a distinct change in tone (fall in pitch) is heard with the tapping sounds.
- Studies have shown that the small stab incisions are entirely invisible postoperatively. The percutaneous lateral osteotomy is simple to learn and execute and allows precise, predictable fractures to be made.

Intermediate Osteotomy

The intermediate osteotomy is used to correct an extreme deviation of the nasal pyramid where one nasal sidewall is far longer than the other. Medial and lateral osteotomies alone in this case could not create bones of equal height and residual postoperative deviation is the norm. The intermediate osteotomy effectively shortens the longer side allowing the nasal bones to be repositioned into the mid line. When performed bilaterally it can be used to narrow a very wide nasal dorsum. The osteotomy is placed along the mid aspect of the lateral nasal wall and it is important to perform it prior to the lower lateral osteotomy as it cannot be done if the lateral wall is mobile.

Nasal Tip Surgery

Surgery of the nasal tip is by far the most complex aspect of rhinoplasty surgery and requires a sound appreciation of the anatomy and aesthetic facial parameters. Preoperative assessment should define what specific anomalies are present and the objectives for correction.

The problems encountered may be thought of as being due to

- volume excess,
- under- or overrotation,
- under- or overprojection,
- width problems, or
- intrinsic tip deformities.

It is beyond the scope of this chapter to describe each aspect of complex tip correction in detail. The basic concepts can be divided into

- volume reduction,
- tip remodelling procedures,
- placement of (usually) cartilaginous grafts.

Projection and rotation of the tip are intricately related and manoeuvres to correct one may well affect the other.

The tripod concept of the nasal tip is a very useful model to predict changes in these parameters with modifications of the alar cartilages, and is detailed later.

Volume Reduction

Where there is isolated volume excess of the nasal tip giving rise to bulbosity, cephalic resection of the lower lateral cartilage may be adequate to increase definition and cause mild narrowing (see Figures 12.9a–12.9d). Access to the cephalic border of this cartilage as previously described may be via a cartilage splitting incision or by retrograde dissection from an intercartilaginous incision. The external approach is not required for isolated cephalic reduction but precise and symmetrical resection is optimal using this technique.

Judgement is critical in ensuring enough cartilage is removed to give a noticeable change in the definition but leaving as much cartilage behind as possible. Overzealous cephalic strip resection can lead to a "visoring" effect due to alar retraction caused by contraction as healing occurs. An absolute minimum of 8 mm width of residual cartilage continuity is recommended but in the presence of an anatomically narrow alar cartilage this may need to be reconsidered. If vestibular mucosa is not preserved, this too can contribute to contracture and promote further retraction.

When employing an endonasal approach, marking in the vestibular area is useful to ensure the incision is made in the correct position — an instrument can be used to make an imprint in the vestibular skin or a needle placed percutaneously in the appropriate place. Symmetrical reduction is essential — both resected cartilages are compared to ensure this is the case.

Following reduction, a small void is created in cephalic region of the lower lateral cartilages. Healing and contracture may cause some upward rotation of the tip to fill the void. Overall this is often a favourable change although care should be exercised in an already overrotated tip. This method cannot be relied upon as a powerful or indeed completely predictable method of causing significant tip rotation.

Rotation Deformities (Figure 12.17a)

Correction of the underrotated tip can be done with various manoeuvres based on the tripod concept. This concept proposes that the conjoint medial crura are one limb of the tripod with each lateral crus representing a separate lateral limb (Figure 12.17b). Manipulation of any part of the tripod can be used to predict changes in the projection and rotation of the nasal tip. The LeFort I maxillary advancement will correct an underrotated tip by advancing the conjoint medial crura and caudal septum. Most rhinoplasty techniques for rotation problems rely on the tripod manoeuvres of the nasal tip.

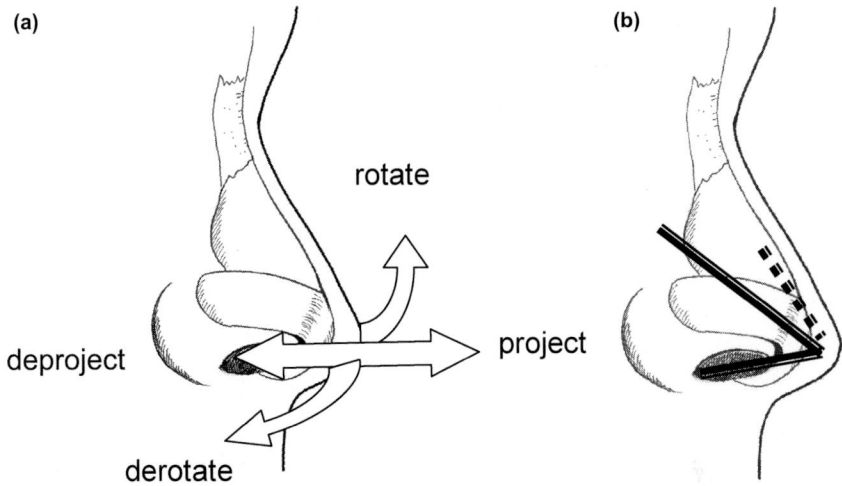

Figure 12.17 (a) Surgical anatomy terminology. (b) Tripod model of lower lateral cartilage dynamics. The tripod limbs represent the two lateral crurae and the conjoined medial crurae as the third limb.

- Thus division and overlay of the lateral crura will produce a marked tip rotation upwards, but will also cause some tip deprojection (Figure 12.18a).
- Lateral crural steal techniques which recruit the lateral crura medially using domal suturing can enhance rotation and also be usefully employed for increased projection (see also projection deformities below) (Figures 12.19a and 12.9b).

An over rotated nasal tip is an unaesthetic "piggy nose". Options for correction are more limited with this situation.

- A graft in the tip/infratip area will give an illusion of counter-rotation and increased length of the nose.
- A caudal septal extension graft also gives a similar effect.
- In order to accomplish counter-rotation in extreme cases, a skin-cartilage composite graft may be needed in space created between the upper and lower lateral cartilages.

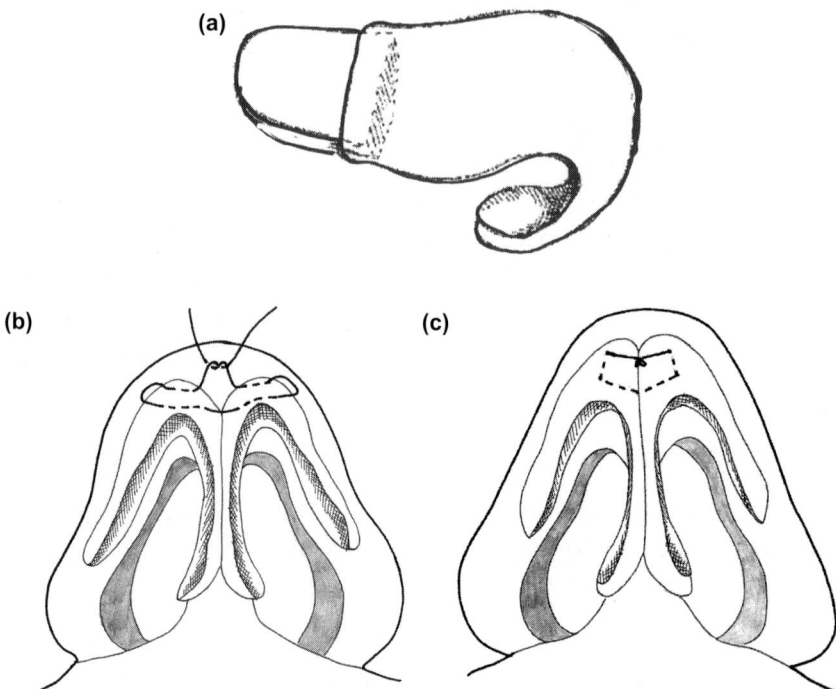

Figure 12.18 (**a**) Division and overlay of lateral crura to cause tip rotation. (**b**) and (**c**) Dome suturing technique.

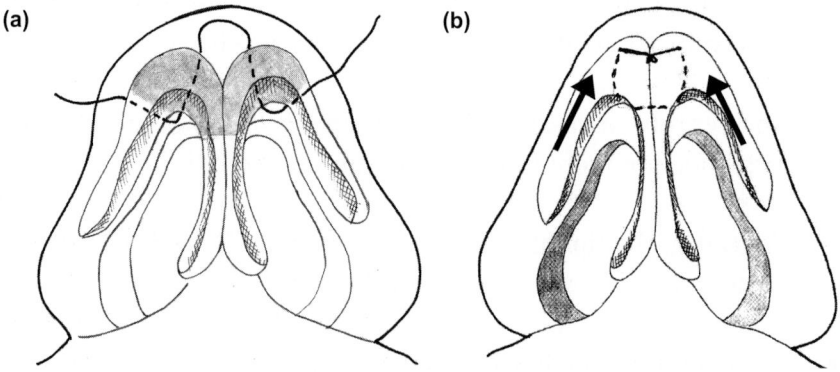

Figure 12.19 (**a**) and (**b**) Lateral crural steal technique to increase tip projection.

- Division and overlap of the medial crurae is another option, although this also deprojects the tip.

Projection Deformities

Increasing the projection of the nasal tip is often desirable in rhinoplasty surgery. As with rotation problems, this can be achieved by reorientation of the alar cartilages or by addition of cartilaginous struts or grafts. Variations of basic techniques are widely described. Commonly performed procedures include the following:

1. *Domal Sutures*

Suture modification of the nasal domal area can refine the shape of the nasal tip into a more aesthetic configuration.

- Domal sutures can convert a "boxy" or trapezoidal configuration of a nasal tip into a more aesthetic triangular configuration (Figures 12.18b and 12.18c). Sutures are placed within an individual dome (intradomal or a single dome unit) and the two domes can then be approximated (interdomal or a double dome unit).
- Mild projection of the nasal tip can also be achieved by transdomal suturing using 6.0 nylon, that causes the domes to be elevated.
- To increase the projection even further, the lateral crus of the lower lateral cartilage is mobilised fully from the vestibular skin. This lateral crus can then be recruited towards the domal area and a new dome created and sutured in a newly projected position — the so-called "lateral crural steal" (Figures 12.19a and 12.19c). This procedure also causes a degree of tip rotation.
- Vertical dome division with resuturing — The Goldman technique is the original and perhaps most well described method of dome division. The many modifications of this technique all

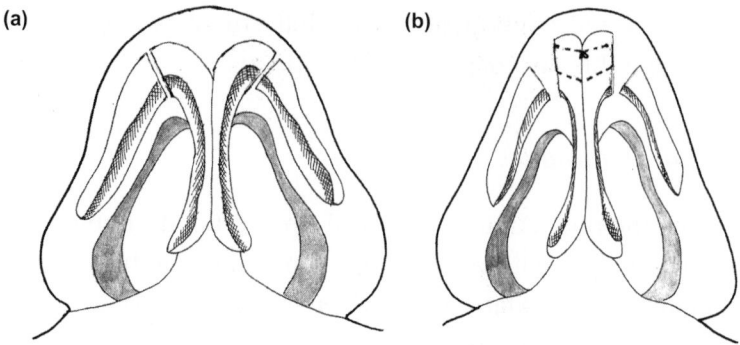

Figure 12.20   **(a)** and **(b)** Goldman technique of dome division.

describe vertical division of the lower lateral cartilage usually 2–3 mm lateral to the existing dome. The medial cut ends of cartilage are then sutured back to back thereby increasing projection of the tip and can be trimmed to the exact height required and if required, can be shortened to deproject the tip (Figures 12.20a and 12.20b). The residual lateral cartilages are left and generally prolapse medially. Vestibular skin may be preserved intact although the original description of this technique suggested incision through this. Current management of the nasal tip has veered away from this technique towards suture modification. Criticisms of its use have included its relative irreversibility and the creation of a very sharply defined, "tent pole"-like appearance to the tip particularly in the presence of thin skin.

These techniques are, however, still very useful and with appropriate selection of patients give excellent form to the tip.

2.   *Grafts and Struts*

Autogenous grafting material is always a preferred source of tissue. Grafts are usually harvested from the quadrilateral cartilage of the septum or auricular conchal bowl (Figure 12.21). Placement on the nasal tip region can cause projection changes. Dependent on the

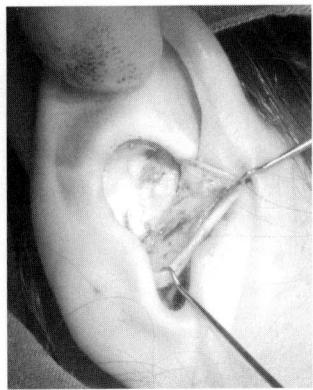

Figure 12.21   Harvest of auricular cartilage via an anterior approach.

area required for projection, various cartilage grafts have been described. Grafts are sutured into place using fine non-absorbable sutures when performing an external approach, or by specific placement in precise pockets if approached endonasally.

The columellar strut is extremely useful in maintaining and to some extent increasing tip projection. With the inevitable loss of tip support with any of the described approaches, ptosis may be anticipated in the postoperative period and placement of a cartilaginous strut between the medial crurae can help prevent this (Figure 12.22).

Placement of grafts in the premaxillary region can be sometimes used to give an illusion of tip rotation and projection.

Deprojection of the tip is less often required and can necessitate a number of manoeuvres based on the tripod concept.

- Division of the medial crural footplate attachment to the caudal septum with an extended full transfixion incision will lose one of the major tip support mechanisms and should cause some deprojection and counter-rotation.
- Vertical division of the alar (lower lateral) cartilages with overlay and suturing of the edges should also decrease projection. Such an overlay can be fashioned in the lateral crurae to give increased rotation and decreased projection.

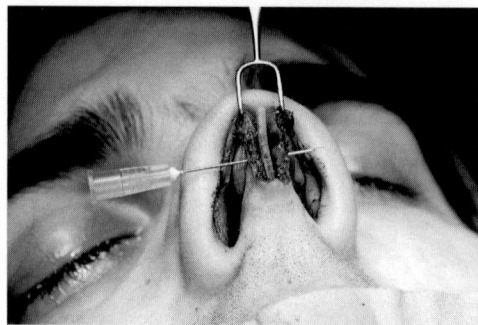

Figure 12.22   Insertion of cartilaginous columellar strut.

Other techniques include:

- Reduction of the nasal spine.
- The previously described vertical dome division with excision of the excess medial crurae and reconstruction with sutures.
- The "tongue-in-groove" technique of septocollumellar suturing remains a further option and is a useful way of establishing both projection and rotation of the nasal tip. A disadvantage of this method is the rigidity and lack of mobility such a procedure imparts to the tip in some patients.

Alar Base Reduction

Assessment of the alar base is made preoperatively and reduction planned if required. Change in tip dynamics may influence the alar base width perioperatively such as in marked deprojection of the overprojected "tension" nose. In this case, the alar base is generally flared as a result of the other corrective procedures and the patient should be told of the possibility of needing reduction.

Alar base reduction is generally divided into correction relating to excess alar flare, excess nostril size or a combination of these. It is universally agreed that alar base reduction is performed as a final step in the operation after all other deformities have been corrected. Conservative reduction is important to avoid the complications of asymmetry and over-reduction which are both difficult to correct.

Nostril Size

Excision of a wedge of skin and soft tissue from the nostril floor alone will reduce the internal dimension of the medial border of the nostril (Figure 12.23a). Subtle alteration of the alar curve can be effected too, but this manoeuvre will not affect the width of the alar bases.

Alar Flare

More marked changes in alar flare are achieved by extension of an incision within the nostril into the alar facial junction.

- The incision is not made within, but rather 1–2 mm above the alar facial crease as this minimises postoperative scarring and visibility. A wedge is removed from this area allowing reduction in the bulkiness of the ala and the width of the base can be narrowed as well (Figure 12.25b).
- If significant alar flare reduction is needed a larger wedge is excised and a small back cut onto the lateral edge of the nostril facilitates adequate medialisation of the alar bases (Figure 12.23c).

Combination

The combination of alar flare and excess nostril size is corrected with a rectangular shaped resection of alar tissue. Symmetrical marking of the excision is critical to diminish the postoperative dissatisfaction of asymmetry (Figure 12.23d).

Eversion of the skin edges with fine non-absorbable sutures (6.0 nylon) are used to ensure an accurate closure.

(a)

(b)

(c)

(d)

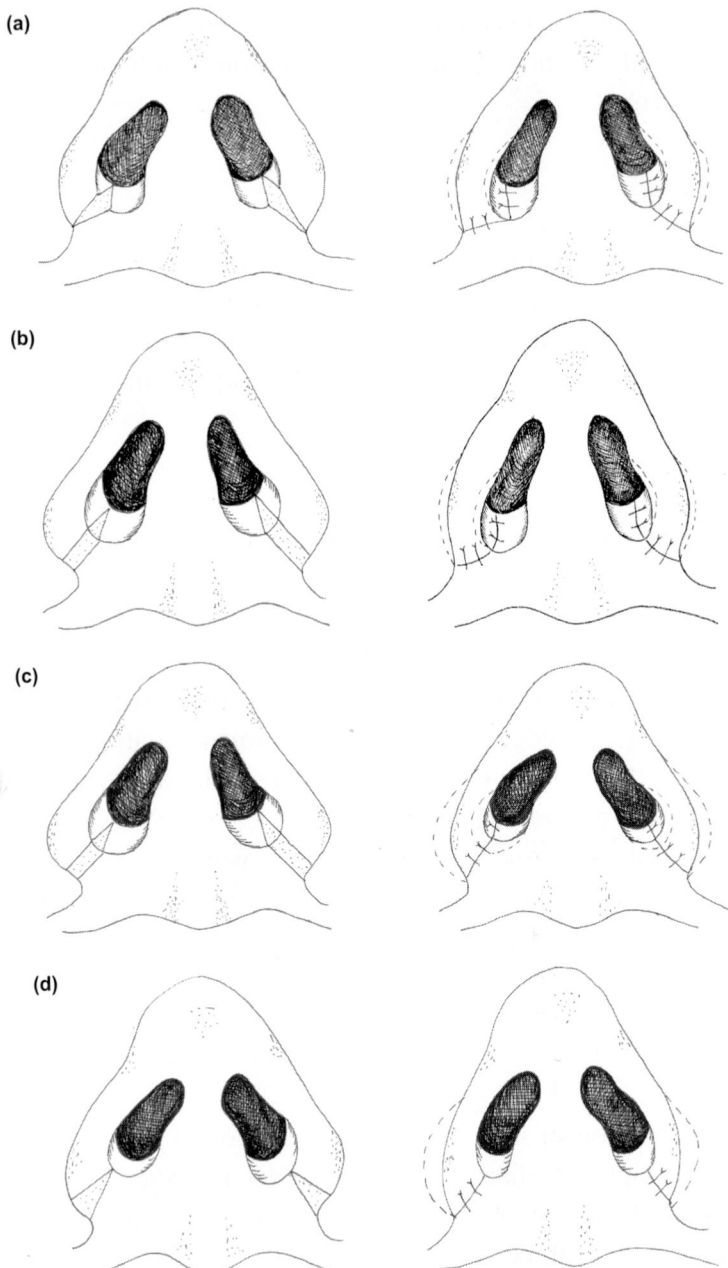

Figure 12.23   **(a)–(d)** Techniques for alar base reduction.

Postoperative Care

Generally, meticulous technique and closure can avoid the need for postoperative nasal packing altogether and this is preferable as the presence and removal of such packs can be extremely uncomfortable. Packing materials, if required, include nasal tampons, ribbon guaze packing that may be impregnated by Bismuth Iodoform Paraffin Paste (BIPP) or non-stick dressings such as Telfa or Melonin. Packing is generally removed a few hours after surgery although can be left overnight.

Intranasal silastic splints are generally not required but are used in patients in whom postoperative synaechiae between the lateral wall of the nose and septum are a risk. Such patients include those with preoperative nasal adhesions from prior trauma or surgery or those who have significant perioperative septal mucoperichondrial tears. Splints are also used routinely after septal perforation closure. Silastic splints are available preformed or may be custom-made from sheets and are sutured to the nasal septum anteriorly. The splints are removed two weeks postoperatively in the outpatient setting.

A dorsal dressing is applied at the end of surgery to stabilise the nasal bones following osteotomies. Initially, steristrips are placed firmly along the dorsum to help re-approximate the dorsal skin and soft tissue envelope to the underlying skeleton. It is important to place one strip across the nasal tip area moulding and holding the tip into a desired position whilst the healing process occurs. Many options for the splint are available including preformed thermoplastic and metallic splints and the author's favoured custom tailored Plaster of Paris. A 5-layer 5 cm × 5 cm triangle of plaster is used. The sharp squared edges are rounded off into gentle curves in particular to ensure the cephalic edge of the plaster does not impinge upon the medial canthus of the eye. The plaster is soaked in warm water and is applied over the steristrips and held firmly whilst it sets and fixes the bony dorsum in the desired position. This creates a small but

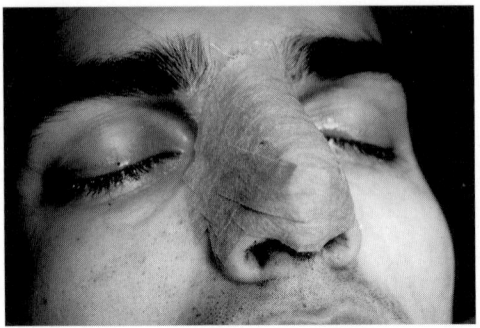

Figure 12.24   Nasal splint.

adequately protective splint that is further secured by taping over the plaster onto the face thereby ensuring it remains in position. Brown coloured micropore is used to act as an effective camouflage of the plaster itself (see Figure 12.24). The dorsal plaster splint is removed a week postoperatively as are any external sutures.

Revision Surgery

Revision corrective procedures remain one the most challenging aspects of rhinoplasty surgery. As techniques evolve, the rhinoplasty surgeon is ever seeking an ultimate postoperative result that will please both the discriminative patient and surgeon alike. New computer-aided preoperative techniques aimed at predicting eventual improvement in cosmesis coupled with the unprecedented number of media articles on cosmetic surgery appear to be increasing patient expectations. The inadequately informed patient is likely to be more critical of postoperative results. Increasing rates of revision surgery may be predicted in Europe, reflecting trends in North America.

The need for revision rhinoplasty may arise from either inadequate or overzealous primary surgery, most often the result of poor judgement by an inexperienced surgeon. Furthermore, postoperative scarring can turn a shorter-term good cosmetic result into a suboptimal one with time. In both cases, the resultant localised loss of contour or deficiency of the support mechanisms may in turn be associated with functional problems.

The revision rhinoplasty patient may further present with psychological issues including the body dysmorphobic disorder, relating to the original surgery and these must be both recognised and addressed during any preliminary consultation. In doing so, the important distinction between a patient-perceived or truly inadequate postoperative result can be made. In the former case it is particularly important not to convey false expectations regarding a revision procedure to the expectant patient. A doctor/patient rapport must be built laying the foundations for extended counselling in order to convey a realistic outcome for any revision surgery. Where a personality disorder is apparent, referral to a clinical psychologist or liaison psychiatrist may be essential.

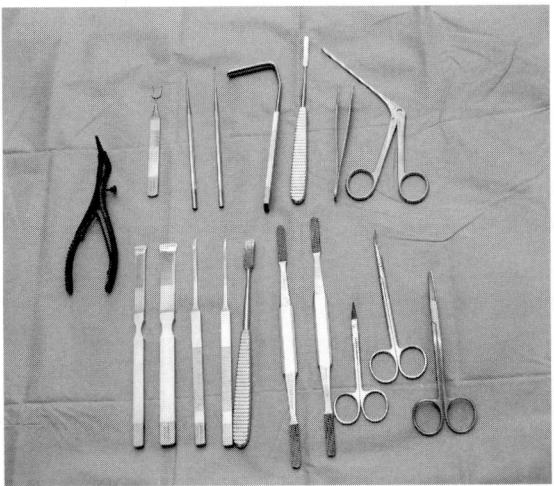

Figure 12.25 Basic rhinoplasty instruments. Instrument list (from left to right), Top row: Cottle's speculum, double pronged wide hook, single/double pronged micro hook, Aufricht retractor, Joseph periosteal elevator, Brown-Adson toothed forceps, Blakesley-Wilde forceps. Bottom row: Osteotomes — 14 mm/10 mm/ guarded 2.2 mm/2 mm, tungsten carbide glabella rasp, tungsten carbide dorsal rasps, Walter scissors, Kilner scissors, Foman scissors.

Retrospective analyses have identified lower-third deformities followed by middle-third deformities as the most commonly encountered problems requiring secondary surgery.

Most authors would agree that revision surgery should not be planned for at least one year following the last operation. This time allows maturing of scar tissue, diminishing the risk of further deformity due to poor tissue healing following subsequent surgery. Whilst this remains a good general guideline, early correction of minor deformities such as an inadequate osteotomy may allay patient anxieties without compromising overall results. Other deformities that may be similarly rectified at an early stage include alar base widening that may be evident following the original surgery, alar retraction and minimal bony dorsal deformities requiring little soft tissue dissection. The majority of revisions, however, are best deferred and a clear explanation regarding the reasoning will usually temper patient pressure. The advantage of soft mature scar tissue during the revision operation facilitates easier dissection. "Shrink-wrapping" of the skin over the structural components is also well established by a year and will identify any irregularities at this stage, although the overall process continues further for some years. However, nasal tip revision surgery may need to be deferred somewhat longer than 12 months as adequate healing and shrink-wrapping may not be complete.

A particular challenge in revision rhinoplasty surgery is the unpredictability of the findings during surgery. Soft tissue contractures and scarring may mimic underlying structural deformity, and even with meticulous planning, the surgeon must remain able to adapt or even change the planned techniques to suit the discovered anomaly. Camouflage grafts are not always predicted for use but should be considered as being required to help correct such unforeseen deformities when formulating the preoperative plan. Experience in a variety of techniques is naturally a prerequisite to undertaking this sort of procedure due the very nature of this unpredictability.

Case Reports

Three cases are presented as examples of the complexity of the rhinoplasty challenge (see Figures 12.25 to 12.27).

Patient Examples

Patient 1 — Dorsal Hump and Tip Ptosis

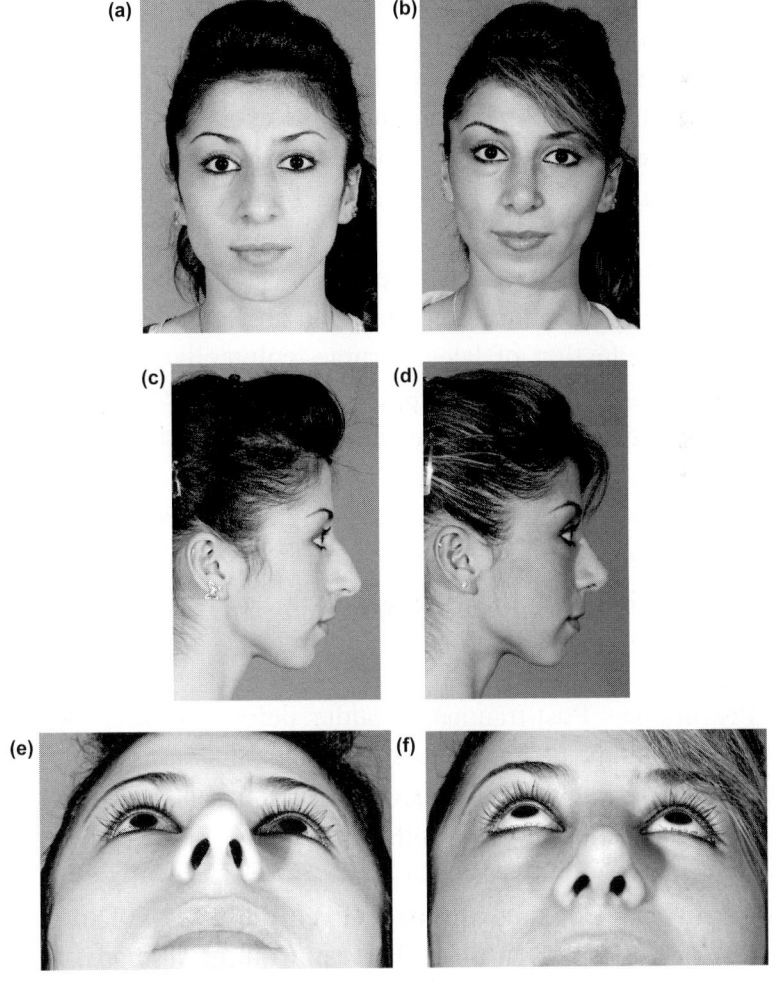

Problems: Dorsal hump, slight deviation of bony dorsum, low take off point of nose from face, ptosis of nasal tip, excess columellar show. Retrognathia — patient not seeking correction of this.

Important Considerations: Large dorsal hump reduction may be the initial intervention for an inexperienced rhinoplasty surgeon. This would lead to a overlong, ptotic looking nose which would be more unaesthetic than the initial presentation. Projection and rotation of the tip here is the key to improving the nasal balance. The "take off point" of the nose is also very low on the face with a shallow nasion — an ideal being approximately at the level of where the upper eyelashes point to on the lateral view. Augmentation of the radix area together with the tip changes mean a much smaller dorsal hump reduction is required.

Surgical Plan: External approach septorhinoplasty; lateral crural steal and suturing to rotate and project tip, minor cephalic volume reduction of lateral crurae, columellar strut harvested from septal cartilage for support, reduction of caudal and membranous septum, dorsal bony and cartilaginous dehump (minor), medial and lateral endonasal osteotomies, crushed radix graft harvested from septal cartilage to augment nasion.

Patient 2 — Post-Traumatic Saddle Deformity

Problems: Post-traumatic saddle deformity, scar overlying dorsum, bony deviation to right, columellar retraction, broad nasal tip (patient unconcerned regarding this). Nasal obstruction with internal nasal valve collapse.

Important Considerations: Given the extent of the saddle deformity, septal cartilage harvest would be impossible and

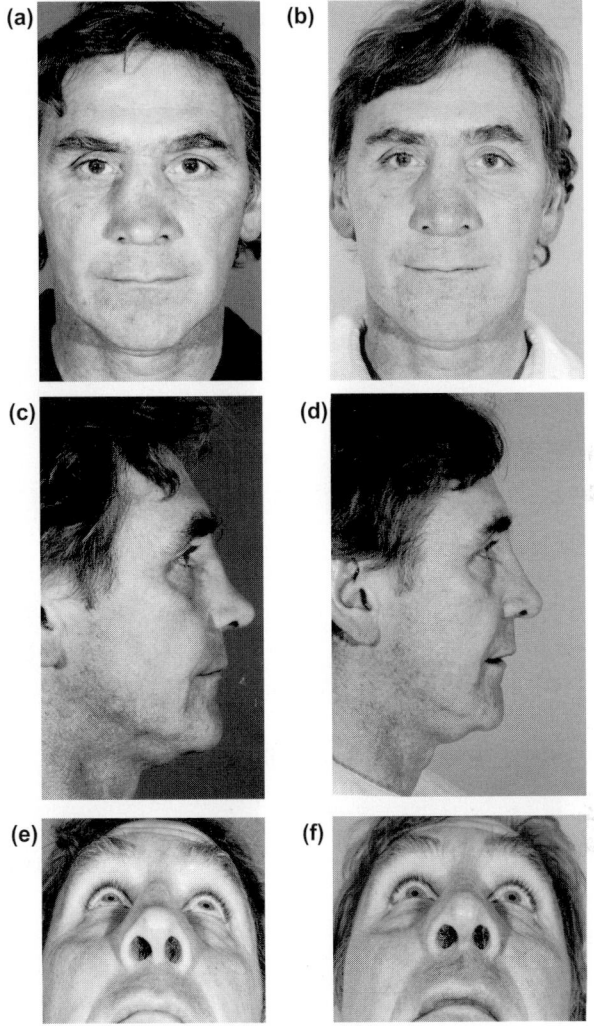

alternative sources are required. Scar revision, if required, should be deferred.

Surgical Plan: External approach rhinoplasty; auricular cartilage harvest for augmentation of dorsum with 2-layer graft, columellar strut and spreader grafts, tip refinement with dome suturing, medial and lateral percutaneous osteotomies.

Patient 3 — Shallow Dorsal Hump and Boxy Tip

Problems: Dorsal hump, wide, "boxy" configuration to nasal tip with excess cephalic volume of lower lateral cartilages. Nasal obstruction with septal deviation and idiopathic perforation.

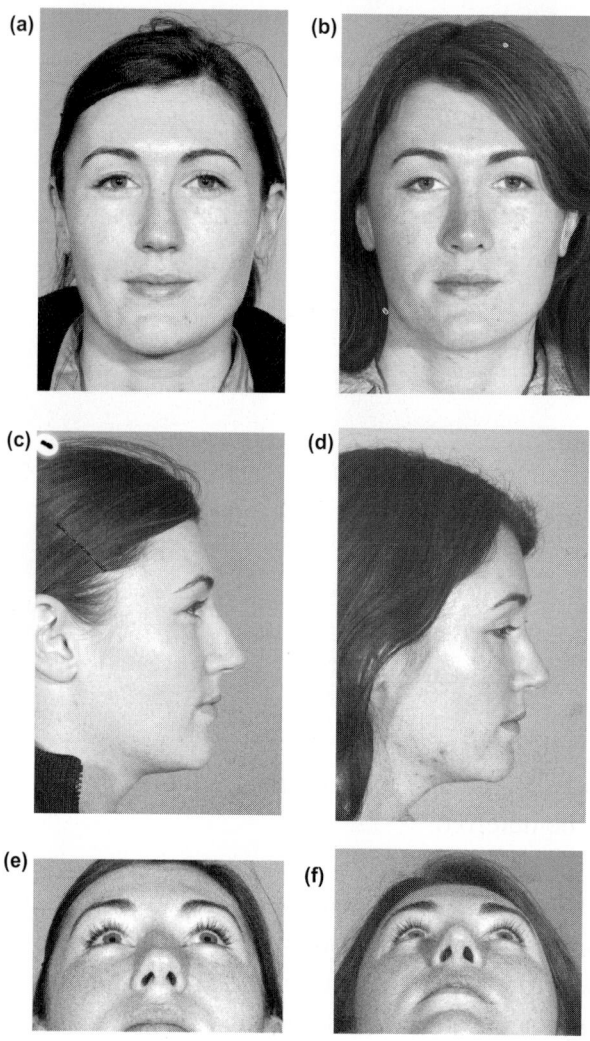

Important Considerations: Subtle improvements are only required here for restoration of cosmesis and improvement of brow-tip aesthetic lines.

Surgical Plan: Septorhinoplasty with closure of septal perforation; minor dorsal bony and cartilaginous dehump, medial and lateral endonasal osteotomies, dome suturing of lower lateral cartilages and volume reduction of cephalic margins. Septal perforation closure with bipedicled mucoperichondrial flaps and interpositional graft.

Conclusions

Rhinoplasty surgery is a complex aspect of aesthetic and reconstructive surgery of the face. Its important relationship to other orthognathic procedures is clear and the principles outlined in this chapter should provide a sound understanding of the basic concepts of this type of surgery.

The wide array of operative techniques involved in rhinoplasty necessitates a thorough understanding of the anatomy of the osseo-cartilaginous vault and septum, surgical principles and healing processes associated with these operations.

13

Ankylosis of the
Temporomandibular Joint

Introduction

There are many causes of limited mouth opening which may be classified as follows.

Intra-articular (intracapsular)

- Closed lock due anterior displacement of the meniscus without reduction.
- Osseous or fibro-osseous ankylosis, secondary to trauma, infection or osteoarthritis.
- Fibrodysplasia ossificans progressiva (formerly myositis ossificans).
- Ankylosing spondylitis, juvenile rheumatoid arthritis.

Extra-articular (extracapsular)

- Trismus.
- Disuse muscle atrophy, contractures secondary to intra-articular ankylosis or psychogenic trismus.
- Post-radiotherapy and thermal scarring.
- Post-traumatic scarring.
- Oral submucous fibrosis.
- Post-cancrum oris scarring.
- Fibrodysplasia ossificans progressiva (formerly myositis ossificans).

414

Only the management of intra-articular ankylosis with its marked disturbance in facial skeletal growth will be considered here.

Aetiology

Although most causes of extra-articular ankylosis are self-evident the aetiology of intra-articular ankylosis is obscure. It is uncommon in the West and the prevalence seems to be higher in tropical and sub-tropical countries although there is no reliable epidemiology.

Certain factors are significant; extra- and intracapsular joint trauma are common in children and adults but ankylosis is very rare (Figures 13.1a–13.1e). Experimental ankylosis is very difficult to produce in animals without inserting a bone graft.

Removal of the meniscus produces a condylar overgrowth similar to the ankylosis deformity but without fusion (Figures 13.2a–13.2c).

However the rare fibrodysplasia ossificans progressiva which has an unexplained short first toe (Figure 13.3) and widespread heterotopic bone formation, is associated with an excess of the bone morphogenetic protein 4 (BMP 4) gene which may be due to a deficiency of the BMP inhibitor genes, curiously named gremlin (DRM) and noggin. Also the progressive ankylosis gene ank produces intra-articular and peri-articular joint fusion in man and mice.

The outcome of such a localised abnormal genotype could be a deficiency of RANKL (receptor activator of nuclear kappa ligand) a key messenger responsible for osteoclastogenesis, when the affected structures are challenged by trauma or infection.

The natural history is usually infantile and pre-adolescent loss of the meniscus due to:

- birth trauma with displacement of the meniscus;
- juvenile joint infection — middle ear, mastoid or haematogenous; and
- juvenile rheumatoid arthritis (Stills disease), plus the unexplained tendency for local ectopic bone formation (see BMP 4, noggin, gremlin and ank above).

(a)

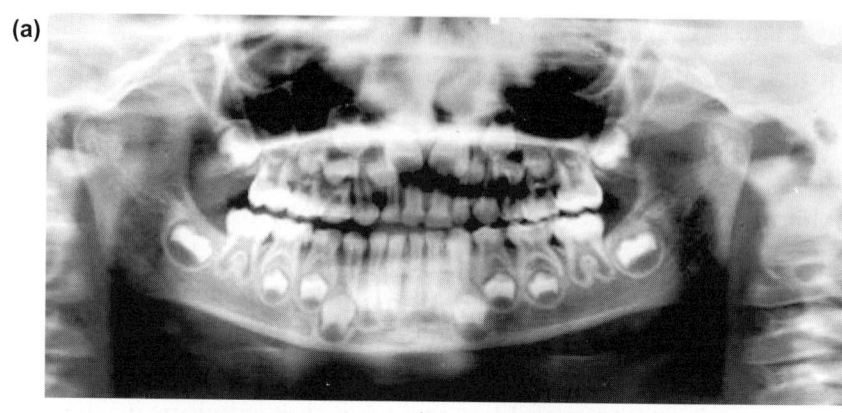

(b)

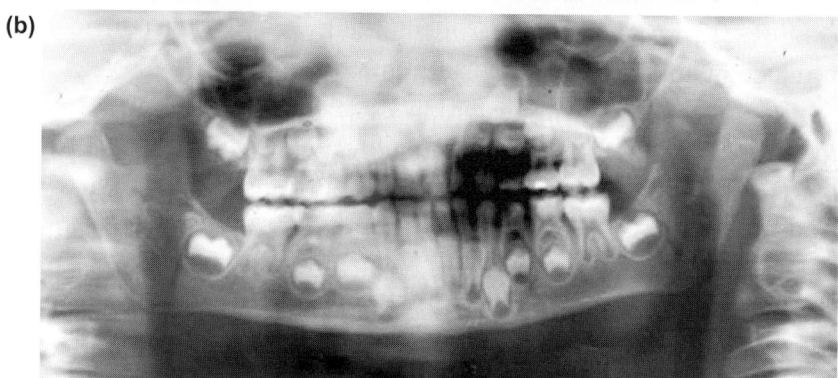

(c)

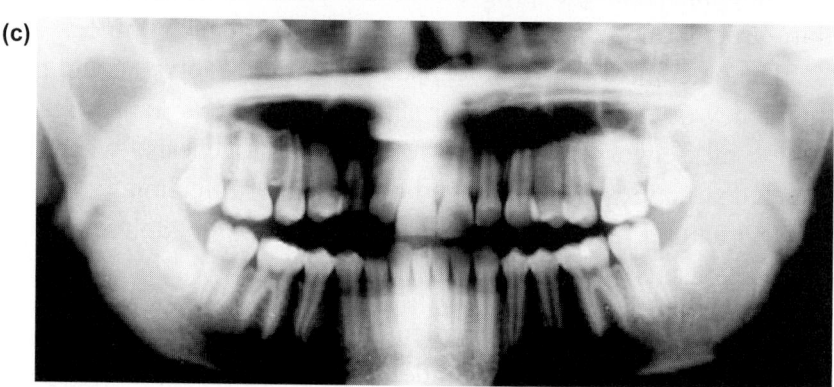

Figure 13.1 **(a)** Radiograph showing bilateral intracapsular fractures at 6 years. **(b)** Condylar remodelling 6 months later. **(c)**, **(d)** and **(e)** Normal growth without ankylosis at 14 years.

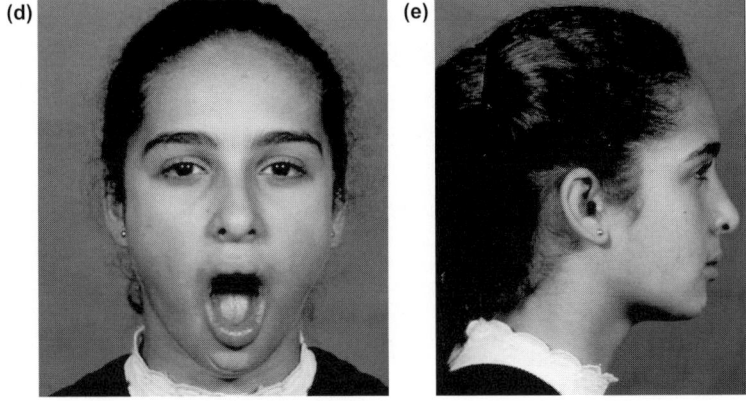

Figure 13.1   (*Continued*)

The idiopathic intracapsular bony fusion appears to arise through the following sequence of events.

i)   Condylar damage and loss of meniscus due to traumatic displacement, inflammmation or infection.
ii) Irregular reparative condylar overgrowth with varying degrees of mechanical, fibrous and bony ankylosis with ossification of the joint capsule.
iii) Extra-articular ankylosis due to masticatory muscle contracture.

The same pattern is less frequently seen in adults following trauma, ankylosing spondylitis or osteoarthritis.

Presentation

Ankylosis in children produces impaired mandibular growth with bilateral deformity in all dimensions. This deformity is asymmetrical in unilateral cases with a straight small hemimandible on the ankylosed side, and a marked contralateral bowing deformity. Retrognathia and retrogenia (Figures 13.4a–13.4c) become more apparent with age. This produces an occlusal cant down to the normal side. In rare bilateral cases the mandible is short but symmetrical. In all cases the inter-incisal opening can be up to 10 mm even with total

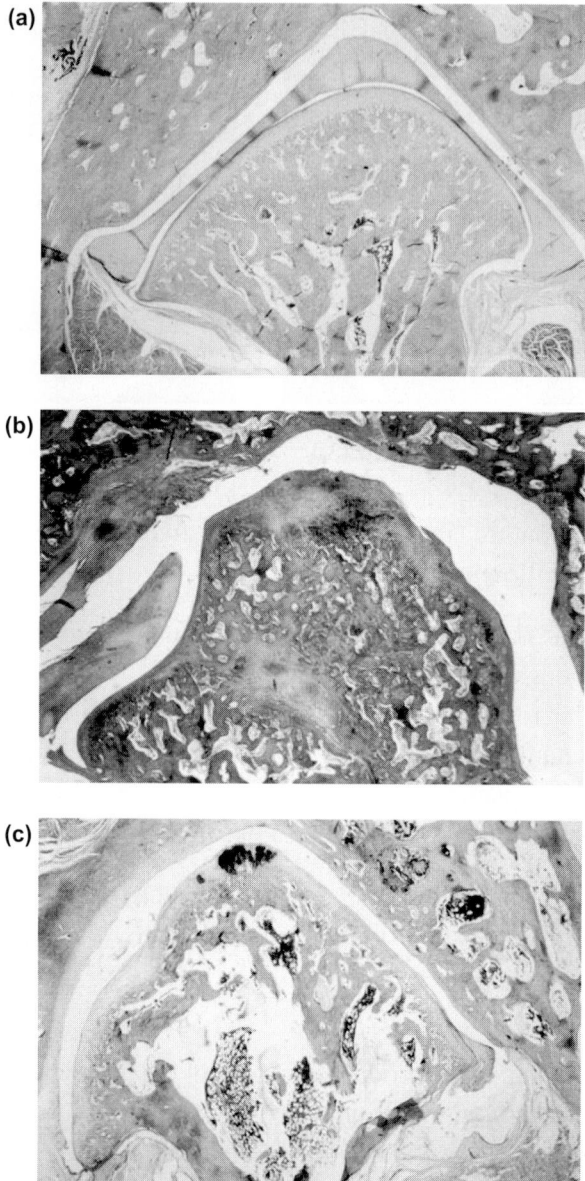

Figure 13.2 **(a)** Normal rabbit condyle and meniscus. **(b)** Hemi-condylar over-growth following partial meniscectomy. **(c)** Total meniscectomy showing condy-lar overgrowth with mechanical but not bony ankylosis, illustrating a modelling role of the meniscus on condylar growth (loaned by Dr. Rudolph Sprintz).

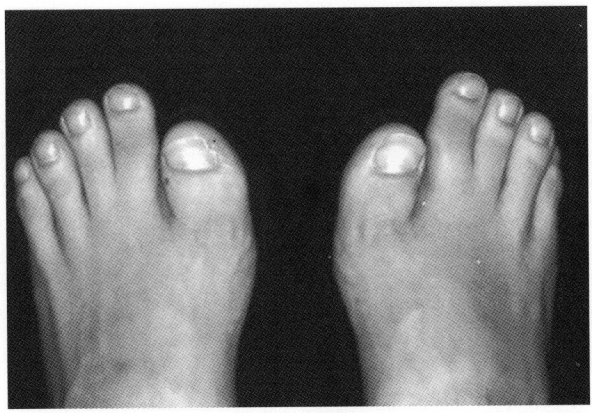

Figure 13.3 Short great toe characteristic of fibrodysplasia ossificans progressiva.

bony fusion reflecting the bone elasticity within the masticatory system. There appear to be two causes of the impaired growth pattern.

i) The loss of the condylar fibrocartilage.

Although the condylar growth cartilage is not considered to be the primary growth centre for the entire mandible, it makes a significant contribution to the height of the condylar head, neck and the ascending ramus including the angle of the mandible. This can be seen very clearly after perinatal ankylosis following birth trauma when the dental lamina has to extend backwards into the ascending ramus due to the lack of local alveolar bone at the angle (Figure 13.4f). The contralateral intact condylar growth centre continues to grow down and forwards towards the affected side producing the characteristic bowing deformity.

ii) The loss of function.

Persistent impaired function of any bone inhibits its linear and cross-sectional growth as can be seen in the ankylosed mandible in Figures 13.5a–13.5d. However this is avoided when the mandibular body is freed early before the adolescent growth spurt and function is restored. Figure 13.4 shows the natural history of a childhood ankylosis treated with a costochondral graft from the age of 4 through to 27 years.

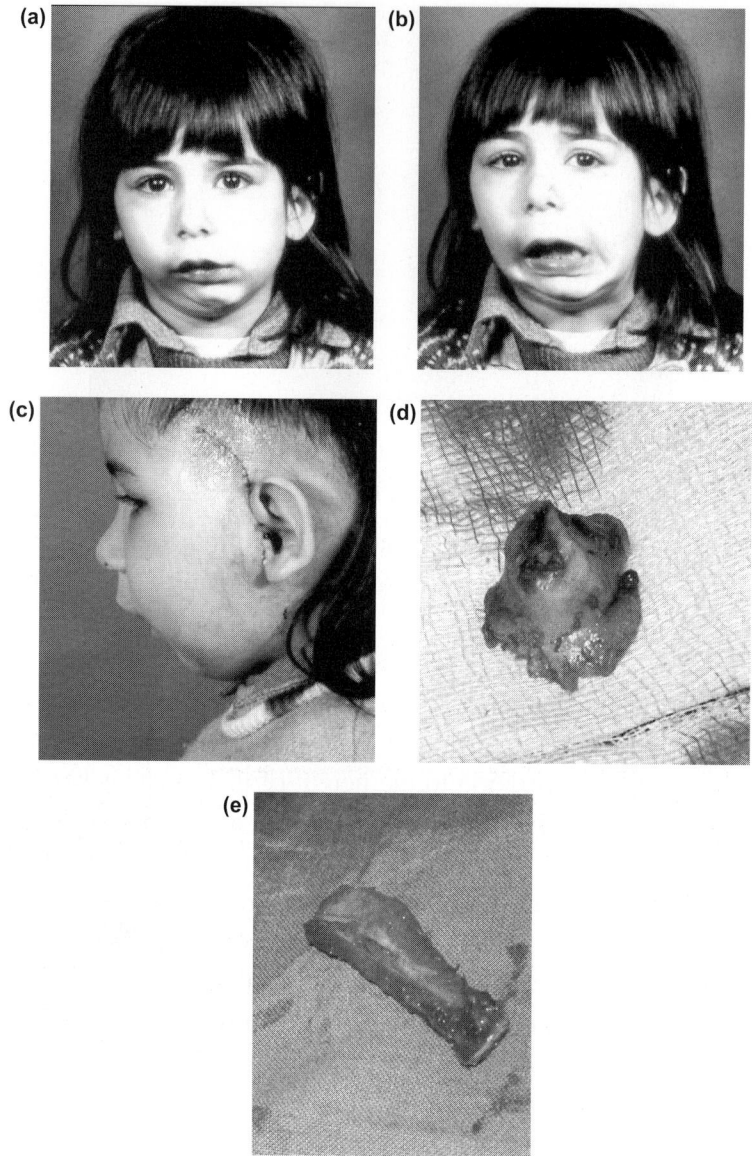

Figure 13.4   Left TMJ ankylosis following birth trauma showing characteristic facial deformity at 4 years **(a)**, **(b)** and **(c)**. Excised ankylosed condyle showing the wide adherent margin **(d)**. Costochondral graft **(e)**. The radiograph shows inverted mushroom ankylosis and extension of the dental lamina into the shortened ascending ramus.

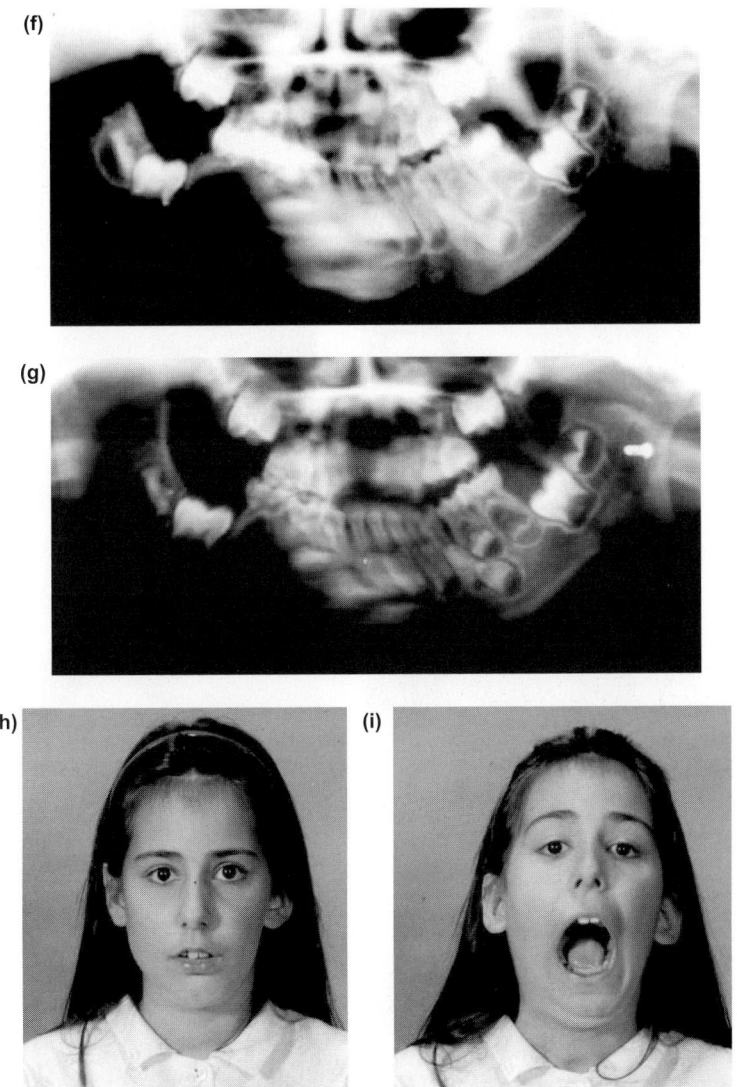

Figure 13.4 (*Continued*) (**f**) and (**g**) Following division of the ankylosis, ipsilateral coronoidectomy and costochondral graft. Early pre-adolescent arthroplasty allows catch-up growth and remodelling at 13 years (**h**) and (**i**), 19 years (**j**) and (**k**) and at 27 years. (**l**), (**m**), (**n**), (**o**) Inadequate growth of the costochondral graft is seen as deviation of the chin at rest and on opening, with a secondary limitation of the ipsilateral maxilla producing inclination of the occlusal plane. The ankylosis defect or surgery has also produced winging of the left ear.

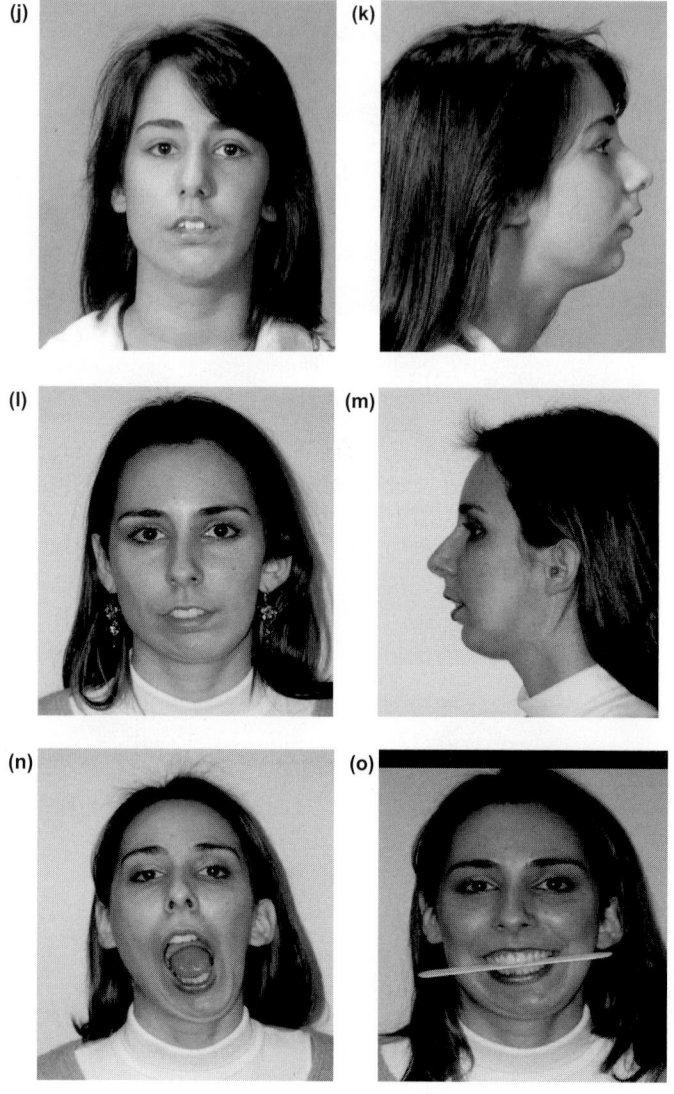

Figure 13.4   (*Continued*)

However it is interesting to compare this with the outcome of a simple gap arthroplasty where the mandible can develop normally even without a condylar growth cartilage replacement (Figure 13.6).

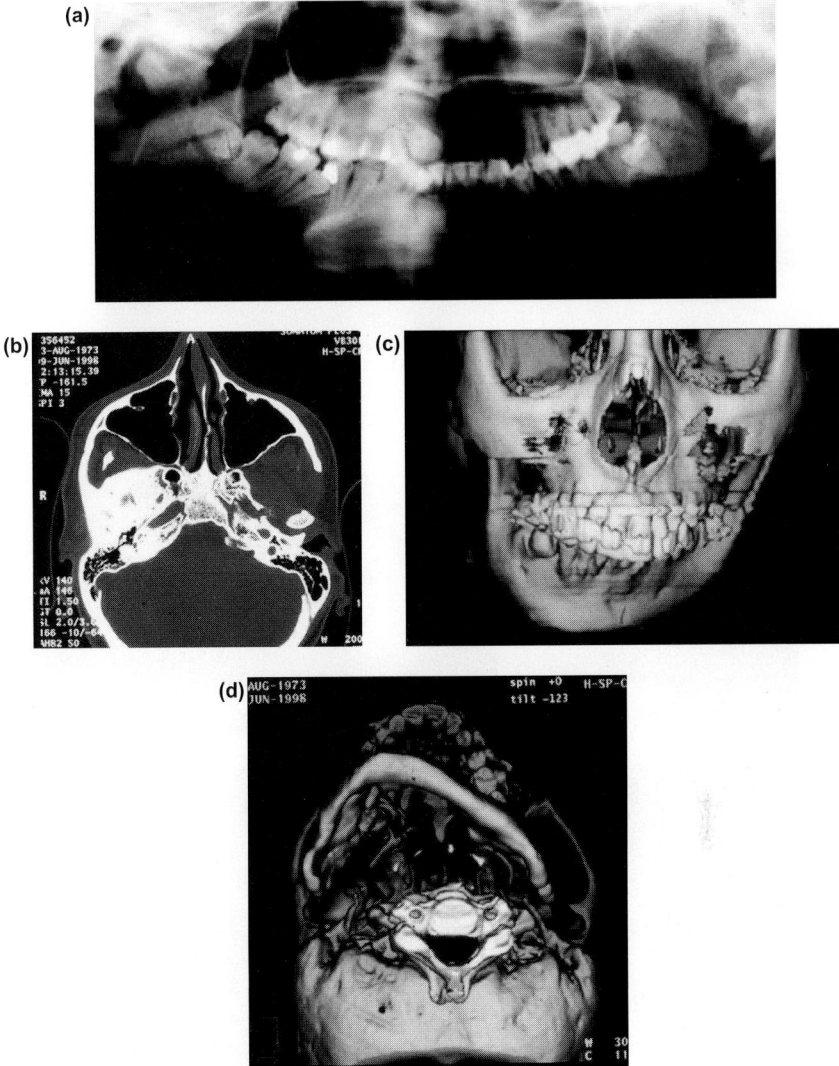

Figure 13.5   Imaging showing **(a)** apparent fibrosseous ankylosis of right TMJ but **(b)** shows complete fusion with base of skull. **(c)** 3D CT shows straight ankylosis side with deformed growing contralateral side with occlussal cant and **(d)** lower border of mandible shows impaired growth in all dimensions (case of Kieren Coghlin).

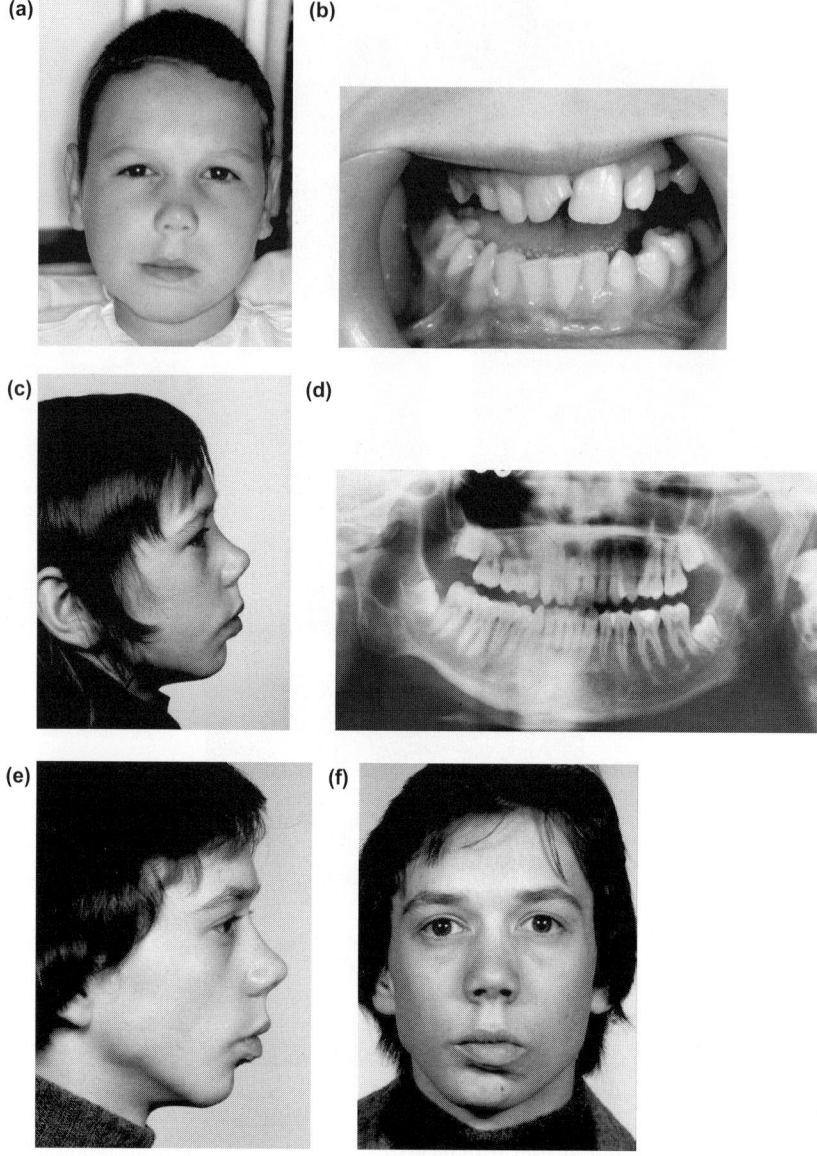

Figure 13.6   Post-traumatic right TMJ ankylosis at 10 years **(a)** and **(b)** treated with only a wide gap arthroplasty. **(c)** and **(d)** Facial growth and a functional pseudarthrosis. Normal growth and function at 19 **(e)** and **(f)** and 26 years with excellent opening but asymmetry limited to the loss of the condylar head and neck height **(g)–(i)**.

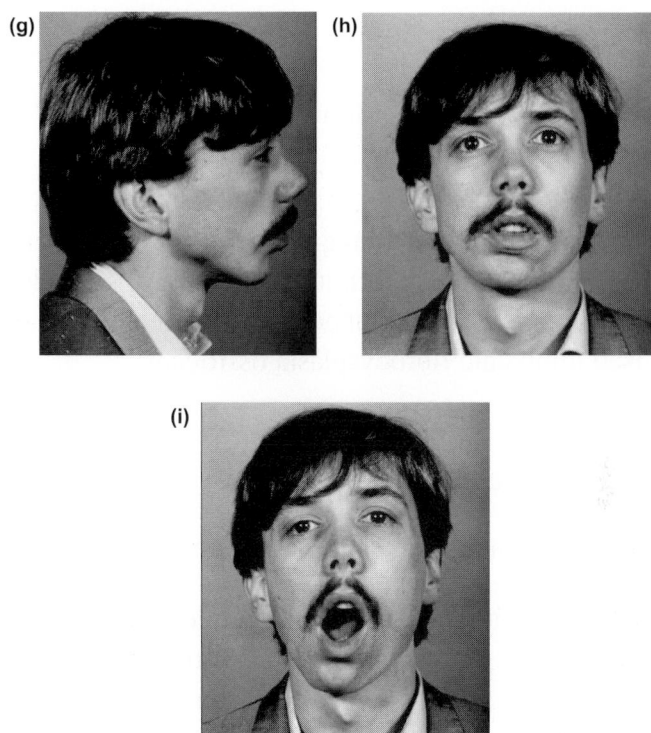

Figure 13.6 (*Continued*)

It has been estimated that from 3–16 years the ascending ramus grows approximately 2 cm in height and the body of the mandible 2.5 cm in length. The aims of treatment are to:

- restore the ramus height and its growth potential as early as possible,
- release the functional growth of the mandibular body, and
- prevent secondary deformity.

Treatment Principles

- Excise the bony fusion as early as possible.
- Reconstruct.

- Prevent recurrent ankylosis.
- Restore function.
- Correct the secondary deformity.
- Correct the occlusion.

There are many treatment strategies depending on the age of the patient the duration of the deformity and degree of secondary deformity, but in all cases, success depends on preventing recurrence of the localised idiopathic fibrodysplasia ossificans.

Treatment Choices

1. Pre-adolescent ankylosis presenting in childhood.

   a) Excision with the insertion of an interpositional temporalis myofascial peninsular flap and reconstruction with a costochondral growth centre to restore function and ramus growth.
   b) Bilateral coronoidectomies (coronoidotomies).
   c) Or excision of the ankylosis creating a simple gap arthroplasty with an interpositional temporalis myofascial peninsular flap followed by distraction osteogenesis (see below and Chapter 10).

The anteroposterior deficiency and asymmetry in childhood is usually self-corrected with catch-up growth.

2. The pre-adolescent ankylosis presenting during or post-adolescence.

   a) Excision with the insertion of an interpositional temporalis myofascial peninsular flap or a sialastic "membrane" and reconstruction with a costochondral graft to restore function and ramus growth if early enough.

b) Bilateral coronoidectomies (coronoidotomies): the earlier the restoration of function the more spontaneous growth and remodelling will be achieved in adolescence.

c) Or as the alternative to the excision of the ankylosis, simply creating a gap arthroplasty with an interpositional temporalis myofascial peninsular flap and the addition of distraction osteogenesis (see point 5 below and Chapter 10).

3. Pre-adolescent ankylosis presenting after the completion of facial growth.

a) As 2 above, with a rotational advancement genioplasty.

b) Marked retrognathia will require a sagittal split or inverted L osteotomy.

4. Late ankylosis in adults with no interference with facial growth.

a) Division of the ankylosis conserving ramus height, sculpting the condylar head with the interposition of an articular membrane such as a temporalis myofascial peninsular flap, a 2 mm sialastic membrane or the retrieved meniscus (Figures 13.7a–13.7d).

b) Bilateral coronoidectomies (coronoidotomies).

In all cases the tendency for localised fibrodysplasia ossificans to produce a recurrent fusion must be inhibited by a 7-day pre- and 2-month postoperative course of bisphosphonate, which is currently alendronic acid 10 mg a day in the morning.

5. Distraction osteogenesis (see Chapter 9).

There is now evidence that

- division of the ankylosis,

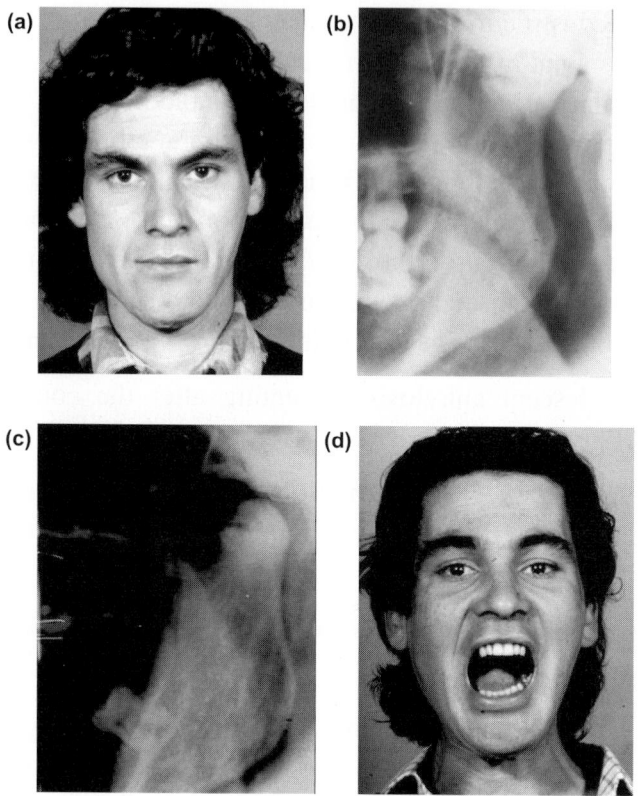

Figure 13.7 **(a)** Left TMJ ankylosis following adult trauma does not impair facial growth. **(b)** Linear radiolucency within the fused "golfball exostosis" is site of failed division of bony mass. **(c)** Separation at skull base, with insertion of sialastic membrane and coronoidectomy, provides function. **(d)** Without loss of ramus height.

- bilateral coronoidectomies (otomies) to free temporalis contractures,
- a myofascial interpositional arthroplasty, and
- distraction osteogenesis

restore movement and function and simultaneously elongates the deformed mandible. As bisphosphonates delay bone formation their role in distraction osteogenesis is as yet unpredictable.

Preoperative Imaging (Figure 13.5)

- OPG.
- True lateral skull.
- CT scan with 3D reconstruction.
- Standard orthognathic photographic series.

Timing

Resection of the ankylosis should be carried out as early as possible to enable normal growth and avoid secondary deformity. The exception is any extra-articular jaw osteotomy which should be deferred until facial growth has ceased.

Surgical Approach

The preoperative preparation differs from the standard orthognathic workup in several respects.

1. The anaesthetist must be skilled in the intubation of patients who are unable to open their mouths. This has been been made easier by the use of fibreoptic intubation but still represents a challenge especially in cases with marked retrognathia. The facilities for a tracheostomy should always be available.
2. The temporal area must be shaved and cleaned before the patient is taken into theatre. This facilitates the incision and prevents hair straying into the operative field.
3. The face and mouth are cleaned with aqueous povidone iodine and draped, exposing both ears for access and orientation. A small piece of sterile petroleum jelly gauze (tulle grasse) is inserted into the depths of the external auditory meatus. A large piece will work its way out within minutes of starting the operation.
4. The incision is marked with a surgical pen, from the temporal area (2 cm above and 2 cm anterior to the tip of the pinna)

diagonally downwards and backwards to the attachment of the ear, and then following the junctional contour to the upper end of the tragal cartilage. It then follows the crest of the cartilage down to the lobe and then skirts behind it (Figure 13.8a).

5. The whole length is infiltrated with bupivocaine and adrenaline to achieve local vasoconstriction.

6. Incise the skin with a No. 15 blade from above downwards, retraction with skin hooks will reveal the superficial veins which are coagulated with bipolar diathermy and divided. The incision along the crest of the tragus will reveal but preserve the cartilage. With fine tooth forceps the skin is dissected forwards off the cartilage and then the attachment of the lobe can be divided from front to back. The length and depth of this incision are crucial for comfortable exposure of the deeper structures (Figure 13.8b). This "parotid" incision gives excellent access to the acending ramus, eliminates the need for an additional submandibular approach and leaves a totally discrete scar.

7. By keeping the temporal incision well back, the orbito-frontal branches of the facial nerve will be safe in the upper anterior flap. The main trunk of the VII nerve emerges from the stylomastoid foramen one and a half fingers breadths below the tragal cartilage (the external auditory meatus) and passes forward 1–2 cm beneath the skin surface deep to the superficial lobe of the parotid gland, and so remains safely enclosed in the depths of the lower anterior flap. The auricular temporal vessels will be encountered but should be readily controlled with bipolar diathermy and 3/0 vicryl ties.

8. After arresting all bleeding points, the incision is deepened through the temporalis fascia down to muscle and down to bone at the root of the zygomatic arch. A small vessel at this point must be coagulated. Below the arch there is a natural vertical cleft in the deeper tissues that can be opened with the blade along the anterior surface of the cartilaginous

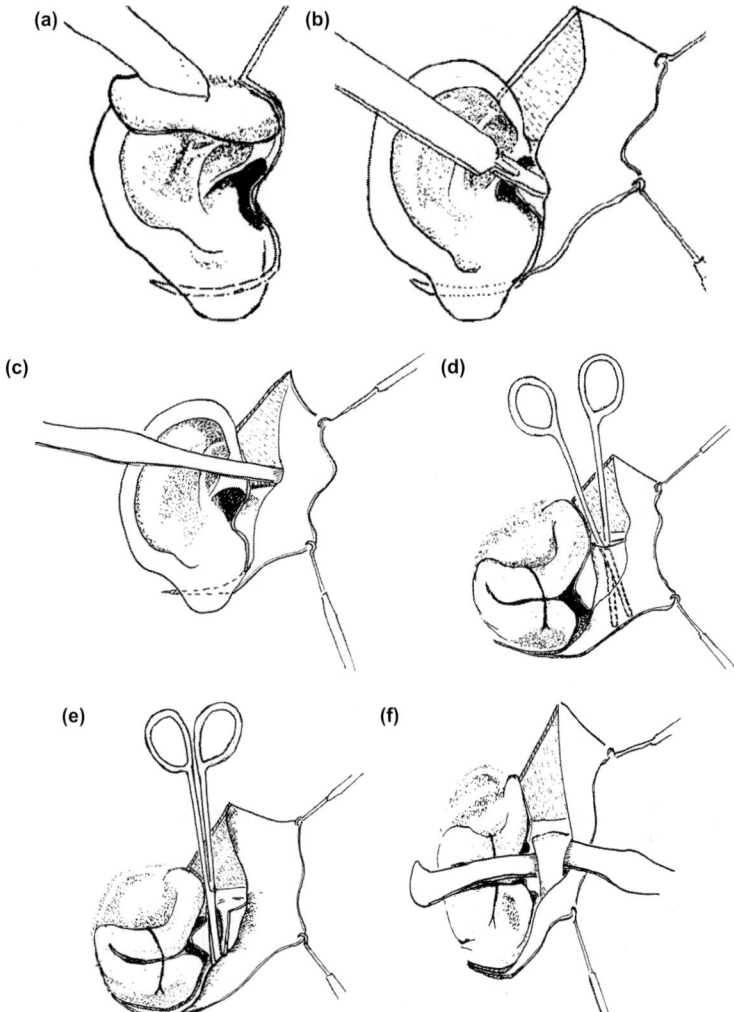

Figure 13.8 (a) The temporal pre- and sub-auricular incision. (b) Dissection along tragal cartilage to open pre-auricular cleft. (c) Sub-periosteal elevation along zygomatic arch. (d) Creation of vertical pocket in the plane of the root of zygoma and the ankylosis. (e) Dividing the posterior partition of the pocket to expose the ankylosis. (f) Isolating the ankylosis with retractors. (g) The bony fusion has been separated with a bur and fine osteotome, the condylar neck has been divided together with a coronoidectomy. The ramus decortication is for the costochondral graft. (h) Division of the ankylosis with preservation of ramus height in an adult without facial deformity. (i) A sialastic interpositional membrane suspended from the glenoid fossa.

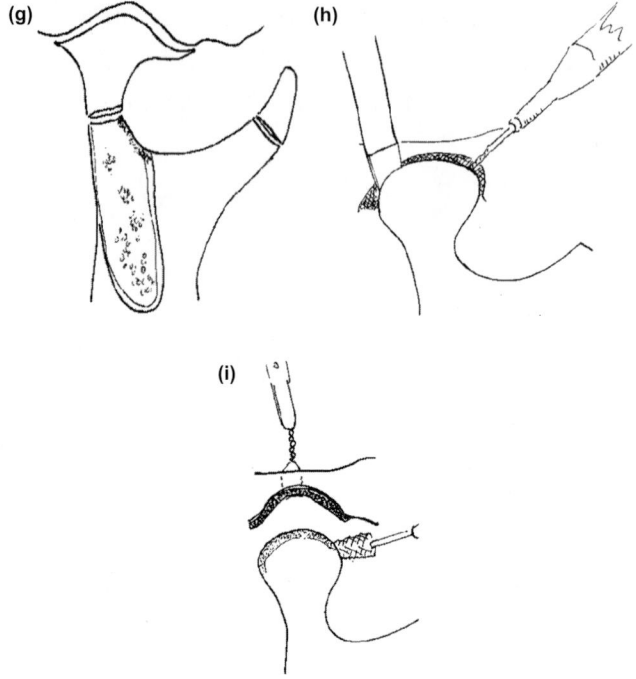

Figure 13.8   (*Continued*)

external auditory meatus and then with Macindoe scissors
(Figure 13.8b).

9. Confirm the periosteal incision on the root of the zygomatic
   arch is down to bone with the rasp end of a Howarth periosteal
   elevator, reverse it and insert the elevator firmly forward along
   the surface of the arch. This will raise a tent of fascia both
   above and below the arch which must be released with scissors
   at both ends of the incision (Figure 13.8c). Posteriorly it is
   convenient to fold the ear and suture the lobe to the pinna with
   2/0 vicryl.

10. The operative plane below the arch is now developed obliquely
    downwards and forwards with a periosteal elevator and then
    Macindoe scissors from the surface of the root of the zygoma
    onto the surface of the ankylosis (Figure 13.8d). This creates a

pocket overlying the ankylosis with a posterior partition separating it from the vertical pre-auricular cleft. This partition must be divided with scissors to create a free peri-articular area to work in (Figure 13.8e).

11. It is now possible to expose the arch as far forward as the zygomatic bone itself. Where the flap can be held with a small Langenbeck retractor.

12. In all cases the joint capsule has been ossified and has disappeared so that sub-periosteal exploration down from the arch will immediately expose the lateral aspects of the ankylosis.

13. Carefully but firmly push the elevator distally around the condylar neck and leave it or a malleable strip against the deeper aspect of the bone as a retractor. Repeat this on the anterior surface of the condylar neck area. With marked loss of ramus height, the space below the arch may be tight admitting only a narrow instrument such as a Frear elevator as a retractor (Figure 13.8f).

14. The child's ankylosis differs morphologically from the fusion occurring in an adult. In the child the fusion resembles an upturned mushroom (Figure 13.8g) whereas adult cases tend to be a proliferative golf ball. The line of fusion should be visible or estimated and is explored by firmly tapping a 5 mm osteotome progressively deeper into its depth at three or four points. It should now be possible to lever the bony mass away from the skull base. The mass is separated by a bur cut at the base of the condylar neck (Figure 13.8g).

   Sub-periosteal dissection forward to the anterior border of the ramus can usually enable the coronoidectomy (otomy) to be done through the pre-auricular incision.

15. There are two forms of adult ankylosis:

   (i) simple bony fusion following osteoarthritis or ankylosing spondilitis and

(ii) those following trauma with an exostotic mass continuous with the zygomatic arch and skull base.

Both have no loss of ramus height, and simply require a line of cleavage. The former is usually apparent and can be separated with a narrow osteotome. The exostotic form has to be estimated and cut deeply with a tungsten carbide fissure bur. A sturdy 1 cm osteotome is then necessary to lever this bony mass from the overlying skull base preserving it to be sculpted into a new condyle with an acrylic bur (Figure 13.8h).

16. In the adolescent and adult the temporalis and its tendon and to a lesser extent the other elevator muscles have undergone a degree of contracture which must be released with a bilateral coronoidectomy or otomy. This can be done on the ankylosis side by extending the sub-periosteal exposure forward over the ascending ramus and retaining access with an Obwegeser channel retractor passed around the anterior border. The lower bur cut instead of just sectioning the neck can be extended simultaneously forward just below the sigmoid notch to the anterior border of the ramus to include the coronoid process (Figure 13.9a).

17. At this point it is essential to inspect the specimen and also explore the depths of the wound on the ankylosis side as the fusion of a fractured condylar neck to skull base can be wrongly assumed to be the complete ankylosis, whereas the medially displaced condyle is often fused with the skull base above and to the medial aspect of the ascending ramus below. If this is the case the aberrant condyle must also be separated and removed (Figure 13.9b). In post-traumatic cases the exploration should also attempt to locate and retrieve the meniscus.

18. A contralateral coronoidectomy or otomy is essential to give maximum opening. This is done intraorally after stretching the mouth open with a Featherstone or similar self-retaining gag. Two blade (Lacs) retractors are required and are pressed, one on

(a) **(b)**

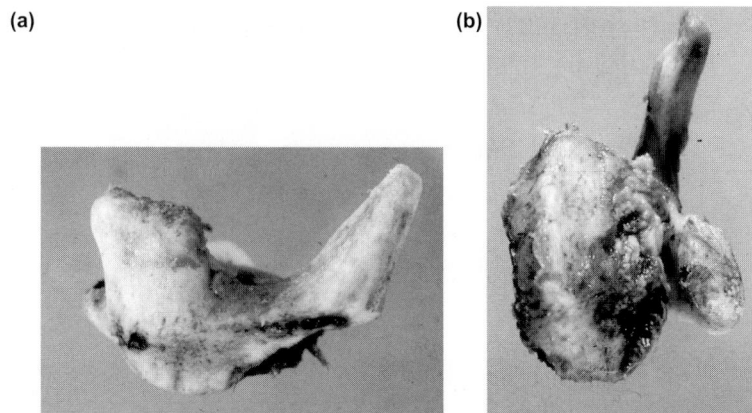

Figure 13.9 **(a)** and **(b)** Combined excision of ankylosis and coronoid showing the major restraint to opening was the concealed medially displaced condylar head which was fused to both the skull base and ascending ramus.

each side of the anterior border of the ascending ramus. Incise downwards between them through the mucosa and muscle to the bone. Elevate the periosteum and muscle layer on both sides of the ascending ramus and insert the blade retractor (Lacs) in each pocket, then using the forked Langenbeck retractor, the coronoid is exposed and grasped with curved Kocher forceps and divided obliquely at its base with a bur. The last remaining bony bridge which is the anterior rim of the sigmoid notch is fractured with an osteotome inserted in the bur cut and twisted. As the coronoid process is elongated its removal can be difficult and is probably unnecessary. The stretched opening of the mouth can now with effort be doubled (Figures 13.10a to 13.10c).

19. Reconstruction using the costochondral graft.

   • Where growth or ramus height are required a costochondral graft is harvested and trimmed to provide a suitable articular surface (Figure 13.11).

   • A groove is prepared on the lateral surface of the ramus by superficial decortication with a bur and an osteotome.

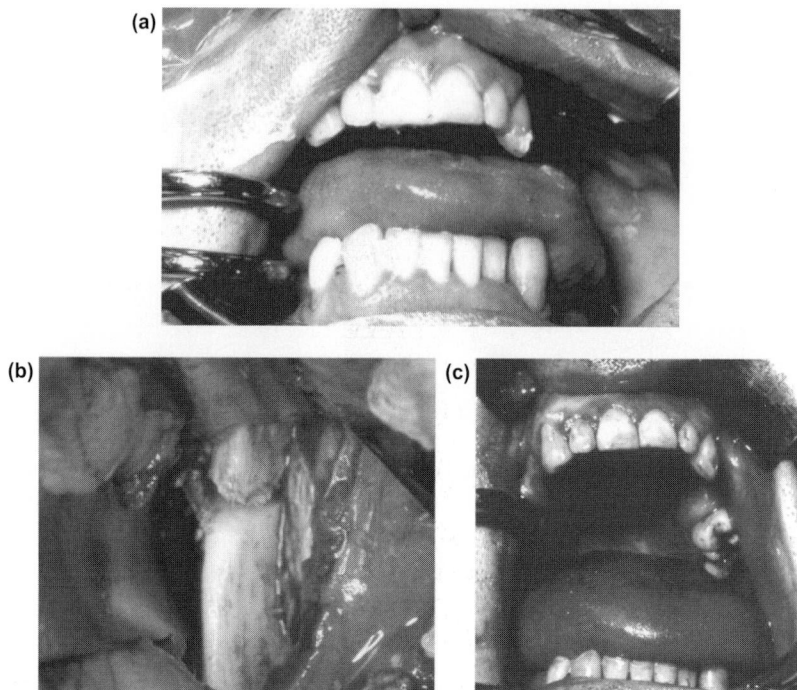

Figure 13.10   **(a)** Opening after resection of fused condylar head and coronoidectomy. **(b)** Intraoral contralateral coronoidotomy and **(c)** significant increase in mouth opening.

- The bite is propped open 10 mm in the ipsilateral molar area with a folded tonsil swab side and the rib placed on the groove with the costal cartilage extending up against the glenoid fossa and 2 screws inserted to fix it.
- The meniscus is replaced if it can be localised from a medial fracture displacement. Otherwise the choice is a temporalis myofascial peninsula flap or a 2 mm sialastic membrane.
- The 2 cm broad myofascial flap is outlined postero-superiorly as shown with its base at the origin of the arch. It is incised down to the calvarium, elevated and firmly pulled (and pushed) down and under the zygomatic arch with a heavy suture passed through its mobile distal end. This

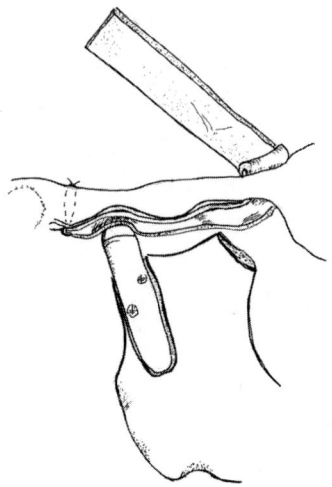

Figure 13.11 Costochondral graft with temporalis myofascial peninsular flap rotated downwards through the zygomatic arch and backwards to act as a meniscus.

suture can be passed down through the arch with a wire "pull" loop, a pair of curved Kochers or Adsons right angled forceps. It is then pulled backwards into the condylar fossa and anchored with a heavy suture passed upwards through a drill hole, done from above through the most distomedial point of the roof of the glenoid fossa (Figure 13.11). This procedure is much easier with the condyle subluxed from the fossa by maximally stretching the mouth open and then reduced to sit beneath the flap.

- Of the many autogenous and alloplast materials used as alternative interpositional membranes, 2 mm sialastic has proved to be ideal for this role suspended by 0.5 wire from the glenoid fossa. The margins must be carefully trimmed to avoid overextension (Figure 13.8i).

20. Reconstruction preserving the condyle.

    This is useful in late onset ankylosis where there is a proliferative fusion and no loss of ramus height. The bone is

sculpted into a neocondyle and the fossa trimmed to accommodate it with an acrylic bur. In these cases a myofascial flap or
2 mm sialastic sheet are used as an interpositional membrane as
described above (Figures 13.8h and 13.8i).

21. Reconstruction with a prosthetic joint. With the many autogenous alternatives, prosthetic total joint replacement is rarely
required but may be essential in the older osteoporotic or
rheumatoid patient. The principles are the same as the costochondral graft with the exception that the occlusion has to be
carefully defined. Alloplastic joints do not remodel and have to
be accurately placed to avoid morphoincompatibility where
function will erode the tense overlying tissues leading to exposure and infection.

22. Post-adolescent cases require an augmentation and rotation
genioplasty (Figures 13.12a to 13.12c). In a bilateral case, if an
advancement osteotomy (or distraction osteogenesis) is
required, ideally this follows preparatory orthodontics. The
osteotomy is not usually necessary when the ankylosis is
treated before adolescence especially with a costochondral
graft or with distraction osteogenesis.

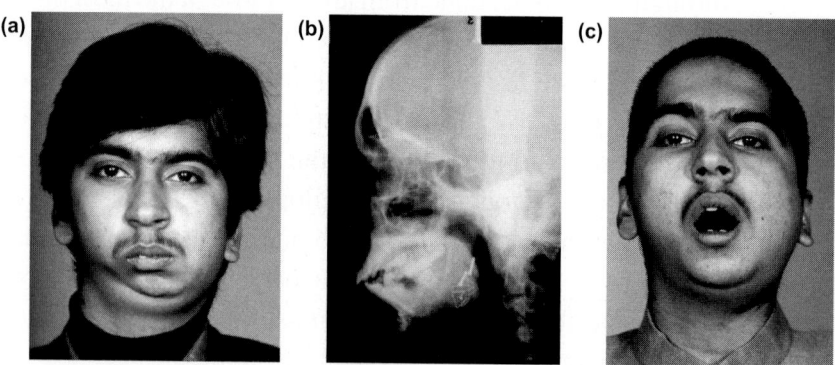

Figure 13.12 (a) Characteristic adult asymmetrical retrognathia from left TMJ
ankylosis in childhood. (b) and (c) After costochondral graft arthroplasty and
rotation advancement genioplasty.

23. Vacuum drains are inserted, and the wounds closed with sub-cutaneous 3/0 vicryl and 5/O prolene for the skin. A firm turban pressure dressing is applied, ensuring that gauze or wool is placed behind the pinna of the ear to avoid compression ischaemia.

24. Postoperative care. Analgesics and antibiotics are prescribed as usual with the addition of daily alendronic acid 10 mg in the morning for 2 months. This is taken 30 minutes before break-fast when upright to avoid oesophagitis. A fluid and soft diet is essential to achieve a compromise between rest and func-tion to be followed by stretching exercises with a modified laboratory chemistry clamp (Figure 13.13) at least 3 times a day for 6 months.

25. The closure of the maxillary cant can be facilitated by taking impressions and a squash bite as soon as possible (intraopera-tively is inappropriately messy) and the models mounted to enable a maxillary plate with a lateral bite wedge to keep open the ipsilateral buccal occlusion until an orthodontic assessment and the insertion of a functional appliance to level the occlusion (Figures 13.14a to 13.14c).

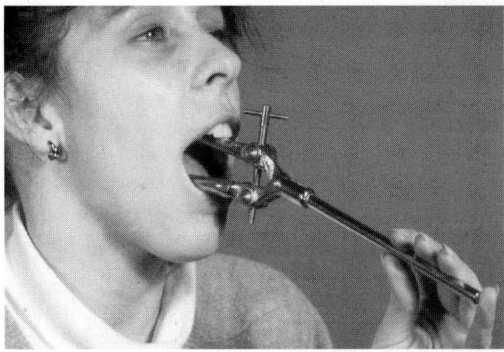

Figure 13.13 Modified laboratory retort (chemistry) clamp with plastic tubing to protect teeth, provides well controlled stretching exercises.

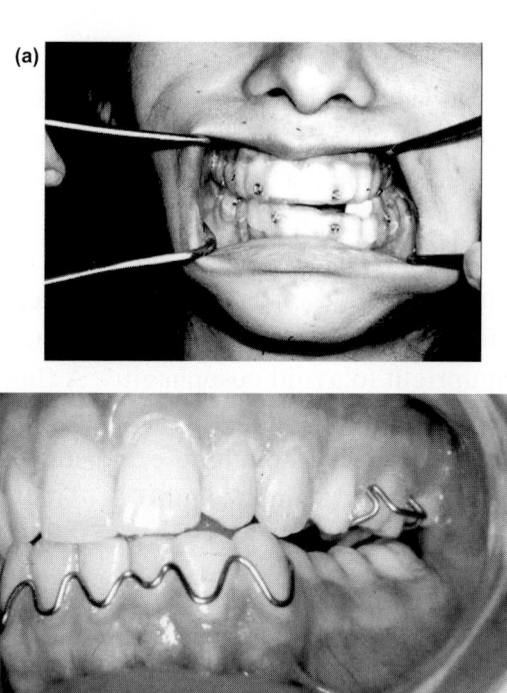

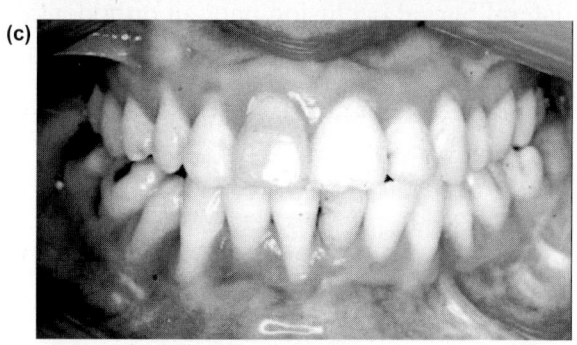

Figure 13.14 **(a)** Acrylic wedge to maintain postoperative lateral open bite and ramus height. Another patient to show **(b)** functional appliance to facilitate closure of postoperative lateral open bite **(c)** closure achieved.

Complications

- Damage to the orbital and frontal branches of the facial nerve is to be avoided by careful flap design.

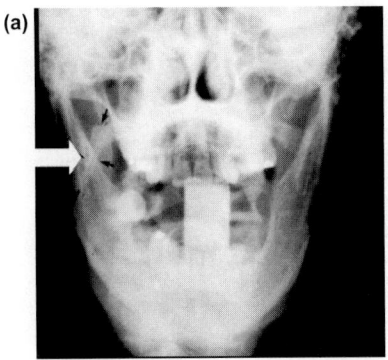

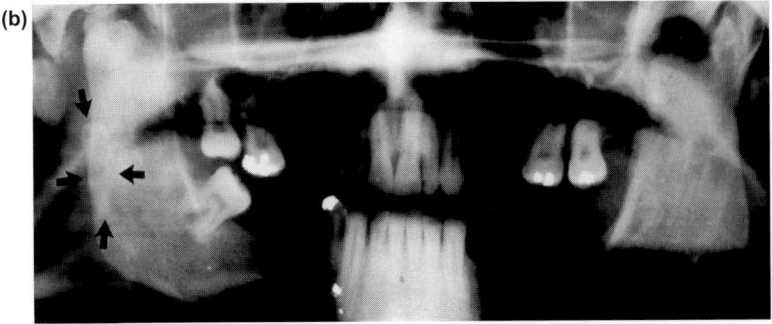

Figure 13.15 (a) and (b) Gradual postoperative onset of impaired opening due to fibrodysplasia ossificans of the medial pterygoid muscle. Treated with 3 months bisphosphonate and stretching.

- Limited opening due to inadequate bone removal especially on the medial aspect of the condylar neck — will be revealed by a CT scan and requires a repeat arthroplasty.
- Persistent limited opening due to a failure to do a bilateral coronoidectomies or otomies. These may be done intraorally but must be supplemented by stretching exercises and bisphosphonates.
- Postoperative fibrodysplasia ossificans in the medial pterygoid and masseter can occur and will also require bisphosphonates and stretching exercises for 2–3 months (Figures 13.15a and 13.15b).

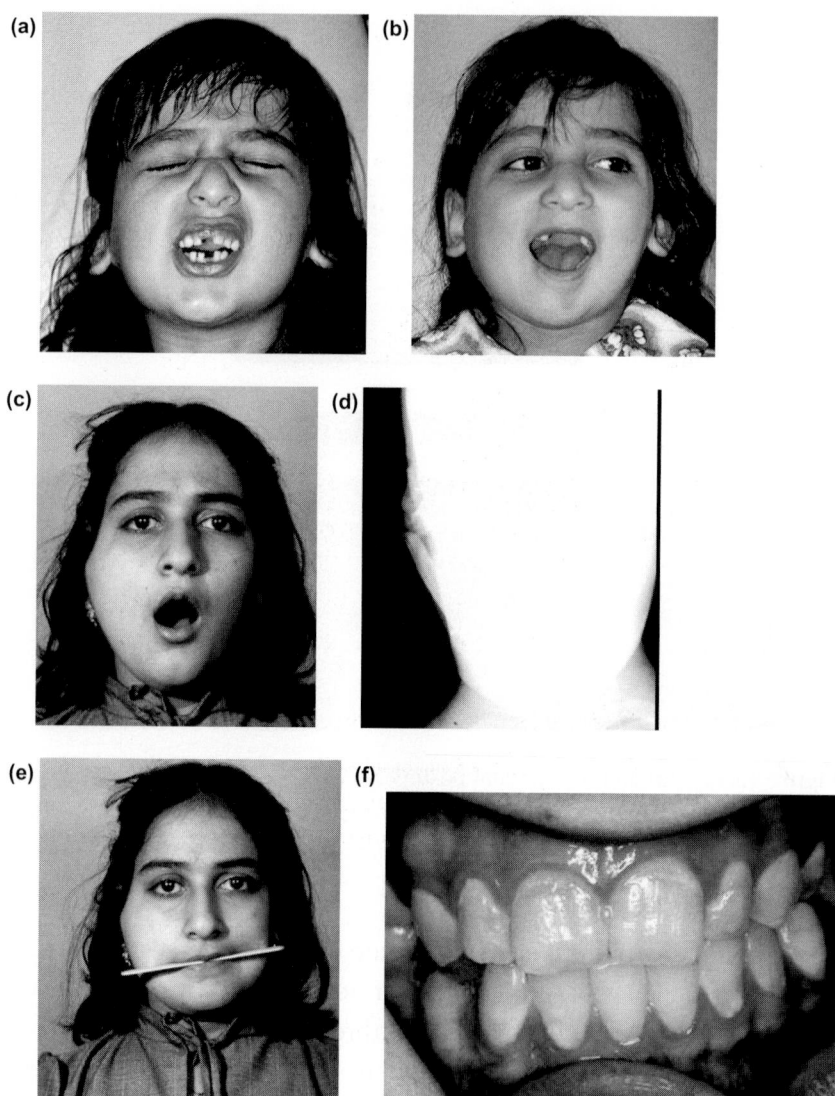

Figure 13.16 (a) Ankylosis in a 5-year-old. (b) Postoperative opening. (c) and (d) Pseudohemimandibular hyperplasia due to costchondral overgrowth at 12 years with lateral displacement of overgrown graft. (e) and (f) Occlussal cant.

- Marked malocclusion will require orthodontics and an osteotomy.
- Failure of the costochondral graft to grow. With function this acts as an interpositional arthroplasty enabling mandibular growth. Asymmetry is rarely great can be corrected by an osteotomy or distraction osteogenesis when mandibular growth has completed.
- Fusion of the graft with re-ankylosis requires a repeat arthroplasty and bisphosphanates or distraction osteogenesis.
- Excess growth of the graft with a pseudohemimandibular elongation can be corrected by trimming the articular end of the graft and levelling the occlusal plane orthodontically (Figures 13.16a–13.16f).
- Pneumothorax (see Complications and Emergencies section).

Summary

The excision of the ankylosis, joint reconstruction with a costochondral graft and bilateral temporalis myotomies remain the most common management. However there is evidence that restoration of growth and function may also be achieved with an interpositional arthroplasty as described for the adult case, and distraction osteogenesis as an alternative to a costochondral graft (see Chapter 9).

14

Emergencies and Complications

Introduction

Problems will vary from the orthognathic to those of a more general nature, which can be life threatening. Although orthognathic surgery is usually carried out on young fit adults, life-threatening complications may arise. Careful technique, and expertise in the management of serious emergencies are essential. This includes the understanding the mysteries of medical monitoring.

Medical Monitoring (Figure 14.1)

ECG: a basic knowledge of abnormal PQRST complexes and arrhythmias is essential for interpreting the ECG. "Three-lead" monitoring gives an interpretable rhythm-strip but is no replacement for a full "12-lead" ECG assessment when acute cardiac problems are suspected.

Heart rate (HR): derived from the ECG and the monitor can be set to detect bradycardia and tachycardia.

Arterial blood pressure (ABP): is measured by direct cannulation of the radial, brachial, dorsalis pedis or femoral arteries. The mean arterial pressure (MAP) is denoted in brackets. Non-invasive monitoring (NBP) is done with an appropriately-sized pneumatic cuff placed either around the upper arm or lower leg.

Central venous pressure (CVP): is useful as an indication of right ventricular preload. Serial readings (i.e. the trend of CVP measurements) are far more useful than single readings. The normal value is 2–6 mmHg. Respiration (RESP): is normally 14–20 a minute.

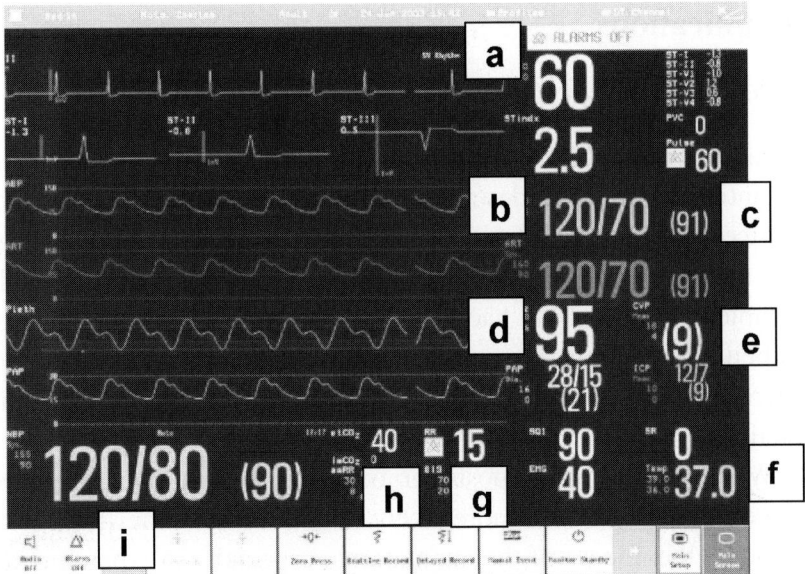

Figure 14.1   Intensive Care Monitor (by courtesy of Panasonic). (**a**) Heart rate. (**b**) Continuous invasive blood pressure (BP). (**c**) Current mean arterial pressure. (**d**) Oxygen saturation. (**e**) Central venous pressure. (**f**) Temperature. (**g**) Respiratory rate. (**h**) End tidal CO_2. (**i**) Non-invasive cuff BP.

Oxygen saturation of arterial blood (SpO_2): is usually measured by a digital pulse oximeter based on the light absorptive properties of oxygenated and deoxygenated Hb. Oxygen saturation monitoring, which assesses oxygenation, not ventilation, is no substitute for arterial blood gas assessment as there are both extrinsic and intrinsic reasons why the reading may be inaccurate.

Carbon dioxide: is expressed in a graphic form by the capnograph. Capnography is an indirect monitor that not only helps in the differential diagnosis of hypoxia, but also provides information about CO_2 production, alveolar ventilation and respiratory patterns.

Temperature: can be monitored by mouth, axilla, tympanic membrane, oesophagus and rectum. Rectal and oesophageal measures are the most accurate.

Complications

1. *Oedema and Infection*

Oedema is reducible with pre- and postoperative dexamethasone and antibiotic cover as described earlier. Contrary to some popular practice vacuum drains can dramatically reduce the swelling arising from mandibular osteotomies, and the minivacuum drain is equally valuable for infraorbital haematomas following dissection through a subciliary incision. The same applies to the iliac crest donor site. Where possible leave drains for at least 24 hours after they cease to function.

Where there is gross postoperative swelling and pain, the presence of a haematoma is more likely than oedema alone. Treatment should be the release of the haematoma, especially if expanding, as it may be the presenting feature of a persistent arterial bleed, which needs to be identified and arrested.

There is some dispute as to whether clean operations require more than one pre- and postoperative antibiotic bolus. However prospective trials have shown that a five-day course produces less postoperative infection at the sagittal split site.

2. *Bleeding Problems*

a) *Minor Haemorrhage*

Even with previously healthy patients not receiving any medication which would predispose to excess bleeding, intraoperative blood loss is significantly reduced by the administration of an antifibrinolytic agent such as tranexamic acid 25 mg/kg orally or 0.5–1 g by slow intravenous injection pre- and postoperatively.

Tearing the periosteum on the medial aspect of the ascending ramus whilst exposing it for a sagittal split may produce a troublesome bleed, which can be controlled with a hot wet tonsil swab and pressure for 3 minutes. Damage to the facial vessels through the base of the subperiosteal pouch prepared for the mandibular buccal cortex cut responds to the same pressure and patience. Rarely the maxillary, tonsillar or lingual arteries may be damaged, giving rise to prolonged serous haemorrhage. Again, packing firstly with a swab, and secondly with a large piece of oxidised cellulose (Surgicel) should be sufficient, assisted by 0.5–1 g t.d.s. tranexamic acid (Cyclokapron, Kabi) given intravenously. If vigorous bleeding persists the external carotid may need to be tied off, as described below.

b) *Persistent Haemorrhage*

Failure to control bleeding despite efficient conservative measures may be due to the following.

i)　A patent damaged artery, either the maxillary or tonsillar that require identification and ligation. Do not delay ligation of the external carotid if significant bleeding persists despite local ligation, packing and antifibrinolytic therapy for more than 30 minutes. This should allow time for investigation.

ii)　A rare manifestation of a latent coagulation defect or defibrination. In both cases there is an evident lack of clot formation on the drapes and the wound oozes "watery blood".

c) *Management — General*

Ensure early that adequate blood is available for replacement; if not, send venous samples for full blood count, cross-matching and a clotting screen which must include the thrombin time, prothrombin time (PT or INR), thromboplastin generation test, fibrin degradation products and a platelet count. In rare cases of acute defibrination there are prolonged prothrombin time (PT), activated partial thromboplastin time (APPT) and thrombin time (TT), increased fibrin degradation products and reduced platelets. The increased fibrin degradation products tend to have an anticoagulant effect.

Maintain the circulation with crystalloid solution until type specific or fully cross-matched blood is available. Remember the circulating blood volume in an average adult is around 5000 ml (75 ml/kg), and transfusion is required after a 20%–30% loss. In a child the circulating blood volume is equal to the weight in kilogrammes × 80 ml, and therefore a relatively small absolute volume will give a 20% loss.

d) *Ligation of the External Carotid Artery*

Clean the neck with detergent and iodine. Resist the temptation to use an aesthetic skin crease incision, as this will limit access if the neck is distended with blood. Always incise obliquely along the anterior border of the sternomastoid muscle (Figure 14.2a). Remember the carotid bifurcation is just below the level of the hyoid bone. Therefore incise obliquely downwards from two fingers' breadth below the angle of the mandible to the level of the prominence of the thyroid cartilage along a line drawn from the mastoid process to the sternal notch. Deepen the wound through fat, platysma and fascia using a No. 10 or 20 blade until the anterior border of sternomastoid muscle can be felt and seen.

The sternomastoid must be retracted firmly with a broad Langenbeck. The carotid triangle contains fine filamentous fascia, unless it has become infiltrated with oedema due to prolonged bleeding into the neck.

The carotid sheath fascia overlying the internal jugular vein is picked up with toothed forceps and incised along the vessel with McIndoe scissors. A nylon tape is passed around the internal jugular, once revealed, and attached to artery forceps; the vein is retracted distally with the sternomastoid muscle (Figure 14.2b).

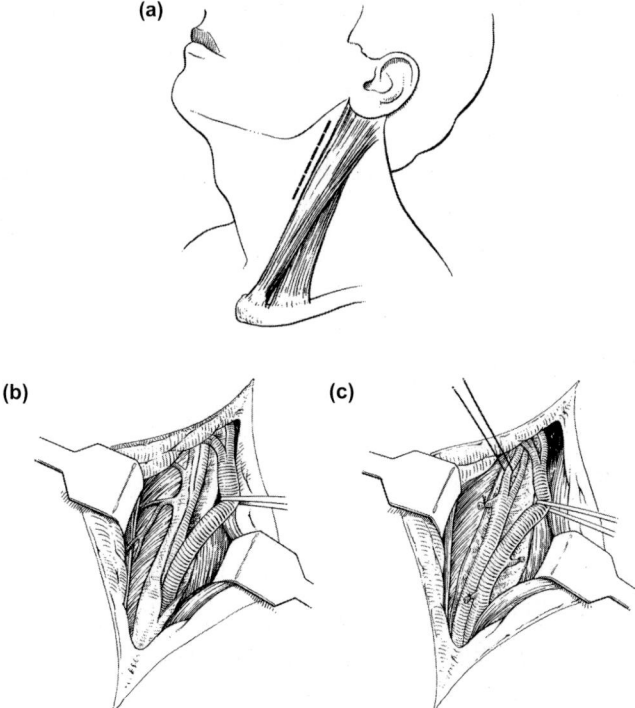

Figure 14.2 (a) Skin incision at upper anterior border of sternomastoid. (b) Opening of carotid sheath with retraction of internal jugular vein to reveal the carotid artery. (c) Ligation of external carotid artery.

The carotid will now be palpable and partially visible; again, fascia will need to be divided to expose the bifurcation. This may be obscured by one or more small veins, which must be tied with 3/0 polyglycollate or linen and divided. The external carotid is anteromedial to the internal carotid and can be identified by its branches. The superior thyroid artery often arises at the bifurcation and has to be ligated with a black silk or linen and divided to gain access to the main trunk. Ligatures are more easily passed around the vessel with small Adson's artery forceps as they have a more pronounced right angle curve. Rather than search for a specific vessel it is better to tie the external carotid at its base. There is no need to divide it (Figure 14.2c).

A vacuum drain is inserted and sutured to the skin with 3/0 black silk and the wound closed in three layers using 3.0 polygly-collate for the platysma and subcutaneous layers and 5/0 interrupted Prolene sutures for the skin.

An absorbent non-adhesive dressing is then secured with adhesive tape.

e) *Coagulation Defects*

Persistent bleeding despite local and carotid ligation indicates either a factor deficiency (the most common unsuspected defect being von Willebrand's disease) or disseminated intravascular coagulation (DIC). By now the laboratory results should be available. A prolonged thromboplastin generation test suggests a missing clotting factor. The prothrombin time (INR) will not be of value unless this is an anticoagulant or advanced liver disease problem, which is unlikely in an osteotomy patient. If however, there are also raised fibrin degradation products and deficient platelets, DIC should be assumed to be the problem. Management should be as follows.

i) Maintain tissue perfusion and oxygenation with intravenous fluid support and supplemental oxygen.

ii) Fresh frozen plasma (FFP), which contains clotting factors as well as the natural anticoagulants antithrombin III and protein C, is given in doses of 15 ml/kg. Cryoprecipitate is given along with FFP to replace fibrinogen if levels are less than 80 mg/dl.

iii) Platelet transfusion, 1 unit/10 kg body weight, should be considered once platelet counts drops below 50,000/cu mm and also packed cells to replace erythrocytes.

iv) Antifibrinolytic agent (tranexamic acid 0.5–1 g IV) must be used to arrest the fibrinolytic process and conserve the clotting factors. However once this process has been recognised it is essential to consult a clinical haematologist for advice.

v) Any patient receiving a large volume of blood replacement (1–1.5 of the circulating volume within 24 hours) will require FFP, cryoprecipitate and platelets. At this stage a clinical haematologist should guide all blood product prescribing. Recombinant activated Factor VII is being increasingly trialled as a treatment for persistent bleeding but its use is currently restricted by the small evidence base and the high costs (£5000 for a single 4.5 mg vial).

vi) The patient has by now been infused with 5–10 litres of fluid, much of which will be distending the bladder. This will require an indwelling catheter (see below), not only to decompress the bladder but also to help calculate the state of fluid balance and renal perfusion.

vii) Continued bleeding into the tissues may fill the soft palate, the lateral wall of the pharynx and the neck, constituting a serious threat to the airway postoperatively. Blood will also have passed the throat pack into the larynx and almost certainly into the stomach. The airway can be managed by prolonged endotracheal intubation but this will be dependent on skilled postoperative intensive care. If support is not available, an early decision should be made to carry out a tracheostomy, which not only guarantees the airway but also prevents aspiration into the lungs of blood or gastric contents and allows aspiration of accumulated secretions from the bronchi.

viii) Remember to administer metoclopromide 10 mg and erythromycin 250 mg intravenously to promote gastric emptying of swallowed blood. Metoclopromide is a dopamine antagonist, which stimulates gastric emptying, and small intestinal transit whilst also enhancing the strength of oesophageal sphincter contraction. Erythromycin and related 14-member macrolide compounds act directly upon motilin receptors in gastrointestinal smooth muscle and, therefore acting as motilin receptor agonists, and also accelerate gastric emptying, increase the frequency of smooth muscle contractions, and shorten orocaecal transit time.

ix) Before the patient leaves the theatre a Ryles nasogastric tube should be passed to aspirate the blood and bile reflux from the stomach. Gastric acid reduction as a prophylaxis against aspiration may also be achieved by giving a proton pump inhibitor such as omeprazole 40 mg by slow intravenous injection. Under normal conditions the effects of proton pump inhibitors are enhanced if the drug is given the evening before surgery and again 2 hours prior to surgery commencing. However this is not possible in cases of surgical emergency.

f) Secondary Haemorrhage

The patient may suddenly bleed profusely postoperatively in the ward, or even at home. The common causes are a partially divided large vein or untied artery in the depths of a mandibular osteotomy wound. Occasionally an undetected coagulopathy such as von Willebrand's is the underlying problem, especially when the bleeding is repeated.

The management must commence with pressure applied to the bleeding site with swabs, and rapid transfer to theatre for exploration and haemostasis, as described.

As with all severe haemorrhage up to 10 mg intravenous morphine should be given immediately by slow intravenous injection as a sedative analgesic, together with tranexamic acid 0.5–1 g intravenously to help conserve clotting factors and clot in favour of haemostasis.

g) Gastric Haemorrhage

The chance of stress-induced gastric erosion is small, even after prolonged orthognathic surgery. However, the combination of a

patient with a history of peptic ulceration, a stressful surgical procedure, anti-inflammatory steroids and analgesics can produce a
gastric bleed. Abdominal discomfort, tachycardia, true melaena
and/or haematemesis and a fall in haemoglobin (a late sign) should
alert one to this possibility. Initial treatment should include intravenous fluid support and administration of a proton-pump inhibitor
(omeprazole), first as an intravenous bolus dose (40 mg), then as an
intravenous infusion for 72 hours. Early endoscopy should be considered after consultation with a gastroenterologist so that the
bleeding point can be injected or banded.

The aim of drug treatment is to raise gastric pH to above 4, thereby
stabilising any clots that may have formed at the bleeding site. This is
the reasoning behind the use of proton pump inhibitors over H2 receptor blockers such as ranitidine, which have a lesser effect on pH.

With vulnerable patients a regular prophylactic proton pump
inhibitor, such as omeprazole or lansoprazole, should be administered as well as eliminating both steroids and non-steroidal anti-
inflammatory analgesic drugs from the intraoperative and
postoperative regimen.

3) *The Airway*

After an uneventful operation, the airway should be maintained
with a nasopharyngeal tube, which is sucked out throughout the
postoperative 12–18 hours at 30-minute intervals. Unless the nurse
ensures that the fine suction catheter passes beyond the end of
the nasopharyngeal airway tube, the end will gradually become
blocked with blood clot and will become an efficient airway obstruction (Figure 14.3a) the same can occur with a tracheostomy tube
(Figure 14.3b). Some anaesthetists leave an endotracheal tube *in situ*
which with modern closed suction units can be kept unobstructed
with minimum effort and nursing intervention.

A facemask with 40% oxygen at a flow rate of approximately
5 litres/min ensures adequate tissue perfusion. In intensive care or

(a)

(b)

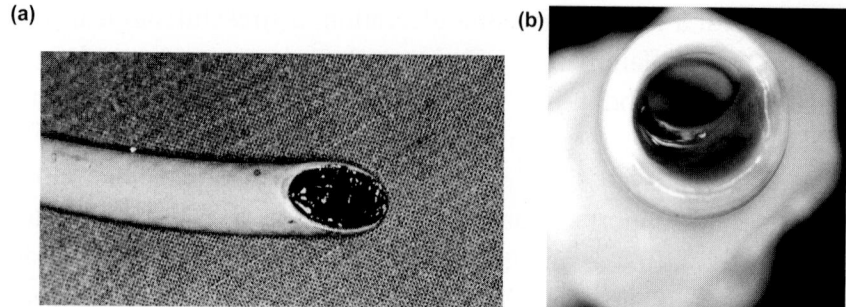

Figure 14.3   Clot obstructing (**a**) endotracheal tube and (**b**) tracheostomy tube.

high dependency units an intra-arterial line may have been inserted to monitor blood gases and invasive blood pressure is displayed on the cardiac monitor as a continuous arterial pressure trace. But this is not an alternative to the provision of a good airway by careful suction and good nursing. Continuous monitoring via a peripheral oxygen saturation probe will give early warnings of evolving airway obstruction and hypoxia.

Nasal obstruction with blood clot and mucous crusting can be prevented by steam inhalations containing Friar's Balsam or some similar aromatic vapour.

Occasionally an asthmatic patient develops acute bronchospasm and airway obstruction despite the dexamethasone cover. This may be resolved by a salbutamol nebuliser; 2.5–5 mg of salbutamol in a pre-prepared solution via a nebuliser mask on 8 litres oxygen per minute repeated as required, with 500 mcg of ipratropium bromide (an antimuscarinic bronchodilator) added 6-hourly. In addition intravenous magnesium (2 g in 100 ml normal saline) over 30 minutes is now an accepted part of The British Thoracic Society Guideline for severe acute asthma management. Magnesium induces relaxation of bronchial smooth muscle in acute asthma by interfering with calcium transport mechanisms and intracellular phosphorylation.

With these basic conservative measures, emergency tracheostomies are rarely needed.

h) *Emergency Airway Procedures*

Acute upper airway obstruction is more likely to follow trauma then operative procedures. In the non-intubated patient, obstruction secondary to haemorrhage into the neck tissues may prevent the clinician from inserting an endotracheal tube through the cords to establish airway patency. In such cases needle cricothryroidotomy and surgical cricothyroidotomy may be used to maintain ventilation and oxygenation whilst formal endotracheal intubation is attempted.

i)   Needle cricothyroidotomy and jet insufflation can provide supplemental oxygenation for around 20–30 minutes, the time constraint being carbon dioxide retention, as only minimal expiration is possible through the obstructed airway via this method. This relatively simple technique buys time to perform more definitive airway procedures by a clinician skilled in difficult and emergency situations.

Technique

Attach a 12–14 gauge cannula to a 10 ml syringe.

With the patient in a supine position extend (neutral in acute trauma) the patient's neck whilst controlling the head.

Palpate the cricothyroid membrane and then stabilise the trachea between thumb and forefinger of the nondominant hand to prevent lateral movement.

Puncture the skin in the midline with the cannula needle directly over the membrane, directing the needle at a 45° angle caudally.

Insert the needle through the lower half of the membrane, aspirating as the needle is inserted.

Aspiration of air indicates entry into the tracheal lumen, at which point the catheter can be carefully advanced into the lumen whilst withdrawing the needle.

Oxygen tubing attached to a Y-connector or with a hole cut into the side is attached to the hub of the catheter.

Intermittent insufflation can be achieved by occluding the open limb of the Y-connector or the hole in the tubing with a finger for 1 second and releasing for 4 seconds, during which oxygenation and then some passive expiration can occur. Expiration is limited as it occurs through the partially obstructed airway and not through the lumen of the inserted catheter.

Oxygen flow is commenced at 10 litres per minute and increased in increments of 1 litre until chest wall movement is observed during the period of hole occlusion.

As well as allowing oxygenation via jet insufflation, needle cricothyroidotomy can be used to carry out a retrograde intubation. After initial insertion of the needle through the membrane has been confirmed by aspiration of air, a guide wire is passed through the needle cephalad. This wire should pass upwards into the pharynx and then grasped with forceps to be brought out through the mouth. An endotracheal tube can then be passed over the wire into the larynx. The wire is removed once the tube reaches the level of the membrane and the tube is then passed further into the trachea.

ii)   Surgical cricothyroidotomy involves the insertion of a small endotracheal tube or tracheostomy tube through the cricothyroid membrane. Using this method the patient can be successfully oxygenated and ventilated with a bag valve system with supplemental oxygen until intubation or retrograde intubation is achieved. This technique is not recommended for children under 12 years of age in whom damage to the cricoid ring is likely.

Technique

Place the patient in the supine position with the neck in a neutral position.

Prepare the skin and anaesthetise the area if the patient is conscious.

Identify the cricothyroid membrane between the thyroid and cricoid cartilages.

Stabilise the thyroid cartilage with the non-dominant hand to prevent lateral movement.

Carefully make a transverse skin incision over the membrane and then incise through the lower half of the membrane.

Open the airway by using either a haemostat, a tracheal spreader, or by inserting the scalpel handle through the incised membrane and rotating it through 90°.

Insert the endotracheal or tracheostomy tube through the incised and opened membrane, directing it distally into the trachea.

Inflate the cuff and secure the airway using either sutures or ribbon ties.

Attach a bag valve system that is connected to a high flow oxygen source to the tube and ventilate the patient, observing for chest wall movement to indicate lung inflation.

iii) Tracheostomy: The need for elective tracheostomy has diminished with improved anaesthetic techniques and emergency care. However, the emergency tracheostomy, especially where there has been marked uncontrolled blood loss into the tissues, is still essential for untroubled postoperative care if prolonged endotracheal intubation cannot be adequately supervised. It provides an assured airway with reduced dead space, easy access for the aspiration of secretions from the bronchi below and prevents aspiration into the bronchi from above.

Technique

Place a sandbag between the shoulders and maximally extend the head on the neck to elevate the trachea (Figure 14.4a).

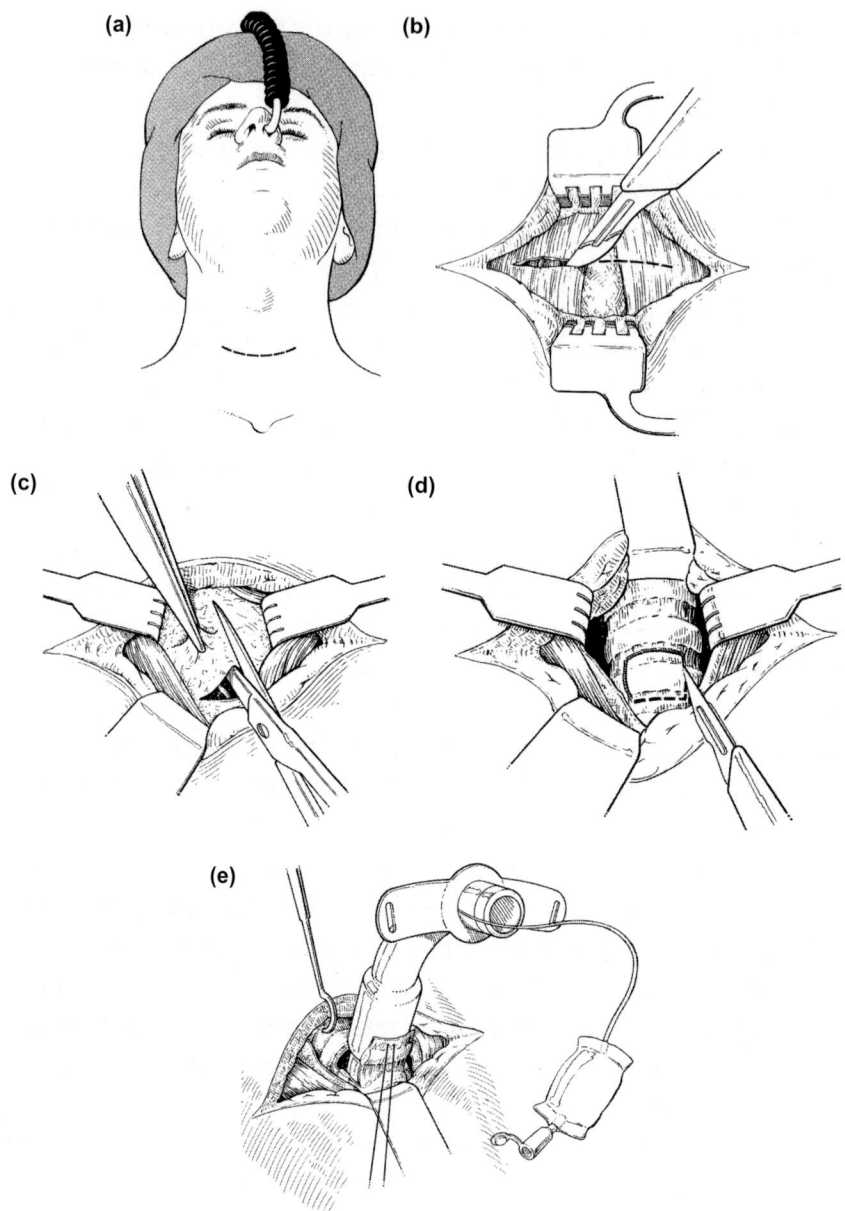

Figure 14.4   Tracheostomy technique, details on pages 457, 459 and 460.

Prepare the skin from the lower border of the mandible to below the clavicles with povidone-iodine. If there is no hurry, mark the incision and infiltrate it with a vasoconstrictor solution.

A horizontal 5 cm incision is made halfway between the prominence of the thyroid cartilage and the sternal notch with a No. 10 blade. Incise through the fatty superficial fascia and platysma down to the muscle layer, revealing the anterior jugular veins on both sides. These may be divided and tied, or undisturbed and ignored if there is any urgency. Retract the flaps with cat's paws or a self-retaining retractor (Figure 14.4b).

Incise vertically in the midline with a knife or scissors, separating the intramuscular fascia and revealing the pretracheal fascia.

Retract the strap muscles laterally.

Lift up the pretracheal fascia with toothed forceps and incise upwards with scissors to reveal the isthmus of the thyroid, and then downward, avoiding if possible the centrally placed inferior thyroid vein (Figure 14.4c). If the thyroid isthmus is large it may be retracted upwards with a broad Langenbeck. Occasionally it may be necessary to clamp the isthmus with long curved haemostats and divide it. To prevent bleeding, the margins should be carefully tied with 2/0 polyglycollate before releasing the clamps.

Re-position the retractors inside the pretracheal fascia on either side of the trachea. If time allows, or if using local analgesia, infiltrate between the second and third tracheal ring with 1 ml 2% lignocaine containing 1:80,000 adrenaline for haemostasis, then inject another 1–2 ml into the lumen. This anaesthetises the mucous membrane and helps to suppress the violent cough reflex when inserting the tube.

Make a horizontal slit between the second and third tracheal ring with a No.15 blade and extend it downwards bilaterally. The trachea may be steadied by passing a tracheal or skin hook beneath the upper ring and gently elevating. The simplest technique is now to remove a circular disc of trachea and then pass a 1/0 black silk stay suture around the lower ring and clip it outside the lower wound margin (Figure 14.4d).

Some surgeons prefer a Bjork flap, which is an inverted U hinged inferiorly (Figure 14.4e). The upper margin of the flap is sutured to the skin surface. This enables re-intubation if the tracheostomy tube is displaced or removed. However, the tracheal defect tends to be larger and there may be a greater incidence of post-tracheostomy stenosis.

Choose a suitable size of tracheostomy tube, 33 to 39 for small to large individuals, and test the cuff by inflating with air.

Insert the tracheostomy tube gently as the anaesthetist withdraws the endotracheal tube, carefully sucking all blood from the area. Inflate the cuff with a 20 ml syringe, noting whether it is self-sealing or requires clamping and sealing with its own spigot (Figure 14.4e).

The endotracheal tube is now completely removed and the anaesthetic hose connected to the tracheostomy tube

Suture the skin margins beneath retaining flanges with interrupted 3/0 Prolene or silk as far medially as possible. Cover the wound margins with an acriflavine-impregnated gauze swab or Telfa pad which has been prepared with a T-shaped cut to fit around the tube.

Tie the tube flanges behind the neck with tapes to prevent displacement.

Postoperative Care

Secretions must be sucked out regularly every half hour, and more frequently if necessary, with a fine catheter and using an aseptic technique

The tracheostomy oxygen must be warmed and humidified.

High volume, low-pressure cuffs no longer need to be released at intervals to prevent ischaemia of the tracheal mucosa but the cuff pressure should be checked.

A chest radiograph must be taken postoperatively to exclude pleural damage and pneumothorax. Note: surgical emphysema of the neck may be dramatic but is of no consequence.

Daily physiotherapy is essential, with gently catheter suction and warm saline to loosen the secretions.

Once the oral and cervical swelling has receded and the chest radiograph is clear, the tracheostomy should be removed. The skin is cleaned with detergent (Savlon) and the tube is sucked out with the patient upright and is then withdrawn. Steri-strips may be used to close the margins of the wound, which is then covered with a dry gauze adhesive dressing and is left unchanged, and sealed for 10 days. Complete spontaneous closure usually takes place in a week. If there is any delay, swabs taken from the wound will show gross antibiotic resistant contaminants. Avoid the temptation to use exotic antibiotics when local cleansing with 0.05% hibitane or povidone-iodine dressings is all that is required.

As osteotomy cases do not require a prolonged tracheostomy, replacement of the tube does not arise.

4. *Drainage of a Pneumothorax*

Occasionally, despite every care on removing a rib graft, there is a breach in the pleura and the patient develops a pneumothorax. The presenting signs are breathlessness and tachypnoea with absent breath-sounds over the area. The typical radiographic appearance where the visceral pleura is breached is a demarcated peripheral area devoid of lung markings — here seen on the left side (Figure 14.5a). However Figure 14.5b shows a mottled oval opacity of surgical emphysema in the right lung field overlying a pneumothorax where both visceral and parietal pleura have been breached following costochondral graft removal.

The most convenient, comfortable and cosmetically pleasing site for drainage is in the fourth or fifth intercostal space in the mid-axillary line. To achieve this, the patient must be comfortably positioned,

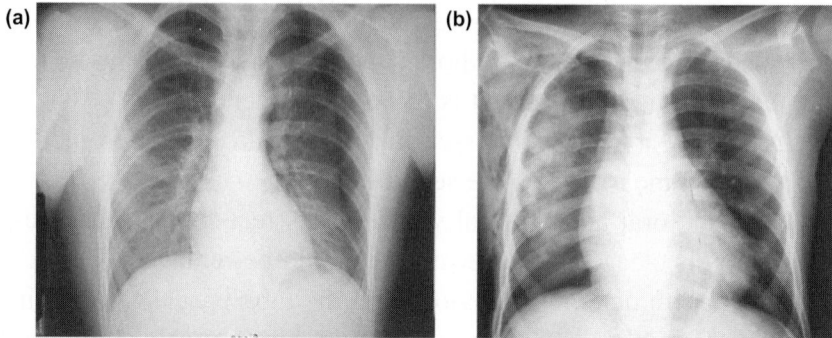

Figure 14.5   **(a)** Left pneumothorax due to breach of visceral pleura producing a demarcated peripheral area devoid of lung markings. **(b)** Oval mottled opacity of surgical emphysema overlying right pneumothorax due to breach in parietal and visceral pleura.

either reclining on the bed with the ipsilateral arm behind the head to expose the axilla, or leaning forward, with folded arms resting on a pillow on the bed-table. The surgeon should scrub, gown and put on gloves. The skin is prepared with povidone-iodine and, with sterile towels to isolate the area, is infiltrated with 1% or 2% lignocaine. Then with a 21-gauge needle (green hub) the chest wall is infiltrated to the pleura (up to 3 mg/kg), at which level air can be aspirated. Always keep to the upper rib border to avoid the intercostal neurovascular bundle that runs along the inferior border of the rib. A small skin incision is made and then blunt dissection used through the superficial fascia and intercostal muscles to the pleural space.

Small calibre chest drain sets (8–14 F) come with a Seldinger technique insertion kit. The method involves passing dilators of increasing size into the pleural space over a guide wire that has initially been introduced through a hollow needle. This creates an almost bloodless and atraumatic tract into the space required, through which the chest drain can be passed prior to connecting it up to an underwater drainage system. The use of the rigid trochar is contraindicated for all sizes of drain due to the risk of intrathoracic injury.

Two sutures are routinely inserted, the first to assist closure of the wound after drain removal, usually a mattress suture, and the second, a stay suture to secure the drain. "Purse-string" sutures are no longer recommended due to the less pleasing scar and increased pain whilst *in situ*.

The catheter position and pneumothorax are then checked with an anteroposterior chest radiograph. The catheter may be removed 24 hours after radiographic evidence that the lung is fully inflated. The drain should be removed whilst the patient performs either Valsalva's manoeuvre or during expiration. Provided aseptic techniques have been used, there is no role for prophylactic antibiotic administration for chest drain insertion.

Vomiting

Postoperative vomiting in patients with intermaxillary fixation was a well-recognised problem. Predisposing factors are blood escaping intraoperatively and postoperatively into the stomach, where partial digestion together with bile reflux creates an irritant stagnant mixture. An additional factor is the emetic effect of opiate analgesics.

Prevention

i)   Avoid intermaxillary fixation by using internal rigid fixation.
ii) A 12–16FG nasogastric tube passed at the time of the anaesthetic induction enables postoperative aspiration of gastric contents. The tube is attached to a bile bag to create a closed collecting system for any spontaneous reflux. As the patient is monitored throughout the postoperative night the stomach should be aspirated hourly and the fluid loss noted. Initially flushing the tube with 20 ml water before aspiration prevents the end becoming clogged with clot.

The administration of an antiemetic, e.g. metoclopromide 10 mg intravenously at the end of the operation, and with any required opiate analgesics, reduces drug-induced emesis (up to a maximum of

30 mg/24 hours). Metoclopromide 10 mg intravenously should also be given at any other time if vomiting is anticipated. 5HT antagonists such as ondansetron block the action of 5HT in the intestine and CNS, which also has an antiemetic effect. This is introduced after the administration of metochlopramide. With a fully conscious patient it is often the nasopharyngeal airway that provokes the problem.

Management

The patient who is being nursed in a 45° sitting position should be sucked out immediately through both sides of the nose with a broad-core catheter. The buccal sulci will also require clearing.

Contrary to popular belief, cutting intermaxillary fixation — if used, is neither essential nor the most efficient way of managing the vomiting patient.

Paradoxically, nasal suction is more efficient than opening the mouth and attempting to clear the oropharynx of vomitus in a conscious patient.

5. *Iliac Crest Problems*

The removal of bone from the iliac crest for orthognathic purposes is becoming less popular. However, the inverted L osteotomy may require a substantial amount of corticocancellous bone to correct a very small mandible.

Postoperative pain is the most frequent complication and can be reduced by drainage and analgesics. Some surgeons leave a fine cannula for infusion of a long acting local analgesic such as bupivacaine (Marcain). It is difficult to be certain if this is of significant value.

If a large graft has been removed near the anterior superior iliac spine, this may fracture with sudden movement once the patient is mobilised (Figure 14.6). No treatment is required apart from reassurance, rest, analgesics and physiotherapy.

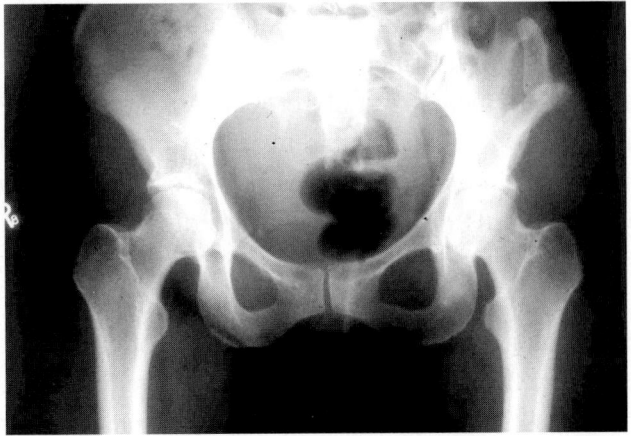

Figure 14.6   Fracture at the base of the anterior superior iliac spine with collapse of the preserved iliac crest lid.

6. *Catheterisation*

Catheterisation is necessary for prolonged surgical procedures, especially where large quantities of fluid have been infused. This is uncommon with orthognathic cases except where there has been unexpected major blood loss. Another occasional indication is the patient, usually male, who has postoperative urinary retention. This may be due to opioid-induced sphincter spasm, diffidence in using a urinal, or a combination of both, leading to gross distension. Any associated agitation will resolve with catheter insertion and bladder drainage and does not need to be controlled with intravenous benzodiazepines.

Technique

As with all separate aseptic procedures, each area must be freshly prepared and the surgeon re-gloved and gowned.

Clean the external genitalia carefully with sterile saline and towel the area. Place a receiver between the abducted thighs. A No. 14 or 16 Foley catheter is the optimum choice; its retaining balloon can be tested by inflating with air. Note: if there is obstruction, try a smaller gauge (10–12 FG) or a firmer, curved Coudé catheter.

With males the penis is held vertically in sterile gauze. Sterile lubricating gel with lignocaine is instilled into the urethra. After giving the lignocaine a minute to work the catheter is then passed vertically downwards to the lower border of the pubic symphysis. With continued pressure on the catheter the penis is rotated downwards (caudally) so that the catheter may traverse the angle at the penoscrotal junction in the bladder. In cases of prostatic enlargement or stricture this may be difficult and will require expert help.

With females it is important to part the vaginal labia to reveal the external urethral orifice within the vestibule. The inexperienced attack the base of the clitoris, which is above the urethral orifice, with the catheter tip.

Once the catheter is in the bladder, urine will pass into the receiver. Gentle aspiration may be required initially to clear obstructing gel from the tip of the catheter. Push the catheter in maximally and fill the balloon with 10 ml sterile water (always check the balloon volume first); a gentle pull should indicate its retention. Attach the catheter to a collection bag to complete a closed drainage system; monitor urinary outflow, which should exceed 30 ml/h. Remember to change the bag every 24 hours if it is retained. Remove the catheter as soon as possible.

7. *Deep Vein Thrombosis*

This is a rare event in orthognathic patients, usually occurring unexpectedly in young women. As a precaution, all women should cease taking oestrogen containing contraceptive pills 4 weeks prior to surgery. If this has been overlooked, subcutaneous low molecular weight heparin prophylaxis should be considered, i.e. Dalteparin Sodium 5000 units preoperatively followed by a daily injection for 5–7 days. Both high and low risk patients benefit from elasticated thromboembolic-deterrent stockings being worn during the operation.

Any complaint of postoperative calf tenderness must be taken seriously, especially when there is an increase in circumferential measurement and/or local erythema. Lower limb Doppler ultrasonography should be carried out and if this is positive (or not possible) the patient is anticoagulated to prevent extension of the thrombus and embolism.

An oral anticoagulant such as warfarin should also be started at 10 mg/day for the first 3 days, or as guided by your local anticoagulation clinic. A baseline prothrombin time is recommended prior to anticoagulation if any liver disease is suspected. Subsequent prothrombin times (INR) should be 2–2.5 times normal and taken on the second and third days of treatment and then weekly to confirm a stable ratio. Follow up in the anticoagulation clinic should be organised prior to discharge from hospital. The usual maintenance dose of 3–9 mg is taken at the same time each day for 3–6 months. The patient should continue on daily subcutaneous injections of low molecular weight heparin until full oral anticoagulation with warfarin is established or on daily heparin injections only if pregnant.

8. *Fixation Problems*

These are infinitely varied but fortunately become uncommon with experience.

  i) Infection may occur around screws and plates. Miniature plates are an essential part of the osteotomy and surprisingly in the maxilla rarely get infected. If drainage and a course of antibiotics do not suppress the infection, the plate and screws have to be removed. Similarly, uninfected bone plates may become palpable subcutaneously or submucosally and also require removal.
 ii) Incorrectly placed screws and plates may displace the bony parts. This occurs more commonly in the third molar area with the sagittal split operation, but is also with Le Fort I procedures where maxillary displacement can distort the nasal septum.

Less commonly plates break. Whenever displacement or loss of control takes place, the patient should be taken back to theatre for correction. Pious hopes that the problem will go away or will be correctable by postsurgical orthodontics always prove to be futile.

iii) The use of screws or buccal plates for rigid fixation of the mandible can create occlusal discrepancies if it is not appreciated that the osteotomy is carried out with the patient anaesthetised and supine. If the condyle is pushed to the back of the fossa when temporary intermaxillary fixation is put on to facilitate the insertion of the bicortical screws or buccal plate, on its release, with the patient conscious and upright, the condyles will tend to recoil downwards and forwards. This is favourable for the Class 2 Division I mandibular advancement but gives a postoperative prognathous malocclusion with the Class 3 setback. To avoid these artefacts (a) the model surgery should be based on a conscious supine centric relation squash bite and (b) the ascending ramus proximal fragment should be displaced backwards for Class 2 advancements but pulled forwards prior to fixation with the Class 3 mandibular setback.

Such problems were less likely to happen with a loose interosseous wire loop at the osteotomy site and prolonged intermaxillary fixation for 6 weeks. This enabled the ascending ramus proximal fragment to achieve an optimum condyle-meniscus-fossa relationship by functional adjustment brought about by swallowing and speech.

iv) Disturbed muscular proprioception and intracapsular oedema may also give a transient deranged postoperative occlusion when using rigid fixation. In these cases, light elastics for 7 days will help to restore the occlusion to the planned relationship. The final occlussal wafer is often left *in situ* even where there is no occlussal problem. This is very uncomfortable for the patient and there is no evidence that it helps. However, if after this elastic "proprioceptive regimen" there still appears to be marked displacement and malocclusion — re-operate.

9. *Relapse*

Relapse is any unanticipated postoperative change in the planned or achieved dental or skeletal relationships. Most arise from inadequate planning or inappropriate surgical technique. The former have been discussed in Chapter 4 on Planning Data Transfer. The latter may be roughly divided into two overlapping groups: those arising from (1) operative structural causes and (2) postoperative functional causes.

a) *Operative Structural Causes of Relapse*

Inadequate bone, cartilage or periosteal separation. Osteotomy cuts and soft tissue dissection must provide absolute freedom of movement of the parts and allow effortless repositioning. Tight bone plates will not correct reluctant anatomical components but will cause some malalignment elsewhere. Common sites are as follows.

i) Inadequate separation of the proximal mandibular bone and the medial pterygoid muscle from the buccal plate when doing a sagittal split. A finger firmly inserted to the depth of the split is used to remove the restraining periosteum and muscle fibres, which hold the two cortices together at the lower border.

ii) Inadequate bone removal from the posterior wall of the antrum or separation of the pterygoid plates in a Le Fort I impaction can also create problems.

iii) The untrimmed nasal septum will create a buckling effect and either displace the maxilla and disturb the occlusion, or displace the nose and produce an asymmetric tip deformity, and obstruct the airway. Late correction will require a rhinoplasty.

iv) Where a mandibular osteotomy has been done with the pious hope of eradicating temporomandibular joint pain in a patient with a meniscus displacement, the osteotomy may not only give rise to more pain initially but may create intracapsular adhesions and limited opening postoperatively.

v) Occasionally lower lip sag may follow a bone graft procedure to increase the chin depth by augmentation, or a mandibular forward movement with a genioplasty. It is difficult to be sure whether it is due to inadequate freeing of the periosteal pouch and overlying soft tissues, or failure to re-attach the mentalis high enough on the anterior mandibular surface, or abnormal muscle activity. The last cause would be inadequate orbicularis tone or decreased mentalis elevated activity.

The lip sag should be avoided by the creation of a large loose periosteal pouch to accommodate the enlarged chin, carefully suturing the divided mentalis to the deep muscle fibres on the alveolar surface, and the application of a firm pressure dressing overlying the labiomantal groove. Once formed it can be eliminated in some cases by vigorous exercising of the lower lip, i.e. the lip is actively stretched upwards over the incisor edges. If this fails, it will be necessary to deglove and reposition the soft tissues upwards using heavy polyglycollate (Vicryl) sutures to elevate the soft tissues of the chin.

vi) Tooth damage may occur with the bone cuts of segmental osteotomies, either apically or laterally. Avoid the former by marking the estimated apical site with a shallow bur hole prior to the section. Lateral root damage arises when burs are used interdentally. Only the buccal and lingual (palatal) bone should be cut with a bur and the actual division should be made with a fine osteotome or saw.

Although root damage often appears to be self-limiting and most teeth survive, occasionally the exposed dentine undergoes progressive resorption. An attempt may be made to preserve the tooth by root canal therapy with calcium hydroxide. However, should root loss progress, extraction and an implant or bridge will be required to salvage the situation.

Segmental cuts in the older patient with incipient periodontal disease may also create intractable bony pockets unless anticipated. The cuts must be done carefully with a fine osteotome after prior periodontal therapy followed by postoperative oral hygiene instruction.

b) *Postoperative Functional Causes of Relapse*

i) The most notorious is the recurrent anterior open bite following attempted correction with a mandibular osteotomy. This will occur in patients with a high mandibular-maxillary plane angle where the low posterior facial height reflects a short pterygomasseteric sling. This is stretched as the mandible is rotated around the fulcrum created by the occluding molar crowns when the anterior teeth are brought into occlusion to close the gap. The inelastic ligaments and the return of postoperative muscular tone may even produce a relapse despite internal fixation. This is avoided by a posterior maxillary impaction equivalent to the anterior open bite to be corrected.

ii) Postoperative tooth movement can be favourable, especially with the spontaneous or assisted closure of lateral open bites. However, unfavourable tooth movements may arise.

- Repositioned lower incisors are proclined by a large or "anteriorly postured" tongue.
- Upper incisors are proclined by the lower lip after a maxillary segmental pushback procedures is carried out on a marked Class II, Division 1 patient without a mandibular forward correction to an edge to edge relationship.
- Continued eruption (occlusal drift) of the lower incisors will follow an anterior segmental setdown unless they are placed in a stabilising contact with the cingula or incisive edges of the opposing teeth.

- Expansion of the maxillary premolar and molar segments may tilt those teeth buccally. Subsequent palatal drift will produce intercuspal contact on closure with the creation of an anterior open bite. Major expansion of the palate should be done surgically with a midline osteotomy to avoid dental relapse.
- Idiopathic periapical and internal resorption may occur in teeth adjacent to an osteotomy cut, even without untoward bur contact. The cause is unknown but may be due to a vascular response to the adjacent surgery.
- Orthodontic depression of lower incisors in adults, before surgery, may cause proclination with alveolar dehiscence and gingival recession. Furthermore, the proclined incisors may then upright spontaneously once fixation is removed.

If, after a considerable input of time and energy if both surgeon and patient, are agreed something has gone seriously wrong with the operative correction — start again!

c) *Nerve Damage*

i) It is important to warn the patient preoperatively of impaired sensation that may arise in the mental or mylohyoid nerve distribution of the lower lip and chin following a sagittal split or anterior segmental operation, and in the infraorbital area following a maxillary osteotomy. The former usually recovers in 2–6 months, although some patients have a permanent deficit, which is less noticeable if the operation is otherwise successful.
   When the inferior dental nerve is exposed and torn during the sagittal split, it may be possible to hold the separated ends together with a 6/0 Prolene suture prior to fixation.

ii) Facial nerve damage with weakness can be localised following external incisions for a subsigmoid (subcondylar) osteotomy but will involve a wider distribution of the facial nerve if it is damaged near its main trunk. This can occur with a sagittal split pushback or an intraoral subsigmoid (subcondylar) operation. The cause is probably traumatic instrumentation. They prognosis is usually very good, with gradual recovery over 6–8 weeks.

iii) The lingual nerve is rarely damaged during an osteotomy. However, persistent impaired lingual sensation after 6 weeks requires open exploration and repair. This is most easily done by removing the overlying sublingual salivary gland.

iv) A rare disturbance is nasal vasomotor hyperfunction, which may occur after a Le Fort I osteotomy. The patient develops continuous rhinorrhoea, which simulates a cerebrospinal fluid leak. The cause is uncertain and may be either loss of sympathetic vasomotor control or damage to the sphenopalatine ganglion with enhanced stimulation. There is no satisfactory treatment.

10. *Emotional and Psychiatric Problems*

These vary from postoperative depression, often manifested as a refusal to take food or medication by mouth, to more dramatic states. Many patients would be spared a reactionary depressive state if they had been carefully warned of postoperative problems on admission. Good nursing care and attentive surgical staff are the treatment of choice.

Agitation can arise both from intolerance of intermaxillary fixation or simply nasal airway obstruction. Both can now be avoided. However, not only is it essential to clear the nose by inhalations and suction, but always seek an underlying structural obstruction, such as a displaced nasal septum.

Unanticipated anxiety of an alien environment, especially the intensive care unit, may precipitate postoperative psychotic behaviour. This can be controlled by intravenous antipsychotic drugs such as haloperidol, which can later be given orally.

Emotionally unstable individuals, especially those who have a history of body dysmorphic disorder, may also become aggressive and difficult to control. Again, an antipsychotic drug regimen is essential, together with preoperative and postoperative psychiatric advice. Unfortunately some patients get legal aid to express their illogical complaints through a solicitor. It is wise to report the problem to risk management in an NHS hospital who can if necessary provide legal support. With private patients the surgeon will need to seek the advice of their medical defence society.

Dissatisfaction can be avoided by repeated preoperative discussion about the operative procedure, the immediate and late complications and, most important of all, the patient's aesthetic expectations. All these should be recorded.

Finally an explanatory handout of the operation covering common complications is essential.

15

Feeding and Postoperative Nutritional Support

Introduction

Postoperative osteotomy and fracture patients are often neglected from a nutritional point of view, despite obvious eating and drinking difficulties, pain and orofacial swelling. Malnutrition is a well-recognised problem in hospitals, with 40%–50% of all patients found to be malnourished on admission and 70%–80% on discharge. Although the former statistic is unlikely to apply to orthognathic patients the latter is often the case.

This patient group are by the nature of their surgery at risk of malnutrition owing to raised nutritional requirements and impaired nutritional intake. Consequences of malnutrition for the postoperative patient include decreased wound healing, decreased immune function and increased infection risk which can lead to unnecessary morbidity. Establishing and maintaining adequate intake should be seen as a priority. Patients with inadequate oral intake post-surgery or those requiring modified texture diets on discharge from hospital, should be referred to a dietician for individualised nutritional assessment and advice. Energy and protein requirements vary according to a patient's age and gender, and individualised nutritional assessment ensures optimum daily requirements are highlighted and achieved.

Optimum Daily Requirements

- Men and women average 2000–3000 kcal.
- 0.8 g protein/kg; 65–1000 g protein.
- 2–3 litres fluid.

Immediate Postoperative Feeding

1. *0–24 Hours Post-Operation: Intravenous Fluids*

Having replaced blood loss to within 500 ml, compound sodium lactate (Hartmann's) solution is given to balance vomited fluid, gastric aspirate, urinary output and metabolic needs. The volume will be 2 to 3 litres depending on the patient's weight and the ambient temperature. The patient should also be encouraged to drink a little.

2. *After 24 Hours*

If the patient is well, and the surgical procedure allows, trials of oral fluid should be commenced using a feeding cup, straw or a large bore syringe and quill. Most orthognathic cases can cope, but if oral intake is proving difficult, enteral feeding should be commenced using a fine bore nasogastric feeding tube. This should be carried out under dietetic supervision to ensure the appropriate calorie and protein content, and minimise the side effects sometimes experienced with enteral feeding such as nausea, vomiting and diarrhoea. Supplemental intravenous fluids are often needed until the patient's normal oral feeding rate is achieved and to prevent dehydration and electrolyte disturbances.

3. *After 48 Hours*

Patients who have commenced nasogastric feeding should continue to receive this until the optimum oral intake has been established. Patients who have tolerated oral fluids from the start can progress to a full diet, but with a liquidised texture.

In many cases of bimaxillary surgery involving the lower labial sulcus with impaired mental sensation, adequate oral feeding may not be possible for up to 7 days and need special attention.

A Range of Commonly Used Supplements

- Ensure Plus/Fortisip/Fresubin Energy.
- Enlive Plus/Fortijuce/Provide Xtra.
- Fortifresh/Ensure Plus Yoghurt Style.
- Scandishake/Calshake.
- Calogen.
- Maxijul.
- Protifar.

These are in a variety of flavours for inpatient care, and can be obtained with or without a prescription on discharge.

On Discharge

The patient should have a comprehensive assessment and education regarding food preparation, food fortification and the use of dietary supplements. Patients must be routinely weighed when attending their outpatient review, and any weight loss addressed. In particular, children and adolescent patients need to be stringently monitored to minimise disruption to growth, along with patients with diabetes and food allergies.

Achieving nutritional requirements is difficult whilst following a liquidised diet. Liquids are more filling than solid foods, decreasing the patient's appetite. In addition, where non-nourishing fluids are used, liquidising can have a nutrient dilution effect causing inadequate calorie, protein and micronutrient intake. Choosing high-energy foods and fluids, encouraging small frequent meals and snacks and using food fortification techniques can help to counteract this.

General Guidelines for Patients

- Aim to include as much variety in the diet as possible, no single food will provide all the nutrients needed.
- Liquids are more filling than solids, so more will be needed to prevent weight loss. Small frequent meals including nourishing fluids will need to be taken.
- Aim for weight maintenance.
- Liquidised foods must be thin and smooth enough to pass through a straw or quill.
- Foods are often more palatable if liquidised separately to preserve individuals flavours and colours.
- Milk is a useful source of protein and calories, and can be fortified further by adding dried milk powder; 3–4 tablespoons of any dried milk powder to 1 pint of full cream milk. When whisked well this can be used as ordinary milk — for drinks, to make milk puddings, sauces etc.
- Vitamin C is an important nutrient for wound healing; a glass of pure orange juice or blackcurrant drink should be taken daily.
- Essential utensils are a liquidiser (blender) or food processor, a sieve, a beaker with feeding spout and straws. This should be discussed preoperatively and on the patient's information sheet.

Sample Meal Plan for Patients

Breakfast

- Fruit juice.
- Ready Brek/Porridge/Weetabix made with fortified milk, cream and sugar.
- Fortified milky drink/milky tea or coffee with sugar if desired.

Mid Morning

- Milky or nourishing drink.
- Mousse or smooth yoghurt.

Lunch

- Soup with cream/milk powder.
- Liquidised meat/chicken/fish/beans and pulses.
- Mashed potato with fortified milk/butter/cream/cheese.
- Pureed vegetables with butter and cheese.
- Milky pudding/smooth yoghurt.

Mid Afternoon

- Milk pudding with pureed fruit.
- Nourishing drink.

Evening Meal

- As per lunch.

Bedtime

- Hot milky drink — Horlicks, hot chocolate, ovaltine.

This diet also requires a dedicated oral hygiene regime with a child's soft tooth brush and a chlorhexidine mouth wash after meals to control plaque.

Information on feeding supplements can be found in the British National Formulary published twice yearly by the British Medical Association and the Royal Pharmaceutical Society of Great Britain.

A Handout for Patients Undergoing Orthognathic Surgery

A carefully designed preoperative handout is essential for an elective procedure which will change a patients face, body image and will also risk complications. There are several available, however below is the one to be considered as a useful model.

Orthognathic surgery corrects the relationship of the jaws to give improved jaw function and facial appearance.

Orthodontics

In almost all cases orthodontic treatment is required before the operation for about 18 months in order to ensure that the teeth are in the ideal relationship afterwards. This dental correction also helps to give the best possible appearance, function and stability following the operation.

Fixed braces are the standard means of orthodontic treatment and they are also invaluable during the operation to achieve the correct relationship of the jaws.

The Operation

This is carried out under a general anaesthetic and carries no risk in a fit young adult. In most cases the patient needs to be in hospital from 1–3 days after the operation.

Today, the bones are fixed during the procedure by miniature titanium plates and screws which are left in place without any harm or inconvenience. Occasionally a plate or screw may need to be removed if it is causing discomfort or gets infected. There are rare situations where the jaws need to be fixed together with wire or elastics after the procedure for up 4 weeks.

It is helpful to bring a small, soft tooth brush into hospital to help keep the teeth and wires clean. An antiseptic mouth wash (for example, chlorhexidene — Corsodyl) is important after your last daily meal.

Problems

Postoperative swelling is to be expected, which may give way to bruising over a period of 2 weeks. In most cases, pain is not a problem and can be controlled with mild painkillers. Most patients need to be away from work for 10 days to 2 weeks depending on their job and how they feel.

Numbness of the lower lip, upper lip and palate is possible depending on the operation. More than half of patients have some degree of short term numbness which in most cases gradually recovers. Small persistent areas tend to diminish in time are and generally not noticeable. There is no disturbance in muscle function.

Diet

It is important to keep the teeth free of decay throughout the treatment procedure and a careful choice of diet is essential. You must avoid sweet sticky foods, soft drinks and an excess of fruit juice. Hard foods must be cut up before chewing as they may damage the brace. Tooth brushing twice a day with a fluoride tooth paste is essential. The postoperative diet is initially liquid and then liquidised for 2–3 weeks. The dietician will advise you or a diet sheet will be given with this handout.

Postoperative Orthodontics

After the operation there is usually a short period of orthodontic fine tuning for about 6 months before the braces are removed.

This combination of orthodontics and surgery will improve your appearance, The details will depend on the procedure and must be discussed with the orthodontist and surgeon so that you do not have any unrealistic expectations of improvement.

Most cases take 2–3 years overall for completion. During this time regular appointments with be required to adjust the brace and review progress.

It is also essential that you have regular dental checkups to avoid serious dental decay.

Index